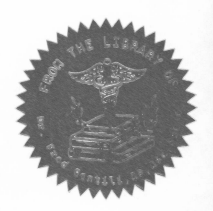

EARLY CARE
OF THE
INJURED
PATIENT

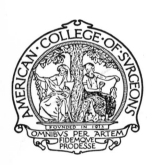

BY THE COMMITTEE ON TRAUMA
AMERICAN
COLLEGE
OF
SURGEONS

W. B. SAUNDERS COMPANY
PHILADELPHIA · LONDON · TORONTO

W. B. Saunders Company: West Washington Square
Philadelphia, Pa. 19105

12 Dyott Street
London, WC1A 1DB

833 Oxford Street
Toronto 18, Ontario

Early Care of the Injured Patient   ISBN 0-7216-1160-5

Print No.:   9   8   7   6   5   4   3   2

Preface

The purpose of this Manual is to improve the quality of the early care of the injured by providing a ready reference for physicians in the care of patients in the emergency department and the early care of patients in the hospital. Thousands of persons receive injuries in the home, on the farm, on the highway, and in industry. Quality early care of these people can reduce death and disability, facilitate rehabilitation, and cut the cost of these accidents.

The American College of Surgeons first published the Manual, *An Outline of the Treatment of Fractures*, in 1931. This paperback pocket manual was written by the Subcommittee on Fractures, from which evolved the Committee on Trauma. The eighth edition of the Fracture Manual was published in 1965. In 1954, the Committee on Trauma published another manual, *The Early Care of Acute Soft Tissue Injuries*, as a paperback pocket manual developed by the Subcommittee on Soft Tissue Injuries. A second edition in 1960 and a third edition in 1965 were developed by the same Subcommittee. In 1960, and again in 1965, the Fracture and Soft Tissue Manuals were combined in a hardcover edition and distributed under the title *The Management of Fractures and Soft Tissue Injuries.*

In 1968, the Subcommittee on the Fracture Manual and the Sub-committee on the Soft Tissue Manual agreed, and the Committee on Trauma approved, that the next edition would be published only as a single manual in a hardback cover. This decision led to the two subcommittees being combined in 1969 as the Subcommittee on Publications, and the decision was made that the next edition would be issued under the title *Early Care of the Injured Patient.*

Rather than a handbook to be carried in the pocket of a house officer, *Early Care of the Injured Patient* is a practical reference book to be used in the emergency department and in the hospital. Although expanded in content, the new Manual remains *a guide* to the early care of the injured patient, not a comprehensive treatise on trauma. The methods described

iii

have proved successful in most circumstances in the opinion of the authors. No implication is intended that other methods would prove less successful or less acceptable. As implied in its title, the Manual does not cover specialized late care that many injuries require. Neither does it cover the less common or all of the more complicated injuries.

This edition of the Manual represents the contributions of many members of the Committee on Trauma, other Fellows of the American College of Surgeons, and other selected authorities on certain subjects who are not surgeons. The Members of the Subcommittee on Publications extend grateful appreciation to the following people for their valuable assistance and contributions to the present edition of the Manual: Doctors Jerome S. Abrams, William A. Altemeier, C. Andrew L. Bassett, Walter P. Blount, C. Eugene Carlton, Jr., Charles T. Fitts, Charles J. Frankel, Nicholas J. Giannestras, Frank E. Gump, Robert P. Hummel, John R. Jones, Raymond H. Kaufman, Herndon B. Lehr, J. Vernon Luck, John B. Lynch, Robert M. McCormack, the late Harrison L. McLaughlin, Joseph S. Redding, Lee H. Riley, Jr., Robert B. Salter, Russell Scott, Jr., Frederick M. Smith, Preston A. Wade, A. Earl Walker, Dabney R. Yarbrough, and Edward E. Yaskovitz, and to Elise Gaston and Alan R. Kamp. We also thank Robert B. Rowan and Albert E. Meier of the W. B. Saunders Company for their splendid cooperation and patience during preparation of this Manual.

THE SUBCOMMITTEE ON PUBLICATIONS

*MERLE M. MUSSELMAN, *Chairman*
*SAWNIE R. GASTON, *Co-Chairman*
*KENT L. BROWN
*ORMOND S. CULP
*ANDREW C. RUOFF, III

CURTIS P. ARTZ, Ex-Officio
H. THOMAS BALLANTINE, JR.,
  Consultant
TRUMAN G. BLOCKER,
  Senior Advisory Member
HAROLD B. BOYD,
  Senior Advisory Member
EDWIN F. CAVE,
  Senior Advisory Member
JOHN H. DAVIS
JOHN D. GERMAN, Consultant

DONALD M. GLOVER,
  Senior Advisory Member
OSCAR P. HAMPTON, JR.,
  Ex-Officio
WALTER A. HOYT, JR.
WILLIAM R. MACAUSLAND, JR.
RUDOLF J. NOER
J. CUTHBERT OWENS, Consultant
LEONARD F. PELTIER, Consultant
HOWARD E. SNYDER,
  Senior Advisory Member

*1971 Subcommittee on Publications

The Committee on Trauma 1972

Curtis P. Artz, Charleston, South Carolina, *Chairman*
H. Thomas Ballantine, Jr., Boston, *Vice Chairman*
Oscar P. Hampton, Jr., Chicago, *Secretary*

Active Members

William W. Babson, Gloucester, Massachusetts
John A. Boswick, Jr., River Forest, Illinois
Kent L. Brown, Cleveland
R. H. Brown (Capt MC USN), Bangor
Chalmers R. Carr, Charlotte
Henry C. Cleveland, Denver
Francis J. Cox, San Francisco
Ormond S. Culp, Rochester, Minnesota
John H. Davis, Burlington, Vermont
A. Campbell Derby, Montreal
Theodore Drapanas, New Orleans
J. D. Farrington, Minocqua, Wisconsin
Sawnie R. Gaston, New York
Robert W. Gillespie, Lincoln, Nebraska
Walter A. Hoyt, Jr., Akron
Francis C. Jackson, Washington
F. R. C. Johnstone, Vancouver
Burton C. Kilbourne, Ripon, Wisconsin
Thomas J. Krizek, New Haven
William R. MacAusland, Boston
Carl D. Martz, Indianapolis

C. Walter Metz, Jr. (Col MC USA), Washington
J. R. Frank Mill, Toronto
Thomas W. Morgan, Gallipolis, Ohio
Merle M. Musselman, Omaha
Alan M. Nahum, San Diego
Charles S. Neer II, New York
Colman J. O'Neill, LaGrange Park, Illinois
James A. O'Neill, Jr., New Orleans
J. Cuthbert Owens, Denver
Leonard F. Peltier, Tucson
Olav Rostrup, Edmonton
William T. Rumage, Jr., Louisville
Andrew C. Ruoff III, Salt Lake City
Roger T. Sherman, Memphis
G. Tom Shires, Dallas
Watts R. Webb, Syracuse
Jack Wickstrom, New Orleans
Chestley L. Yelton, Birmingham

Senior Members

Vernon C. Abbott, Pontiac, Michigan
Alexander P. Aitken, Winchester, Massachusetts

Rufus H. Alldredge, New Orleans
Otto E. Aufranc, Boston
Sam W. Banks, Chicago

Contents

Chapter 1

Primary Assessment and Management of the Injured

Summary

The management of an injured patient admitted to an emergency department must include a workable sequence such as the following:

1. Make a rapid and initial assessment of the patient's condition, including state of consciousness.

2. Establish and maintain a patent airway.

3. Assure effective respiratory exchange (tamponade open chest wounds, stabilize flail chest).

4. Maintain or restore effective circulatory volume.

5. Conduct a methodical, thorough physical examination.

6. Splint all obvious or suspected fractures immediately and avoid flexion of any patient with a suspected spinal injury.

7. Do not move the patient unnecessarily. Hold to an absolute minimum transfers of the patient (i.e., emergency room area to x-ray to ward to operating room).

8. Obtain appropriate consultation in patients with multiple injuries.

9. The surgeon in charge must coordinate priority and timing for correction of specific injuries.

INITIAL EVALUATION

When an injured patient arrives at an emergency department, the responsibility assumed by the first physician who examines him cannot be overemphasized. This responsibility includes: (a) instituting lifesaving procedures when required, (b) diagnosing the injuries present, and (c) providing an orderly sequence of treatment to correct the injuries.

LIFESAVING PROCEDURES

Although a thorough physical examination is mandatory, a rapid initial survey should be made immediately to evaluate: (a) airway and respiration, (b) heart action, (c) active bleeding, (d) state of consciousness, (e) evident shock without active bleeding, and (f) life-endangering injuries (flail chest or sucking chest wounds). Since the maintenance of useful life is dependent essentially upon the flow of oxygenated blood to the tissues the initial priority treatment must be: (1) to assure an airway, (2) to control hemorrhage, and (3) to maintain an effective circulatory volume.

Airway: If the patient is unconscious or has evidence of trauma about the face and neck, the mouth should be examined, and secretions, blood, and vomitus removed. If facial fractures result in instability of the jaws, an oral airway or nasotracheal tube may be required immediately. Open wounds of the chest must be controlled with pressure, and hemothorax or pneumothorax should be evaluated and decompressed immediately. In crushing injuries of the chest, chest-wall stabilization or positive-pressure breathing may be required. Tracheostomy should be reserved for those cases where the nasotracheal tube cannot be inserted instantly (see Chapters 11 and 12).

State of Consciousness: If the patient is in a state of confusion or is unconscious, the cause may possibly be brain injury, blood loss, hypoxia, excessive alcohol intake, or diabetic acidosis. A tentative decision should be reached immediately, particularly if the cause is suspected to be active intracranial bleeding or mechanical airway obstruction.

Bleeding: Simultaneously with the establishment of an adequate airway the patient should be evaluated for external or internal bleeding. External hemorrhage of the extremities can usually be controlled with a properly applied pressure bandage. Tourniquets should be used as a last resort and only in cases of extremely traumatized extremities in which major vessels have been injured. If a tourniquet must be applied to an extremity, it should be maintained until proper provisions have been made to correct shock. Pressure dressings are also helpful for external bleeding of the trunk and face. The patient must be continually watched for evidence of internal bleeding and shock.

Shock: Shock must be anticipated in every seriously injured patient. The first step is to establish an adequate intravenous lifeline, preferably a plastic catheter, which is not as easily dislodged from a vein as the standard intravenous needle. At the time the intravenous infusion is started a blood sample should be drawn for blood type and crossmatching to insure sufficient blood for subsequent treatment. The cause of shock may not be immediately apparent. The patient should be evaluated for internal hemorrhage in the peritoneal cavity, chest cavity, or crushing injuries of an extremity.

MEDICAL HISTORY

The patient must be approached in a calm reassuring manner which will help allay much of his anxiety and apprehension. The physician must not convey a sense of panic to the patient through hasty purposeless actions or an excited tone of voice.

During the course of the initial examination, most of the relevant immediate history can be obtained. Information that is helpful, if it can be obtained, concerns the exact type of accident which has occurred, the position of the patient at the time of the accident, and his subsequent displacement. It is particularly helpful to know if a passenger in an automobile accident has struck any object such as the dashboard, windshield, or rearview mirror. In addition, it is desirable to obtain information relating to the length of time since the injury, and any prior treatment, particularly with narcotics or analgesics, or intravenous therapy that may have been administered before arrival in the emergency department.

In addition to the detailed information about the accident, it is also desirable to survey the patient's past history with particular emphasis on any prior incidence of cardiac or pulmonary abnormalities, renal abnormalities, or associated metabolic diseases such as diabetes. The patient should be questioned specifically about any drugs, such as digitalis, and steroids, that he has taken regularly or recently. A history of excessive alcoholic intake or narcotic usage can provide useful information, if it can be obtained. In addition, it is important to determine whether the patient has received previous immunization with tetanus toxoid and whether or not he has any known sensitivity to drugs, particularly penicillin. Any information relating to previous untoward experience with anesthesia or any past evidence of abnormal bleeding is important. Knowing when the patient last ate is important if anesthesia is to be administered.

Ideally, this information should be obtained from the patient if he is able to give it. If not, as much information as possible should be obtained from the available relatives or friends if any accompany the patient.

EXAMINATION OF THE PATIENT

Once the attending physician has evaluated the patient's state of consciousness, has assured the presence of a patent airway with good respiratory exchange and an adequate circulation, and has attended to any obvious bleeding, his next step is to conduct a thorough and careful physical examination. The patient should be completely undressed; if necessary, scissors should be used. Until the examination is completed injudicious moving of the patient should be avoided, and if there is a suspected fracture of the spine, the patient must be kept flat on the table. If it is necessary to turn the patient for examination or treatment he should be rolled from side to side "like a log" with the spine kept straight—neither flexed nor extended. If the patient complains of localized pain or obvious wounds the examiner's immediate attention should be directed to this area.

After the physician has evaluated the major or obvious injuries he should conduct a thorough methodical examination to avoid overlooking associated injuries. Undiscovered injuries are usually overlooked because a detailed examination of all parts of the body has not been carried out. Too often this means that an extra trip to the x-ray department must be made after a day or two for films that should have been made at the time of admission.

An orderly examination must include the following areas even in the absence of related symptoms: head and neck, thorax, abdomen and pelvis, genitalia and rectum, and the extremities.

HEAD AND NECK

First, the examiner quickly but gently palpates the scalp with both hands in search of previously undisclosed lacerated wounds, depressed fractures, foreign bodies, deformity, swelling, hematoma, tumor, or points of tenderness. In the absence of symptoms the cervical spine is palpated in order to detect pain, tenderness, muscle spasm, limitation of motion, deformity, or crepitus. Any suggestion of a positive finding is an indication for x-ray examination of the cervical spine, including oblique views because of the frequent complaints of "whip lash." Movements of the mandible and occlusion of the teeth are similarly checked.

In the absence of obvious wounds, the neck is examined for venous distention, hematoma, tumor, adenopathy, unusual arterial pulsation, or displacement of the trachea. Paresis of facial muscles and the trapezius muscle or sternomastoid, indicating damage to cranial nerves VII or XI, is recorded. In the oral cavity, evidence of bleeding, deformity, tumor, missing or loose teeth, or paralysis of the soft palate (cranial nerve IX) or tongue (cranial nerve XII) is noted. Extraocular movements and pupillary responses are observed with great care and are recorded. The critical, early eye signs which clearly localize a brain injury may be transient, and the first examiner may be the only one to see them.

THORAX

The rib cage is palpated quickly and carefully for asymmetry, deformity, points of tenderness, fracture, retraction, bulging, or subcutaneous emphysema. Expansion is observed, and the two sides are compared. The precordium is palpated to estimate the impact, rhythm, and rate of the heart beat Then, by percussion and auscultation, the cardiac outline is delineated, and the character of heart sounds, areas of dullness and flatness, rales, and evidence of mediastinal shift are noted. If a sucking wound is present, it is securely covered with a thick pad of sterile gauze to avoid further build-up of intrapleural pressure while the examination is being completed. Finally, the spine can be palpated enough without moving the patient to disclose obvious deformity or points of tenderness and spasm that may give a clue to the presénce of a fracture.

ABDOMEN AND PELVIS

Spine and Pelvic Bones: The examiner continues his palpation of the dorsal and lumbar spine and the sacrum. Palpating the iliac crests and applying gentle pressure over the anterior superior iliac spines may elicit tenderness, suggesting pelvic bone fractures or joint separations. Gentle pressure directly over the pubic symphysis may elicit pain or tenderness, suggesting disruption of the pubic synchondrosis or fractures of the pubic rami.

Indwelling Catheter: If any suspicion of pelvic fracture exists at this point in the examination, a catheter should be introduced into the bladder at once and left in place. The incidence of disruption of the anterior urethra is high with pubic fractures. It is easy to pass a catheter into the bladder soon after injury; a few hours later, edema, hemorrhage, and extravasation of urine may make it impossible. By this simple expediency the surgeon may be saved hours of tedious dissection needed to find the ends of an avulsed urethra, and the patient may be saved much pain and disability (see Chapter 14).

Abdominal Palpation: The abdominal wall and flanks are palpated for hematoma, muscle spasm, localized tenderness, distended loops of intestine, solid viscera, or tumors, and the findings are checked by percussion. Unusual pulsations or vascular thrills are noted and checked by auscultation for presence of audible bruit. Auscultation for peristaltic sounds is time-consuming and unproductive at this stage of the investigation, although it may be significant later.

When the abdomoninal examination has been completed, the observer checks the abdominal and cremasteric reflexes as a part of the neurological survey. If abnormal responses are elicited, a rapid attempt is made to determine abnormal sensory levels on the trunk.

Wounds: Open wounds are not probed during examination. They are protected by sterile dressings or sterile towels. Protruding masses of omentum or intestine are covered with sterile saline dressings and are not returned to the peritoneal cavity until adequate preparations have been made for thorough exploration of the abdomen.

Bleeding: Obviously dangerous bleeding from the wound demands immediate exploration. In rare instances it may be possible for the examiner to control intraabdominal bleeding with fist pressure on the aorta while the surgical equipment is being readied and anesthesia is being induced. This procedure may sometimes be lifesaving. However, it is so exhausting even to the most vigorous surgeon that preparation for abdominal exploration must be made in a matter of minutes.

GENITALIA AND RECTUM

After the abdominal examination has been completed, the genitalia are checked for open wounds, herniation, subcutaneous hemorrhage, or extravasation of urine. A drop of blood at the urethral meatus may represent a significant urethral injury. Since this may be the only early finding it should not be overlooked. A digital examination of the rectum is then carried out to observe sphincter tone, fecal content, presence or absence of tumors or normal pelvic organs. Displacement of the prostate should be evaluated during rectal examination (see Chapter 14). Abnormal contours of adjacent pelvic bones may confirm the presence of a fracture. The finding of gross blood or clots in the rectum may provide a clue to disruption of the rectum or lower colon, which may require immediate surgical intervention. In the female, bimanual pelvic examination is performed.

EXTREMITIES

Upper Extremities: In the absence of obvious deformity or grotesque position which would suggest a fracture, the extremities are examined individually in accordance with the systematic routine. First the examiner flexes the elbow and passively rotates and abducts the humerus through the normal range of motion; then he flexes and extends the elbow and wrist and rotates the forearm through the normal range of pronation and supination. If the patient is conscious and cooperative, these maneuvers are repeated with active movement while the observer exerts passive resistance to the successive muscle groups. Biceps, triceps, and distal radial reflexes are then checked, and any gross abnormality of sensory pattern is noted. The hands are examined simultaneously while the patient goes through the normal movements of the wrist, thumb, and fingers. This simple routine should make apparent any fractures or dislocations, avulsion or weakness of muscle groups, or nerve deficits that had not been disclosed previously. Check the pulses for evidence of injury to the arteries.

Lower Extremities: The lower extremities are similarly evaluated. With the knee flexed, the hip is abducted and rotated passively through its normal range; the knee and ankle are similarly investigated, and the stability of the knee joint is checked. When practical, the extremity is put through the same maneuvers actively, against muscle resistance. Knee jerks, ankle jerks, and plantar reflexes are elicited, and abnormal sensory patterns noted.

Any puncture wound in the vicinity of a joint should be considered a penetrating joint wound until proven otherwise (see Chapter 15).

MEDICATIONS

If pain medication is initially indicated, it should be administered intravenously. The absorption of intramuscular medication is uncertain during periods of shock, and if repeated doses of narcotics are given intramuscularly, the subsequent establishment of adequate circulation may result in absorption of excessive amounts of the drug with undesirable respiratory depression.

ROENTGENOGRAMS

Only after lifesaving measures and a complete physical examination have been performed should roentgenograms be ordered. This avoids the pitfall made by inexperienced physicians of performing a preliminary examination and sending the patient to an x-ray department for examination of the more obvious injuries. After the initial x-rays a more detailed physical examination may reveal additional findings that require a second trip to the x-ray department. Every effort should be made to minimize the number of times a patient must be transferred from a stretcher to an x-ray table.

In many instances, it may be possible to have adequate x-ray equipment available in the emergency department so that most of the necessary examinations can be carried out there. In the event the patient is to be moved to another area, it is imperative that any obvious fractures or suspicious fractures be splinted prior to the time the patient is moved. Of course, splints should be applied immediately and not reserved for transporting the patient. In addition, if a suspected injury of the spine is present, the patient must be handled accordingly (see Chapter 15).

QUESTIONS TO BE ANSWERED BY PRIMARY ASSESSMENT OF THE INJURED

After completing the preliminary survey of the patient, the examiner should be able to answer some of the following questions:

1. Does the patient urgently require immediate surgical treatment?
2. Does the patient require additional supportive therapy, to be followed by a definitive operation as soon as he has been adequately prepared?
3. Are further diagnostic procedures indicated, and, if so, what?
4. Does the patient require additional immoblization or fixation before being moved?
5. How should he be transported?
6. Will an additional period of observation be advantageous before definitive treatment is undertaken?
7. Can he be treated as an ambulatory patient?
8. Is prophylactic administration of antibiotics and tetanus antitoxin or toxoid indicated?
9. What type of anesthesia should the injured person be given?

PATIENT WITH MULTIPLE INJURIES

The patient with multiple injuries presents particularly complex problems of treatment.

First, it is essential that all of the significant injuries be recognized at the onset. The importance of careful and complete examination of the injured patient cannot be overemphasized.

The **second** consideration is priority for treatment of the various injuries. While it is axiomatic that one injury usually dominates the picture, several injuries may be treated simultaneously to the advantage of the patient. For example, with two teams operating at once, a wound of an extremity may be debrided and repaired at the same time that the abdomen is explored. Or, extensive burns of the body and extremities may be dressed while a decompression is being performed for head injury.

The **third** consideration is the amount of supportive treatment required. The patient with multiple injuries usually suffers more profound shock than does the patient with a single injury. He must, therefore, receive more supportive therapy before and during definitive treatment.

The **fourth** consideration concerns who does what and who supervises the overall management of the patient with multiple injuries. This is often a difficult problem. When multiple injuries traverse the field of several specialists, problems of priority or jurisdiction may arise and can work to the detriment of the patient. Where no specialists are available, the decision is simple; the physician who is confronted with the injured patient must make all the decisions and conduct all the treatment. Fortunately, it is relatively uncommon in present hospital circumstances to encounter specialists who demand that injuries in their own field be treated at the expense of other necessary treatment. Nevertheless, it is imperative that the overall supervision of the patient with multiple injuries be in the hands of the surgeon who has the broadest experience and competence in dealing with wounds, hemorrhage, and shock. This surgeon must become the captain of the team in the interest of optimal functional recovery by the patient and to ensure that the patient receives proper treatment regardless of the specialty involved.

GENERAL PRINCIPLES OF OPEN-WOUND CARE

Certain general principles apply to the care of all open injuries, regardless of location. In some instances special precautions are necessary. These will be detailed in the specific chapters. The general considerations are:

1. **Avoid further contamination of the wound.** All inspection and manipulation of the wound are made under aseptic conditions. The surgeon, and all others in attendance, should wear masks to decrease

additional contamination from the nose and throat. Dressing of the wound is carried out with sterile instruments.

2. **Provide suitable anesthesia.**

3. **Cleanse area surrounding the wound and the wound itself.** The wound is covered with a sterile dressing and the area surrounding the wound is first cleansed, and all hair shaved. The dressing is then removed, and the wound is washed gently with fresh materials and irrigated. Practices vary somewhat in the selection and use of the cleansing agent. Many surgeons use plain soap both for cleansing the skin and for cleansing the wound. Others use soap and water for the skin and simply irrigate the wound with large amounts of physiologic salt solution. Most surgeons prefer to use one of the hexachlorophene soaps; however, it should be noted that such agents are too irritating to be used on or near mucous membranes. Copious saline irrigation of open wounds is mandatory but vigorous scrubbing in the wound may produce additional trauma. Regardless of how it is done, cleansing should be carried out with gentleness and care.

4. **Excise destroyed tissues and remove foreign bodies.** The purpose of excision is to remove devitalized tissue and tissue destined to succumb because of the injury it has sustained. Needless sacrifice of viable tissue is to be avoided. The skin, especially, must be carefully conserved. In sharply incised wounds, none of the skin border need be excised. In severe crushes and avulsions, large areas of skin may be nonviable and may require excision.

5. **Repair the deep tissues if this can be done with safety.** For help in determining the plan of action, refer to the chapters dealing with specific injuries.

6. **Close the wound.** In civilian practice, most wounds are amenable to primary closure. There are important exceptions. These include: (1) wounds seen 12 hours after injury, (2) wounds produced by high velocity projectiles, (3) wounds already grossly infected, (4) wounds which are badly contaminated and in which there is extensive muscle damage, and (5) wounds caused by human or animal bites.

In the absence of the above contradications closure is completed by suturing the skin edges if this can be accomplished without tension. If there has been great loss of skin, split-thickness skin grafts may make immediate closure possible. Under some circumstances flaps will be required. If primary flaps are considered for wound closure the length of the flap should not exceed the base for single pedicles. In bipedicle flaps (relaxing incisions) the length of the flap should not exceed 2 times the base. If the surrounding skin is contused or traumatized it should not be used as a flap. As a general rule distal-based flaps should not be used on the extremities. Every effort should be made to close the wound primarily, if the aforementioned contraindications are not present, so as to minimize the amount of fibrosis produced and to achieve maximum function.

Chapter 2

Cardiopulmonary Resuscitation

Summary

Routine for Resuscitation

Condition	Treatment
1. Patient is obstructed, trying to breathe.	Relieve obstruction.
2. Patient is apneic.	Relieve obstruction, ventilate lungs.
3. Patient is pulseless after 30 seconds of ventilation.	Begin external cardiac compression, elevate legs, start venous cutdown.
4. Patient is pulseless after 60 seconds of ventilation and compression.	Epinephrine 1 mg intravenous, intracardiac, or intratracheal, whichever is quickest.
5. Electrocardiogram shows ventricular fibrillation.	External countershock.
6. Patient is still pulseless.	Continue ventilation and compression. Give sodium bicarbonate 44 mEq. I.V. every 5 minutes. Repeat epinephrine or start vasoconstrictor I.V. drip.
7. Electrocardiogram still shows ventricular fibrillation.	Methoxamine 20 mg intravenous. Repeat countershock.
8. Circulation is restored.	Individualize treatment according to patient's condition.

Cardiopulmonary resuscitation refers to those measures used to restore ventilation and circulation in persons in whom these functions have been interrupted. Resuscitation techniques have no value in the management of irreversible disease states. They are intended to revive otherwise healthy individuals who experience some reversible catastrophe that interrupts breathing and circulation.

PATHOGENESIS

Asphyxia is the common denominator in all cases of sudden death. Common causes of sudden death include drowning, electrocution, smoke and gas inhalation, drug or chemical intoxication, stroke, injuries of the head, neck, or chest, coronary occlusion, convulsions, and unconsciousness from any cause.

IMMEDIATE TREATMENT

The measures to initiate artificial ventilation and artificial circulation are the same whether carried out by physicians or lay rescuers and whether performed in a hospital or any other location. Immediate recognition of the need for resuscitation is essential. In most instances, respiration stops before circulation. Respiration should always be checked first, since **resuscitation depends on oxygen transport from air to lung to tissue.** Clinical death occurs when the victim's heart stops beating. Cellular metabolism continues for a limited time thereafter. Unless effective artificial ventilation and circulation are promptly instituted and continued without interruption until they are no longer necessary, irreversible changes occur in the vital tissues.

AIRWAY

Movement of the chest or abdomen indicates that the victim is trying to breathe. **The airway is obstructed if no air can be heard or felt moving in and out of the victim's mouth.**

Foreign material in the oropharynx may be obstructing the airway. Grasp the tongue, using a piece of cloth or a towel clip, look in the mouth, and pass a finger through the back of the mouth and throat to detect and to remove any foreign material. Suction may be used to remove liquid foreign material such as blood or vomitus.

The unconscious state is life-threatening whatever the cause. When the head of an unconscious patient assumes the neutral or flexed position, the back of the tongue comes to rest against the back of the pharynx. This blocks the passage of air into the trachea (Fig. 2–1). Asphyxia follows. This obstruction of the airway by the tongue can be corrected by stretching

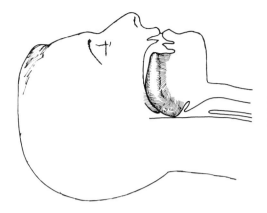

Figure 2-1 With the head in neutral position, the base of the tongue obstructs airflow through the nose and mouth into the trachea.

Figure 2-2 Maximal backward tilt of the head displaces the base of the tongue from the posterior pharyngeal wall. Airway is open.

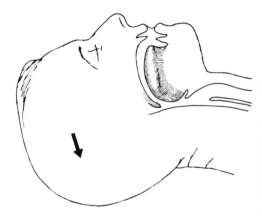

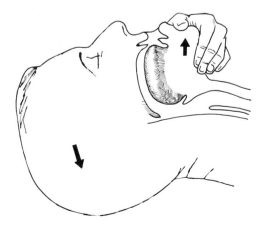

Figure 2-3 Combination of maximal backward tilt of the head and anterior displacement of the mandible provides maximal airway.

the soft tissues of the neck which are attached to the mandible. **In most unconscious patients, maximal backward tilt of the head relieves airway obstruction** (Fig. 2–2). If backward tilt of the head is not followed by free movement of air through the victim's mouth, anterior displacement of the mandible should be combined with backward head tilt. **Lift the jaw forward so that the lower teeth are in front of the upper teeth** (Fig. 2–3).

PULMONARY VENTILATION

If the victim is not making breathing movements, the rescuer opens his own mouth widely, takes a deep breath, and, after pinching the victim's nose to prevent leakage, blows forcefully into the victim's mouth. **Blow hard enough to expand the victim's chest.** If no expansion occurs, the airway is obstructed. In this event the victim's head and jaw should be repositioned, and the rescuer should blow more forcefully. If chest expansion still is not achieved, the rescuer should quickly examine the victim's mouth and throat for vomitus or foreign material and remove it with his fingers or suction equipment (if available).

After successful lung inflation, the rescuer should immediately **feel for a pulse** in one of the victim's carotid or femoral arteries. If a pulse is felt, there is sufficient circulation to permit resuscitation by artificial ventilation alone. If a pulse is not felt, two probabilities exist. First, the heart may have stopped. Second, the heart may be beating so weakly that a pulse cannot be felt. Skilled observers are not able to feel a carotid pulse when the systolic blood pressure falls below 60 mm Hg. If a pulse is not felt, the rescuer should give 3 or 4 more breaths and check again for a pulse. Enough oxygen may be transported to reoxygenate the heart and restore circulation. **If a pulse is not felt after 30 seconds of ventilation, artificial circulation must be started.**

CARDIAC RESUSCITATION

It is most urgent to restore cardiac action at the earliest possible moment to prevent irreversible damage of the vital tissues. The principal function of circulation is to transport oxygen, so artificial circulation and artificial respiration must be used together.

When the sternum is compressed toward the vertebral column, blood is forced out of the heart into the arterial system. When the sternum is released, the normal elasticity of the chest wall allows it to rebound and the heart fills with blood. Although the circulation produced in this fashion is of a lesser magnitude than normal, it is sufficient to reoxygenate the arterial blood when combined with artificial ventilation. Unfortunately, it is usually not sufficient for adequate tissue perfusion, so **the emergency persists after external cardiopulmonary resuscitation has been started.**

Place the victim with his back resting on a firm surface. If two rescuers

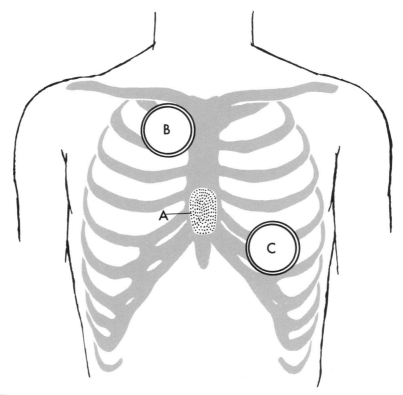

Figure 2–4 Landmarks for cardiopulmonary resuscitation. A, area for pressure during external cardiac massage. B and C, location of electrodes for external electrical countershock.

are present, one should ventilate the lungs at a rate of 12 breaths per minute while the other rescuer compresses the sternum about 60 strokes per minute. Pressure should be applied with the heel of one hand only in the midline over the lower third of the sternum (Fig. 2–4). **The sternum must be compressed with sufficient force to cause pulsation of the carotid artery.** If only one rescuer is present, the best compromise is to deliver 3 breaths followed by 15 compressions of the sternum. **Blow hard enough to expand the chest and compress hard enough to make an artificial pulse!**

DEFINITIVE TREATMENT

The methods just described are the first steps necessary in any attempt at cardiopulmonary resuscitation. **Artificial respiration and artificial circulation must be continued without interruption until the resuscitation attempt is successful or hopeless.** These first steps may be sufficient to restore spontaneous circulation and ventilation. Often additional measures are necessary.

Equipment used in resuscitation is helpful, but not essential, to management of the emergency. Use of equipment requires experience and judgment, thus increasing the possibility of mechanical or human failure. But situations may occur in the course of resuscitation that cannot be satisfactorily managed without specific items of equipment.

AIRWAY

Three basic items are of assistance for maintaining the airway. These are the oropharyngeal airway, the endotracheal tube, and suction equipment. Proper use of an oropharyngeal airway often makes it unnecessary to maintain anterior displacement of the mandible. **However, obstruction may occur with an airway in place if the head is allowed to flex.** The mouth-to-mouth airway is a special variation of the oropharyngeal airway. It is an S-shaped tube, one end of which is inserted into the victim's pharynx; the other end provides a mouthpiece into which the rescuer blows, eliminating the need for direct oral contact (Fig. 2–5).

Insertion of an endotracheal tube is of help in maintaining airway patency. **Use of an endotracheal tube does not ensure an airway since the tube may kink or be displaced.** Endotracheal tubes may be inserted through the nose or mouth into the trachea. This is usually accomplished with the aid of a laryngoscope (Fig. 2–6). Considerable experience is required for rapid intubation. **Unskilled attempts at intubation may be catastrophic.** Other advantages of tracheal intubation include preventing aspiration of gastric contents into the lungs and preventing gastric insufflation during artificial ventilation.

Suction equipment is useful in removing foreign material and gastric content from the mouth, nose, throat, and trachea. Adequate negative pressure and adequate catheter size are necessary in order to remove foreign material of large size or high viscosity.

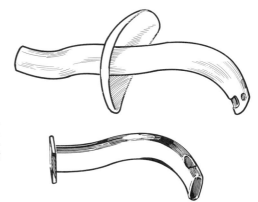

Figure 2–5 Mouth-to-mouth airway (top). Long end is inserted into victim's pharynx. Short end provides mouthpiece for rescuer. Flange helps prevent leakage of air from victim's mouth. Oropharyngeal airway (bottom) used to relieve rescuer of necessity for maintaining anterior displacement of mandible.

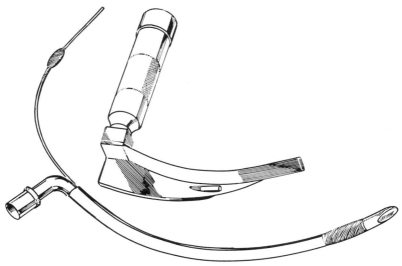

Figure 2–6   Laryngoscope (top) used to displace tongue and soft tissues during insertion of endotracheal tube. Endotracheal tube (bottom) with inflatable cuff and connector in place.

PULMONARY VENTILATION

Several items of equipment are available for use in artificial ventilation of the lungs. The simplest of these is the mouth-to-mouth airway just mentioned. An ordinary anesthesia mask may be used to cover the mouth and nose of the victim and to blow air into the victim's lungs. A number of self-inflating bag-mask units are available that utilize room air for ventilation of the lungs (Fig. 2–7). These do not depend on a source of compressed gas, but do accept oxygen from a tank for enrichment. Effective use of these devices requires, **simultaneously,** maintaining a patent airway, squeezing the breathing bag, and keeping the mask applied so that the air does not leak between the mask and the victim's face. Mechanical resuscitators are available to perform intermittent positive pressure breathing. Properly used, these deliver air or oxygen-enriched air until a set peak pressure is

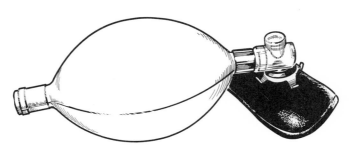

Figure 2–7   Self-inflating bag with non-rebreathing valve and anesthesia mask attached.

reached under the mask. Exhalation then occurs passively through a valve. **The most common error in the use of equipment for artificial ventilation is failure to maintain an airway.**

CARDIAC RESUSCITATION

Equipment: There are two functional types of cardiac arrest. *Asystole* is total absence of myocardial contraction. *Ventricular fibrillation* is a totally disorganized, ineffective quivering of the heart muscle so that no cardiac output results. Cardiac contraction is impossible because various portions of the myocardium are in different stages of depolarization and repolarization; refractory areas prevent simultaneous excitation of the entire myocardium. Unless the heart is exposed to direct vision, distinction between these two types of cardiac arrest must be made by electrocardiograph. **A reliable electrocardiograph or electrocardiographic oscilloscope is an essential item of equipment for the definitive treatment of cardiac arrest.**

The electrocardiographic pattern of asystole may be of two kinds. First, there may be no electrical activity, so that only a straight line is recorded (Fig. 2–8). Second, ventricular complexes, occasionally relatively normal in appearance, may be recorded even though there is total absence of cardiac output. No palpable pulses or recordable blood pressure can be

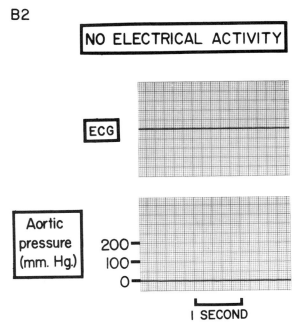

Figure 2–8 Cardiac arrest. Simultaneous recording of aortic pressure and electrocardiogram. No electrical activity of heart and no aortic pressure. (From Redding, J. S.: Cardiopulmonary Resuscitation. Traumatic Medicine and Surgery for the Attorney, 5:323, 1966. Butterworth, Inc., Washington, D. C.)

detected (Fig. 2–9). Therefore, it is essential to remember that **the heart is a pump, not a television station.** Whether electrocardiographic complexes are or are not recorded modifies neither the treatment nor the prognosis. It is not unusual for asystole to convert to ventricular fibrillation during resuscitation as partial reoxygenation of the myocardium causes differing areas of electrical potential.

Ventricular fibrillation is easily recognized by a totally disorganized formless wandering of the electrocardiographic baseline (Fig. 2–10). Distinction between ventricular fibrillation and cardiac asystole is essential since the disorganized activity of the fibrillating heart must be stopped so that the next impulse originating in the sino-atrial node can lead to cardiac contraction.

The only practical method of correcting ventricular fibrillation is electrical countershock. Consequently, **a reliable external defibrillator is an essential item of equipment for definitive cardiac resuscitation.** Two types of external defibrillators are available. Alternating current defibrillators deliver alternating currents of about 480 volts for 0.25 second. Direct current defibrillators deliver a capacitor discharge of 100–400 watt seconds. There appears to be little difference in the effectiveness of the two types for correction of ventricular fibrillation.

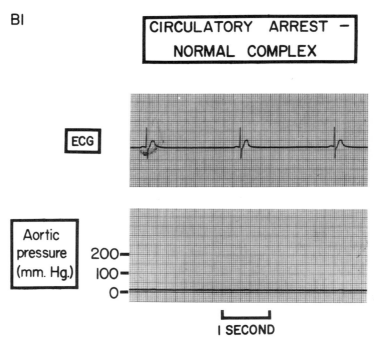

Figure 2–9 Cardiac arrest. Electrocardiogram showing normal sequence of P, Q, R, S, and T waves with total absence of circulation as shown by aortic pressure. (From Redding, J. S.: Cardiopulmonary Resuscitation. Traumatic Medicine and Surgery for the Attorney, 5:323, 1966. Butterworth, Inc., Washington, D. C.)

A4

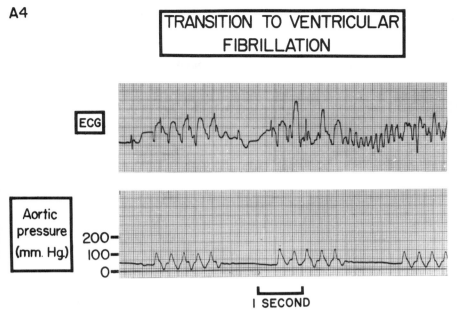

Figure 2–10   Cardiac arrest. Electrocardiogram showing development of ventricular fibrillation. Spikes of blood pressure to 100 mm. Hg resulted from external cardiac massage. (From Redding, J. S.: Cardiopulmonary Resuscitation. Traumatic Medicine and Surgery for the Attorney, 5:323, 1966. Butterworth, Inc., Washington, D. C.)

With either type, electrodes are applied with firm pressure at the locations indicated in Figure 2–4. Countershock is useful in resuscitation only when ventricular fibrillation is known to be present, since shocks applied to the heart in asystole accomplish nothing and are a waste of time. Unless the countershock can be delivered within 60 seconds of the onset of ventricular fibrillation it must be preceded by a preliminary period of artificial ventilation, cardiac massage, and injection of vasoconstrictor drugs to aid reoxygenation of the myocardium. **Electric current applied to the anoxic heart is ineffective.**

Drugs: Recommendations for the use of drugs in cardiac resuscitation have been obscure, conflicting, and based on inference from their actions under other circumstances. Recent evidence indicates that proper drug and fluid therapy greatly increases the effectiveness of external cardiopulmonary resuscitation.

The purpose of drug and fluid therapy in resuscitation from cardiac arrest is twofold: to increase blood flow to the coronary arteries and to minimize the effects of metabolic acidosis resulting from interruption of the circulation.

VASOCONSTRICTORS: The bloodflow resulting from cardiac massage is a fraction of normal and usually is insufficient for adequate tissue perfusion. During cardiac arrest primary concern must be given to restoring adequate spontaneous cardiac activity. Epinephrine (Adrenalin) has been used for many years in cardiac resuscitation. Recent evaluation indicates that it adds greatly to the effectiveness of resuscitation by increasing resistance to the flow of blood to most of the body, consequently increasing perfusion of the coronary arteries. The peripheral vasoconstriction caused by epinephrine is transient, lasting only 3 to 5 minutes, and is followed by rebound vasodilatation. If spontaneous cardiac contractions begin during the vasoconstrictor phase, improved tissue perfusion results during the vasodilator phase. Tachyphylaxis (decreased response to successive doses) is characteristic of epinephrine. Therefore if repeated doses are necessary, they should be given at 3-minute intervals, and another vasoconstrictor drug is advisable after 3 doses of epinephrine. Several other vasoconstrictor drugs, such as phenylephrine (Neo-Synephrine) 10 mg or methoxamine (Vasoxyl) 20 mg, have been shown to be as effective as epinephrine 1 mg in restarting arrested hearts.

Vasoconstriction is as crucial in resuscitation from ventricular fibrillation as it is in resuscitation from cardiac standstill. It would appear that methoxamine 20 mg is more effective than epinephrine 1 mg given prior to attempts at external defibrillation.

There should be no delay in using an appropriate vasoconstrictor, and dosage should be adequate. **Cardiac arrest is no time for homeopathic measures.** Since **the useful action of the drugs is on the peripheral circulation, not directly on the heart,** intracardiac injection is not advantageous over intravenous injection. In fact, when an endotracheal tube is in place and intravenous injection is not immediately possible, **the drugs may be diluted tenfold with water and given down the endotracheal tube.** This produces as quick and effective a response as does either intracardiac or intravenous injection. Unless the drugs are given by the intratracheal route, there is no advantage to dilution before injection.

CARDIAC STIMULANTS: The direct stimulating effect of epinephrine and other drugs on the heart is incidental during attempts to restart the arrested heart since **the arrested heart cannot be stimulated.** Drugs that have their principal effect by cardiac stimulation, such as isoproterenol (Isuprel) or calcium salts that increase myocardial tone, may be useful after the heart is restarted, but they are useless during the period of cardiac arrest.

FLUIDS: Adequate venous return to the heart is essential to maintain cardiac massage. Therefore, the victim's legs should be elevated to improve venous return, and rapid intravenous fluid administration should be started promptly. Unless a needle is already positioned in a vein before cardiac arrest occurs, this usually necessitates **rapid cutdown and positioning of an intravenous catheter under direct vision because during the period of circulatory arrest the veins are usually collapsed.**

SODIUM BICARBONATE: When circulation is inadequate to maintain oxygen delivery to the tissues, anaerobic metabolism causes accumulation of lactic acid and other acid metabolites. Consequently, severe metabolic acidosis develops during cardiac arrest. This increases the susceptibility of the heart to ventricular fibrillation. Also the response to vasoconstrictor drugs is diminished, but not abolished. For these reasons it is recommended that 44 mEq. of sodium bicarbonate be given intravenously every 5 minutes until the heart restarts. Undue preoccupation with giving sodium bicarbonate in excessive amounts should be avoided. **Sodium bicarbonate will not restart the heart and poor tissue perfusion prevents correction of acidosis until adequate tissue perfusion is restored.**

POSTCARDIAC ARREST CARE

Usually the patient's reflexes are absent and respiration and circulation are in precarious condition requiring constant support. Useful measures to preserve cerebral function must be taken without delay.

CIRCULATION

Isoproterenol, to increase myocardial contractility and decrease resistance to tissue perfusion, should be used only when the heart is beating weakly. The same is true for the use of calcium chloride to increase myocardial tone and of lidocaine to control myocardial irritability.

VENTILATION

Artificial ventilation should be continued after the heart is restarted. The possibility of fractured ribs or pneumothorax resulting from the resuscitative effort must be considered. Controlled hyperventilation with a respirator insures adequate ventilation and it causes a respiratory alkalosis that tends to decrease intracranial pressure. Continued ventilatory support necessitates tracheal intubation or tracheostomy.

CEREBRAL FUNCTION

The only factor clearly shown to reduce cerebral damage after resuscitation is prompt restoration of spontaneous cardiac activity.

If the patient's nervous system is obtunded, massive doses of steroids have been recommended to prevent further cerebral edema. Osmotic diuresis has been suggested to reduce existing cerebral edema. Deliberate hypothermia to 30°–32° C has been suggested to reduce oxygen consumption and carbon dioxide production.

METABOLIC ACIDOSIS

Improved tissue perfusion after spontaneous circulation is restored usually leads to mobilization of acid metabolites. Arterial blood pH, PO_2, and PCO_2 should be determined at frequent intervals to guide further administration of sodium bicarbonate and to regulate ventilation and the concentration of inhaled oxygen necessary to prevent hypoxemia.

PROGNOSIS

The patient's state of consciousness is the best indication of the success of the resuscitative effort. The earlier reflex activity returns, the more likely the patient is to recover fully. Steadily progressive lightening of consciousness is more encouraging than early return of partial consciousness which is followed by periods of no further improvement. Successful resuscitation is more likely in young patients with reasonable mental facility before the arrest than it is in older patients or those who originally had marginal intelligence.

Chapter 3

Shock

Summary

1. Obtain initial vital signs and start a chronologic record or flow sheet (Fig. 3-1).
2. Place the patient in Trendelenburg position.
3. Obtain a venous blood sample for type and crossmatch and hematocrit determination.
4. Obtain arterial blood pH, pO_2, and pCO_2, when indicated.
5. Insert a central venous catheter and measure central venous pressure (C.V.P.) at intervals of 15 to 30 minutes.
6. Start a rapid infusion of electrolyte solution via one or more large-bore catheters.
7. Insert an indwelling urethral catheter; record urinary output every 30 to 60 minutes.
8. Start transfusion of crossmatched blood as soon as it is available.
9. The response to fluid or blood replacement is adequate when: (a) pulse rate decreases; (b) arterial blood pressure increases; (c) signs of peripheral vasoconstriction diminish or disappear; (d) C.V.P. rises to normal; (e) urinary output exceeds 30 ml. per hour; (f) metabolic acidosis improves.
10. If oliguria persists despite an improvement in other parameters, consider renal shutdown.
11. A satisfactory but transient response to fluid replacement in a patient with hemorrhage suggests continuing blood loss requiring operative treatment.

A patient is in **shock** when there is inadequate perfusion of oxygen and nutrient materials in his cells, tissues, organs, or entire body. Failure to improve perfusion leads ultimately to the death of the cell, the tissue, the organ, and finally the patient. Shock develops in every patient prior to death, even though it may last only a few seconds.

In some patients, inadequate perfusion can exist for many hours and yet still be reversed. For example, experience in Korea showed that injured soldiers with severe shock secondary to massive hemorrhage (marked hypotension, oliguria, and loss of consciousness) responded dramatically to rapid blood replacement. When therapy was delayed, however, the hemodynamic and metabolic changes were not corrected by simple replacement of lost volume, and, occasionally, the patient would not respond to any therapy, a state termed **irreversible shock.** With each succeeding year, improved knowledge and treatment have extended the period of reversibility.

MECHANISMS

Shock has traditionally been divided into four types: hemorrhagic, cardiogenic, neurogenic, and septic. Recent knowledge suggests that the pathophysiology of shock is better appreciated by understanding the hemodynamic and metabolic changes that occur in patients with blood loss, burns, or extensive trauma. Ohm's law can serve as a basis for this understanding.

Ohm's law of electricity states that E (voltage) is equal to the product of I (current) times R (resistance). Borrowing from that law, one might define arterial blood pressure (B.P.) as the product of the output of blood by the heart (cardiac output or C.O.) times the peripheral resistance in the arterial system (P.R.). In other words, man has a measurable blood pressure because of the volume of blood pumped out from the heart and the intrinsic tone within the arterial tree. Putting this hypothesis in the form of an equation:

$$(1) \text{ Arterial B.P.} = \text{C.O.} \times \text{P.R.}$$

Since cardiac output represents the volume of blood pumped by the heart per minute, there must be two factors involved: the actual volume pumped per beat (stroke volume) and the number of beats per minute (heart rate):

$$(2) \text{ C.O.} = \text{Stroke Volume} \times \text{Heart Rate}$$

At any given moment, substitute stroke volume in equation 1 for C.O.

$$(3) \text{ Arterial B.P.} = \text{Volume} \times \text{P.R.}$$

A fall in volume must be compensated by a rise in peripheral resistance, or blood pressure will fall. A phlebotomy of 500 ml of blood usually produces mild tachycardia, just enough to maintain adequate cardiac output. After withdrawal of 1000 ml of blood, however, the compensatory tachycardia cannot maintain adequate cardiac output, and blood pressure will fall unless there is a corresponding increase in peripheral resistance.

Before considering specific forms of shock, two areas deserve further comment: (1) central venous pressure and (2) adverse effects of a sustained increase in peripheral resistance.

CENTRAL VENOUS PRESSURE

Pressure within the great veins of the thorax and abdomen reflects the pressure in the right side of the heart. This pressure can be measured with a large-bore plastic catheter introduced through a peripheral vein into the superior or inferior vena cava. Using the level of the right atrium (or midaxillary line) as a "zero," the normal central venous pressure (C.V.P.) measures from 5 to 10 cm of saline. The C.V.P. monitors two separate hemodynamic functions: (1) the ability of the heart to pump out venous return and (2) an adequate blood volume in the great veins. A very high C.V.P. means that the heart is unable to pump out the amount of blood returning to it (heart failure). A very low C.V.P. indicates a diminished blood volume (*hypovolemia*). Thus, the initial and serial measurements of C.V.P. provide an essential means of diagnosing and treating shock.

INCREASED PERIPHERAL RESISTANCE

A normal systolic blood pressure above 100 mm Hg may not reflect the state of tissue perfusion. An example of this would be the patient who has sustained a major blood loss. To maintain blood pressure, peripheral resistance rises, leading to decreased perfusion of the skin. A further increase in peripheral resistance reduces perfusion of the kidney, the intestinal tract, and the liver. Inadequate perfusion interferes with the normal state of aerobic metabolism since oxygen is not available to the tissues. Conversion to an anaerobic system produces acids that cannot be excreted by the poorly perfused kidney. Metabolic acidosis develops. Attempts to increase systemic blood pressure with vasopressors (as was done in the past) further increases peripheral resistance and aggravates this cycle. Thus, the patient is in profound shock (and probably will die) despite an apparently adequate systemic blood pressure.

In terms of the four classic forms of shock, the foregoing principles can be applied as follows:

Hemorrhagic Shock: Loss of blood volume → diminished venous return to the heart (*C.V.P. falls*) → tachycardia and a rise in peripheral resistance (vasoconstriction) → decreased perfusion → anaerobic metabolism → metabolic acidosis → further decrease in perfusion → renal failure, and so forth. A sustained increase in peripheral resistance increases the work load on the heart → heart failure (*C.V.P. rises*).

Cardiogenic Shock: Massive myocardial infarction or congestive heart failure (pump failure) → decreased C.O. → tachycardia and a rise in peripheral resistance (vasoconstriction) → decreased perfusion → metabolic acidosis, and so forth. The patient's appearance may suggest hypovolemic shock but the *C.V.P. is normal or elevated.*

Neurogenic Shock: Peripheral vasodilation → a decrease in peripheral resistance → pooling of blood → diminished venous return *(C.V.P. falls).* Inability to increase peripheral resistance → a fall in systemic blood pressure → syncope. Return of normal arterial tone reverses this sequence.

Septic Shock: Recent studies suggest that two forms exist:

(1) **Acute bacterial inflammation** → toxemia → marked fever and fall in peripheral resistance with pooling → inadequate venous return *(C.V.P. falls).* This is similar to neurogenic shock except that (a) compensation is inadequate since an inflammatory lesion with its arteriovenous shunting may require a 2- or 3-fold increase in cardiac output and (b) return of normal peripheral resistance requires control of the infection. An example would be an acute pyelonephritis.

(2) **Acute or chronic inflammation associated with hypovolemia** is the second form of septic shock and may follow the first form or may occur spontaneously, as in pancreatitis. A pattern identical to that shown for hemorrhagic shock occurs with decreased venous return *(C.V.P. is low),* increased peripheral resistance, reduced tissue perfusion, and the development of a severe metabolic acidosis. Correction of the hypovolemia will not reverse the sequence until sepsis is controlled.

TREATMENT

GENERAL TREATMENT

Regardless of etiology, shock, except for simple neurogenic shock, requires aggressive management. Any patient with extensive soft tissue injury, although hemodynamically stable on first examination, may decompensate and develop shock. To treat shock:

1. Establish the baseline pulse and respiratory rate and blood pressure.

2. Obtain a venous blood sample for hematocrit or hemoglobin, type, and crossmatch.

3. Place patient in the Trendelenburg position to aid venous return from the lower extremities and prevent air embolism during insertion of a subclavian catheter.

4. Insert a large-bore intravenous catheter (15–18 gauge) via the upper extremity, neck, or subclavian vein into the superior vena cava to

NAME _Doe, John_ AGE _24_

DATE: _3/30/70_
TIME: _0130_

PROBLEM #1 _Pulmonary Contusion (R) c̄ hemothorax 2° auto acc_
#2 _Deep laceration scalp (R) occip area_
#3 _LUQ injury, R/o ruptured spleen_

TIME	P	R	BP	Temp	CVP	Hb/Hct	Arterial Blood pH	pO₂	pCO₂	I.V. Fluid cc	Tot.	Blood cc	Tot.	In cc	Tot.	Urine cc	Tot.	Other Output cc	Tot.	REMARKS
0130	120	28	90/50	36.5 R	1					T.R.										Cutdown (R) arm for C.V.P.
0145	124	34	100/30		2	38	7.27	90 (40% O₂)	38	200	200			200	200	310	310			#18 Foley #16 tube T+Y
0200	110	32	110/60		4					300	500			300	500	25	335	Chest tube		Chest X-ray
0215	112	24	118/70		5	33				300	800			300	800	30	365	30	30	Chest tube (L)
0230	100	24	118/72		5					300	1100			300	1100	20	385	100	130	Bright Red blood from Chest Tube
0300	100	20	118/90	37.2 R	5	30	7.36	120 (40% O₂)	42	500	1600	500	500	1000	2100	55	440	210	340	Chest Tube
0330	120	22	110/64		3					500	2100	500	1000	500	2600	50	490	300	640	
0400	120	22	108/70		3					500	2600	500	1500	500	3100	40	530	250	890	to O.R.

Figure 3-1 Sample flow sheet.

measure C.V.P. and start an infusion of electrolyte solution or plasma expander. The C.V.P. should be measured at least every 30 to 60 minutes.

5. Insert an indwelling urethral catheter, obtain urine sample, and record urine output every 30 to 60 minutes.

6. Obtain a sample of arterial blood to determine pH, pO_2, and pCO_2 in all patients with severe chest trauma, with respiratory distress, or with profound shock.

7. Initiate a chronological record, as shown in Figure 3-1 (flow sheet), to include: vital signs, C.V.P., urine output, change in physical signs, laboratory data and treatment.

8. Treat the underlying disorder.

HYPOVOLEMIC SHOCK

Hemorrhage: Patients with an uncomplicated loss of blood volume (i.e., external loss from major lacerations, hemorrhage associated with pelvic or femoral shaft fractures) usually present with restlessness, thirst, tachycardia, hypotension, increased peripheral resistance (cool, blanched, moist extremities), a low C.V.P., oliguria, and, if treated shortly after injury, a normal hematocrit and hemoglobin. Unless therapy has been delayed or hypotension is marked, arterial blood pH, pO_2, and pCO_2 will be normal.

Treatment involves inserting a central venous catheter and recording the C.V.P., and then rapidly infusing electrolyte solutions (e.g., Ringer's lactate). A second intravenous infusion catheter may be necessary. There is sufficient clinical evidence that plasma expanders and electrolyte solutions can expand blood volume adequately until type-specific, cross-matched blood is available. On rare occasions, however, the use of un-matched O-Negative blood may be required.

The **goals of therapy** are: (a) to restore the C.V.P. to a normal range; (b) to produce a urinary output of 30 to 50 ml per hour; (c) to restore normal peripheral resistance (extremities become warm and dry).

Confusion sometimes exists relative to the hematocrit following massive blood loss. If a patient's preinjury hematocrit is 40 per cent and he loses 2000 ml of blood, the hematocrit of the blood lost and that remaining in the circulation is still 40 per cent. Hemodilution occurs when extracellular fluid enters the vascular space and may require 4 or more hours to produce an appreciable fall in the hematocrit. Equilibrium may require 24 hours or more.

A second misconception relates to the treatment of the metabolic acidosis that occurs with decreased tissue perfusion due to hypovolemia. Buffer solutions may produce a normal arterial pH but have little effect on tissue perfusion while correction of a volume deficit restores cardiac output to normal, reduces the increased peripheral resistance, improves tissue perfusion, and usually corrects the acidosis. Most patients in hypovolemic shock due to hemorrhage respond dramatically to replacement therapy. When treatment has been delayed, however, resuscitation becomes far more complex (see Complications).

Plasma Volume and Extracellular Fluid Loss: Thermal burns, which are greater than 20 per cent of the body surface area, and peritonitis produce a massive loss of plasma water and extracellular fluid. Management is identical to that for blood volume loss, except that whole blood is rarely required during the acute period of resuscitation. Monitoring the C.V.P. and urine output serves as a guide to therapy. Whereas the hematocrit falls gradually after hemorrhage, hemoconcentration rapidly follows loss of plasma and extracellular fluid. Serial hematocrit determinations may be required every 1 to 2 hours to determine if replacement is "keeping up" with the losses.

Patients with hypovolemic shock due to spreading bacterial and chemical peritonitis (e.g., pancreatitis) simulate those patients with thermal burns and require the same type of aggressive therapy and monitoring. Unfortunately, when proper therapy is delayed, hypovolemic shock may produce the same complications as those described for hemorrhagic shock.

CARDIOGENIC SHOCK

While this type of shock usually follows myocardial infarction, it may also be associated with trauma:

Cardiac Tamponade: Direct cardiac trauma, such as a penetrating injury, can lead to hemorrhage into the pericardium. Acute tamponade of as little as 150 ml will prevent adequate cardiac filling during diastole. Shock appears rapidly with a fall in blood pressure, tachycardia, peripheral vasoconstriction, and a high C.V.P.

Myocardial Infarction: Contusion of the heart by blunt trauma or injury to a coronary artery can produce a myocardial infarct. The patient's appearance suggests hypovolemic shock, but the *C.V.P. is normal.* The intravenous infusion of large volumes of plasma expander or electrolyte solution may precipitate acute heart failure (see Complications).

NEUROGENIC SHOCK

Treatment for neurogenic shock is rarely necessary. However, loss of sympathetic tone following high spinal cord injury can produce significant peripheral vasodilation and can lead to relative hypovolemia that responds to fluid administration.

SEPTIC SHOCK

Sepsis is usually a late complication of soft tissue trauma. As noted earlier, the major hemodynamic defect is (1) relative hypovolemia—inflammation requires an abnormally high cardiac output, or (2) true hypovolemia—large plasma volume and extracellular water loss into the area of infection. **Treatment** is identical to that for hypovolemic shock and must be accompanied by adequate medical (antibiotics) and surgical (drainage, excision of infarcted bowel) therapy.

COMPLICATIONS

CONGESTIVE HEART FAILURE

Overtransfusion or infusion (too much, too fast) may lead to acute pulmonary edema. Careful monitoring of C.V.P. may often, but not always, prevent this severe complication, since C.V.P. essentially measures the function of the right side of the heart but not the left. Clinically, however, it is unusual for acute pulmonary edema to develop without some prior rise in C.V.P.

Treatment consists of:

1. Stopping or reducing the **rate of infusion.**

2. Administering a **digitalis** preparation, e.g., lanatoside C (Cedilanid); 0.8 mg, intravenously, followed by 0.4 mg 4 and 8 hours later, making a full dose of 1.6 mg.

3. Administering a **diuretic,** e.g., furosemide (20–40 mg) intravenously.

4. Inserting an **endotracheal tube** and administering **oxygen.**

5. Considering the possibility of a **phlebotomy,** if necessary.

RENAL FAILURE

Oliguria (less than 30 ml per hour), during massive intravenous infusion therapy, may signal the development of acute renal tubular necrosis secondary to prolonged renal ischemia. Continued volume replacement leads rapidly to pulmonary edema. How do you distinguish between the oliguria of renal failure and that due to inadequate volume replacement? In oliguria due to renal failure, the C.V.P. is normal or elevated; it remains low if the patient is hypovolemic. An intravenous "push" of **mannitol,** 12.5 to 25 grams, will produce a distinct diuresis in hypovolemia but has no effect in renal failure. A positive response to mannitol indicates the need for additional fluid therapy to produce an adequate urinary output. Persistent oliguria, during and shortly after mannitol infusion, confirms the presence of renal failure. Fluids must be limited to meet maintenance requirements; dialysis may prove necessary.

COAGULOPATHY

In some instances, patients, after receiving 5000 ml of whole blood or more, develop diffuse bleeding from mucous membranes, cut-down sites, and the like. Standard clotting tests are usually normal and no definite coagulation deficiency has been described. Improvement may follow correction of the abnormal hemodynamic and metabolic states of shock, suggesting that the coagulopathy represents vascular deterioration with diffuse hemorrhage secondary to poor perfusion and metabolic acidosis.

IRREVERSIBILITY

As noted earlier, delay may markedly alter the response of the patient to fluid replacement. Hypotension, oliguria, peripheral vasoconstriction — shock — persist. The C.V.P. rises rapidly leading to pulmonary edema even though plasma and extracellular fluid deficits remain. Renal shutdown and death are inevitable. Several drugs, particularly vasodilators and corticosteroids, may prevent and, on occasion, reverse this course (see next section).

ANCILLARY TREATMENT

DIGITALIS PREPARATIONS

These have been discussed previously.

VASOPRESSORS

Since a major part of the pathophysiology of shock is due to excessive vasoconstriction, the use of vasopressor drugs is generally contraindicated, particularly in patients in hemorrhagic shock. Hypotension due to peripheral vasodilation, as in sepsis or following spinal cord injury, should be treated by fluid expansion rather than by pressors.

VASODILATORS

If vasoconstriction is bad, why not reverse the rising peripheral resistance that develops in hypovolemic and cardiogenic shock? Two types of drugs have been used clinically: alpha-adrenergic blocking agents, e.g., phenoxybenzamine (Dibenzyline) and beta-stimulating agents, e.g., isoproterenol (Isuprel).

Dibenzyline: The drug specifically blocks vasoconstrictor receptors in arteriolar smooth muscle and has no direct effect on the myocardium. The response to a single intravenous injection of 1 mg/Kg may last up to 24 hours. When administered to a hypovolemic patient, the compensatory vasoconstrictive mechanism is abolished and blood pressure may literally disappear. Therefore, administration of this drug must be accompanied by the rapid intravenous infusion of fluids in a volume equivalent to 50 ml/Kg or more. Great care and judgment plus careful monitoring of systemic blood pressure (preferably by intra-arterial cannula) are mandatory. Dibenzyline remains an experimental drug and cannot be recommended for general clinical application.

Isuprel: In addition to stimulating vasodilator fibers in the arterioles, isoproterenol is a positive inotrope, i.e., it improves myocardial function. Its activity is of short duration and ceases when the drug is withdrawn. It should be administered in a concentration of 1 mg in 250 ml dextrose/water at a rate adequate to reduce vasoconstriction, increase urinary output, decrease C.V.P. (if elevated), and maintain or raise arterial pressure. Unfortunately, Isuprel is also a chronotrope and may have to be discontinued if a severe tachycardia or an arrhythmia develops.

CORTICOSTEROIDS

Although the exact action of corticosteroids is unknown, massive doses of these drugs (hydrocortisone, 50–150 mg/Kg, dexamethasone, 6 mg/Kg), given as a single injection, have been reported to produce dramatic improvement in patients in "irreversible" shock. This response is characterized by an increase in urinary output, reduced peripheral vasoconstriction, increased cardiac output, and a rise in systemic arterial pressure. Repeat injections should be administered at 2- to 4-hour intervals if a satisfactory response follows the initial injection.

Chapter 4

Infection

GENERAL CONSIDERATIONS OF BACTERIAL CONTAMINATION

Open wounds resulting from accident or violence should be considered contaminated by bacteria with the potential for infection. When infections develop in these wounds, they may have profound effect on mortality and morbidity, as well as on the ultimate result of the injury. Some bacteria which contaminate wounds may be highly virulent while others are less so. The presence of bacteria in wounds may or may not be followed by infection, depending upon certain factors that influence the growth of bacteria and determine the development of the septic process. Wounds may be contaminated by exogenous bacteria and foreign bodies. Agents which may serve as a source of exogenous or external environmental contamination are clothing, soil, dust, wooden splinters, water, oil, chemicals, or whatever medium surrounds the wound at the time of injury.

Wounds may also be contaminated by bacteria from endogenous sources. Injuries complicated by penetration of the abdominal and thoracic cavities with perforation of the alimentary, genitourinary, or respiratory tracts may have significant endogenous bacterial contamination.

DEGREE OF CONTAMINATION

Conditions which influence the degree of contamination and promote the growth of bacteria in wounds, resulting in the development of infection, include the following:

Nature and Velocity of the Wounding Agent: An appreciation of the type of damage caused by high velocity missiles is essential for proper debridement and care of traumatic wounds if serious local infection is to be avoided.

The Virulence, Types, and Numbers of Contaminating Bacteria: Infection is the unfavorable result of the equation of bacterial dose multiplied by virulence and divided by the resistance of the host. The mere presence of virulent bacteria in the wound does not mean that infection will definitely occur. The physiologic state of the tissues within the wound before and after treatment seems to be more important than the presence of bacteria per se. The synergistic activity of bacteria present in the wound may also determine the nature and severity of the infection.

Nature, Location, and Duration of the Wound: Extensive wounds containing large amounts of devitalized tissue furnish excellent culture media for bacteria. Wounds produced by crushing injuries and associated with heavy contamination are frequently characterized by extensive tissue destruction, severe shock, and early virulent infection. The location of the wound is important because various tissues in the body have differing degrees of resistance to infection.

Patients with multiple wounds may not receive early adequate debridement, and because of associated severe shock or hemorrhage, the local treatment of wounds may assume a minor role in relation to the general treatment of the patient. If the period of time required for resuscitation and general treatment exceeds 6 to 8 hours, infection may have occurred before local definitive treatment can be started.

Amount of Devitalized Tissue and Impairment of Local Circulation Within the Wound: These two factors deserve special emphasis. Unhealthy or dead tissue in a wound invites and supports the growth of bacterial organisms since the tissue has little power of resistance to their growth. On the other hand, healthy tissues possess a remarkable capacity to kill bacteria and withstand their effects.

Presence of Foreign Bodies: These materials may carry large numbers of bacteria into a wound and further the probability of infection by causing local irritation to the tissues.

Type and Thoroughness of Treatment: Of primary importance is the surgical excision of all dead tissue and foreign bodies within the wound, preferably within the first 4 to 6 hours after injury.

Local and General Immune Response of the Patient: Local immunity depends to a great degree on the type of tissue injured and its vascularity. General immunity resides in the body as a whole, particularly the globulin fraction of plasma, the cells of the reticuloendothelial system, and the protective action of the lymph nodes.

General Condition of the Patient: The presence of such conditions as dehydration, shock, malnutrition, uncontrolled diabetes, and anemia may lower the patient's resistance sufficiently to allow bacterial invasion. Drug therapy, such as steroids and immunosuppressive agents, may also render the patient susceptible to infection. General exposure to irradiation may result in spontaneous infections.

Other special circumstances which may modify treatment and therefore predispose to wound infection are lack of medical facilities and personnel to carry out adequate debridement (as in disaster conditions) and any sensitivities or drug intolerances which may affect the patient's response to drug prophylaxis.

PROPHYLACTIC TREATMENT OF
SURGICAL INFECTIONS

Wound care should be planned so that prompt primary healing of wounds can occur with a minimum opportunity for bacterial colonization, invasion, and sepsis. Since delays in treatment increase the likelihood of infection, treatment should be started within 6 hours of injury. Primary closure is usually contraindicated in wounds which have not been treated within 6 hours (except under special circumstances).

CLEANSING AND SURGICAL DEBRIDEMENT OF WOUNDS

Adequate debridement of traumatic wounds consists of meticulous removal of all dead or devitalized tissue, detached fragments of tissue, foreign bodies, and debris which might provide favorable media for bacterial growth, thereby increasing the potential for infection and impeding the healing process.

In wounds of the face and hands conservative debridement should be the rule since both areas include essentially irreplaceable structures that are necessary for proper function and appearance. Simple shaving and cleansing of skin, gentle irrigation of the wound with saline, conservative trimming of ragged edges, and removal of fragmented tissue may be all that is required.

Massive wounds of the extremities, on the other hand, may require extensive debridement and painstaking removal of detached bone fragments, foreign bodies, and every bit of muscle that is necrotic or ischemic. Occasionally when it is obvious that one extremity is irreversibly damaged, amputation may be the only effective form of debridement.

IMMOBILIZATION

The traumatized part of the body should be placed at rest as much as possible. After the wound is cleansed and debrided, a bulky dressing is usually applied to place the damaged structures at rest thereby decreasing the danger of further hemorrhage and dissemination of bacteria by muscle movement. The bulky dressing also conserves heat and may increase the circulation in the wounded area. In the case of extremity wounds, thoughtful elevation may be helpful in aiding the patient's comfort, reducing local swelling, and favoring wound healing.

ADJUNCTIVE SURGICAL PROCEDURES

Operative procedures may be employed to minimize contamination, thereby decreasing the likelihood of infection. Proximal colostomies in wounds of the colon will divert the fecal stream and greatly decrease the bacterial flora which might otherwise pass through the site of perforation and cause continuing contamination with resulting infection. Adequate drainage of areas, such as the retroperitoneal space, contaminated as a result of traumatic wounds, as well as drainage of traumatic wounds of the liver, biliary tree, and pancreas will frequently prevent widespread infections. Early debridement and skin grafting of third-degree burns will greatly reduce the bacterial contamination of the burn wound and help prevent sepsis.

PROPHYLACTIC ANTIBIOTIC THERAPY

Since all accidental wounds are assumed to be contaminated, the advisability of instituting antibiotic therapy at the onset of treatment must be considered in each instance. The following general principles should be kept in mind:

1. Foremost, a history of sensitivity or drug idiosyncrasy is sought. When the patient gives a clear history of sensitivity reaction to one or more antibiotics, it is well to consider an effective antibiotic which has not been previously used or to which the patient is known not to be sensitive.

2. Almost all patients with extensive wounds should be given antibiotics, preferably aqueous penicillin G and preferably intravenously, as part of their preoperative resuscitation. This becomes more important when primary treatment has been delayed or is likely to be delayed.

3. Minor wounds of the face, not including the buccal cavity, usually do not require antibiotics.

4. However, minor wounds in patients with diabetes, extensive vascular disease, or debilitating conditions of any origin, require antibiotic therapy.

5. Visceral injuries of the abdomen or chest require large doses of antibiotics.

6. Patients with massive wounds which afford ideal sites for anaerobic growth (see sections on Tetanus and on Clostridial Myositis and Clostridial Cellulitis) should receive large doses of aqueous penicillin G and one of the tetracyclines intravenously, as soon after injury as possible; these should be continued until the danger of this type of infection is over.

7. Animal bites, and especially human bites, even when the wounds are small require antibiotic therapy. At the present time, penicillin is the agent of choice.

8. All patients who have been subjected to excessive or extensive radiation should receive antibiotics.

9. Antibiotic therapy should be continued for at least 5 days after all clinical evidence of infection has disappeared. When there is no evidence of infection following administration of prophylactics, the antibiotic may be continued until wound healing is advanced.

10. It is advisable to begin prophylactic antibiotic therapy prior to initiating operative procedures on traumatized patients so that an antibacterial blood level of the antibiotic agent will be present in the tissues and body cavities before and throughout the operation.

11. Cultures should be taken at the time of operation from all contaminated areas so that if resulting infection develops, a more intelligent approach to specific antibiotic therapy will be possible.

SPECIAL PROPHYLACTIC MEASURES

TETANUS

This severe and dreaded infectious complication of traumatic wounds could be almost completely eliminated by universal active immunization during childhood. Tetanus is caused by the anaerobic organism *Clostridium tetani* and its toxins and is characterized by local convulsive spasm of the voluntary muscles and a tendency toward episodes of respiratory arrest. It may occur as a complication in either large or small wounds including lacerations, open fractures, burns, abrasions, and even hypodermic injections. However, the fact that approximately one-third of the patients seen with active tetanus either have no obvious wound or have wounds considered to be insignificant by the patient or his physician, emphasizes the problem of tetanus prophylaxis following unknown or minimal wounds and suggests that the disease will never be eliminated until universal active immunization has been achieved.

GENERAL PRINCIPLES OF TETANUS PROPHYLAXIS

Individual Consideration of Each Patient: For each patient with a wound, the attending physician must determine individually what is required for adequate prophylaxis against tetanus.

Surgical Debridement: Regardless of the active immunization status of the patient, meticulous surgical care, including removal of all devitalized tissue and foreign bodies, should be provided immediately for all wounds. Such care is as essential for the prevention of tetanus as it is for other types of wound infection.

Active Immunization: Tetanus toxoid is the simplest, surest, and cheapest immunologic agent available. Immunization should be started in infancy with DPT shots, sometime between 2 and 6 months of age. Two to three doses given intramuscularly 1 month apart followed by a booster at 12 months is the usual method of immunization. Another booster is administered when the child is 5 or 6 years old, usually when he begins to attend school. Booster injections of tetanus toxoid should be given periodically, but the time schedule has not been definitely established since several studies to determine the need for tetanus boosters are still in progress. Basic active immunization with adsorbed toxoid requires three injections. A booster of adsorbed toxoid is indicated 10 years after the third injection or 10 years after an intervening wound booster.

Each patient with a wound should receive adsorbed tetanus toxoid intramuscularly at the time of injury, either as an initial immunizing dose or as a booster for previous immunization, *unless* he has received a booster or has completed his initial immunization series within the past 5 years. As the antigen concentration varies in different products, specific information on the volume of a single dose is provided on the label of the package.

Passive Immunization: Whether or not passive immunization with homologous (human) tetanus immune globulin should be provided must be decided individually for each patient. The characteristics of the wound, the conditions under which it was incurred, and the previous active immunization status of the patient must be considered. In those patients without previous active (toxoid) immunization, passive immunization is indicated. In the past it was traditionally administered with equine or bovine antitoxin in a dose of 3000 to 10,000 units. Because of the danger and frequency of allergic reactions, as well as the rapid elimination of the antitoxin, and the incidence of delayed serum sickness following the use of equine or bovine antitoxin, passive immunization with these agents has been discouraged and should be discontinued. Instead the safer human tetanus immune globulin (Hypertet) is recommended by intramuscular injection. It should *never* be given *intravenously.* This product (Hypertet) has a much longer half-life of protection of approximately 30 days.

Patient Record: Every wounded patient should be given a written record of the immunization provided and should be instructed to carry the record at all times and, if indicated, to complete his active immunization. For precise tetanus prophylaxis, an accurate and immediately available history regarding previous active immunization against tetanus is required.

Antibiotic Prophylaxis: The value of antibiotic agents in the prophylaxis of tetanus remains questionable. There is no doubt that *Clostridium tetani* is sensitive *in vitro* to penicillin and tetracycline, as well as other antibiotics, but there seems to be some difficulty in delivering an adequate dose of antibiotics to the susceptible bacteria before they liberate toxin. The tetanus-prone wound characteristically has a decreased blood supply and contains necrotic tissue which may prevent high antibiotic blood levels from reaching the infecting bacteria. It is recommended that antibiotic therapy not be relied upon as adequate prophylactic therapy in the place of immunization. In large necrotic wounds, particularly those in which debridement has been delayed or compromised, penicillin and tetracycline have often been employed as prophylaxis against other types of wound infection which may occur, as well as for prophylactic action against tetanus.

SPECIFIC MEASURES FOR PREVIOUSLY IMMUNIZED PATIENTS (TABLE 4–1)

When the patient has been actively immunized within the past 10 years:

1. To the great majority give 0.5 ml. of adsorbed tetanus toxoid as a booster unless it is *certain* that the patient has received a booster within the previous 5 *years*.

2. To those with severe, neglected, or old (more than 24 hours) tetanus-prone wounds, give 0.5 cc. of adsorbed toxoid unless it is *certain* that a booster was received within the previous *year*.

When the patient received active immunization more than 10 years previously and has not received a booster within the past 5 years. (Some authorities advise 6 rather than 10 years, particularly for patients with

TABLE 4–1 PROPHYLACTIC TREATMENT OF TETANUS

| Type of Wound | Patient Not Immunized or Partially Immunized | Patient Completely Immunized Time Since Last Booster Dose | | |
		1* to 5 years	5 to 10 years	10 years +
Clean minor	Begin or complete immunization per schedule; tetanus toxoid, 0.5 cc.	None	Tetanus toxoid 0.5 cc.	Tetanus toxoid 0.5 cc.
Clean major or tetanus prone	In one arm: **Human tetanus immune globulin 250 mg. In other arm: **Tetanus toxoid 0.5 cc., complete immunization per schedule	Tetanus toxoid 0.5 cc.	Tetanus toxoid 0.5 cc.	In one arm: **Tetanus toxoid 0.5 cc. In other arm: **Human tetanus immune globulin 250 mg.
Tetanus prone, delayed or incomplete debridement	In one arm: **Human tetanus immune globulin 500 mg. In other arm: **Tetanus toxoid 0.5 cc., complete immunization per schedule thereafter. Antibiotic therapy.	Tetanus toxoid 0.5 cc.	Tetanus toxoid 0.5 cc. Antibiotic Therapy	In one arm: **Tetanus toxoid 0.5 cc. In other arm: **Human tetanus immune globulin 500 mg. Antibiotic Therapy

*No prophylactic immunization is required if patient has had a booster within the previous year.
**Use different syringes, needles and sites.
NOTE: With different preparations of toxoid, the volume of a single booster dose should be modified as stated on the package label.

severe, neglected, or old tetanus-prone wounds such as may be sustained by military personnel in combat.):

1. To the great majority give a dose of 0.5 cc. of adsorbed tetanus toxoid.

2. To those with wounds which indicate an overwhelming possibility that tetanus might develop:

a. Give 0.5 cc. of adsorbed tetanus toxoid, and

b. Give 250 units of tetanus immune globulin (human), using different syringes, needles, and sites of injection.

c. In severe, neglected, or old wounds, inject 500 units of tetanus immune globulin (human).

d. Consider providing oxytetracycline or penicillin prophylactically.

TREATMENT FOR PATIENTS NOT PREVIOUSLY IMMUNIZED

With clean minor wounds, in which tetanus is most unlikely, give 0.5 cc. of adsorbed tetanus toxoid (initial immunizing dose).

With all other wounds:

1. Give 0.5 cc. of adsorbed tetanus toxoid (initial immunizing dose).

2. Give 250 units of tetanus immune globulin (human). The dose should be increased to 500 units in severe or neglected wounds.

3. Consider providing oxytetracycline or penicillin prophylactically.

Equine or bovine antitoxin. Do *not* administer heterologous antitoxin (equine) except when tetanus immune globulin (human) is not available within 24 hours and ONLY if the possibility of tetanus outweighs the danger of reaction to heterologous tetanus antitoxin. Before using such antitoxin, question the patient for a history of allergy and test for sensitivity. If the patient is sensitive to heterologous antitoxin, do not use it because the danger of anaphylaxis probably outweighs the danger of tetanus; rely on penicillin or oxytetracycline. Do not attempt desensitization because it is not worthwhile. If the patient is not sensitive to equine tetanus antitoxin and if the decision is made to administer it for passive immunization, give at least 3000 units.

CLOSTRIDIAL MYOSITIS (GAS GANGRENE)

TYPES OF WOUNDS WITH INCREASED RISK

Clostridial myositis is most likely to develop in wounds which have the following characteristics:

1. Extensive laceration or devitalization of muscle such as occurs in compound fractures and injuries from high velocity missiles.

2. Impairment of the main blood supply by the injury, a tourniquet, a tight cast, or delayed thrombosis.

3. Gross contamination by foreign bodies such as soil and clothing.

4. Delayed treatment.

5. Inadequate treatment such as incomplete debridement or lack of immobilization.

PREVENTION

Surgery: The most effective means of preventing gas gangrene continues to be early and adequate operation which includes wide incision, thorough debridement of all devitalized and potentially devitalized tissues, removal of contaminating dirt and all foreign bodies, and effective drainage as required. Adequate debridement is especially important in irregular deep wounds in which there are loculations and recesses which favor anaerobic bacterial growth. Dead and devitalized tissue and foreign bodies must be removed at the time of initial operation. In war wounds, in wounds incurred in mass disasters, and in all wounds in which there has been some trauma to the soft tissues, this thorough debridement should be coupled with delayed suture of the wound. The wound should be left open from 4 to 7 days following the debridement, and then delayed suture should be accomplished if the wound has remained clean.

Antibiotic: Antibiotic therapy is of some prophylactic value when combined with proper surgical procedures, but experimental and clinical experience affirms this principle and indicates that antibiotic therapy alone cannot be relied upon to prevent the occurrence of clostridial myositis. The tetracyclines are the most effective agents against the clostridial organisms.

Antitoxin: Prophylactic administration of gas gangrene antitoxin at the time of injury or shortly thereafter is not recommended. The evidence indicates that it has been of little or no practical value in the prevention of clinical gas gangrene. Many physicians, however, continue to give it at the time of injury despite evidence of its ineffectiveness.

Hyperbaric Oxygen Therapy: Hyperbaric oxygen therapy remains experimental and unproven as a prophylactic therapeutic measure in gas gangrene. The experimental evidence indicates that it has little value without adequate surgical debridement. It has been used more effectively in some instances in the treatment of established clostridial infections.

THERAPY OF ESTABLISHED INFECTIONS

GENERAL PRINCIPLES

Successful treatment of surgical infections depends largely upon the physician's realization that the newer antibiotic agents are adjunctive to the employment of old and established surgical principles. Early and accurate diagnosis is of great importance in the control of surgical infections. It is important to obtain information about the infecting microorganism by immediate examination of stained smears of pus and by culture of this material. Biopsy may be helpful in establishing the nature of infection, particularly in chronic infections of a specific nature. Daily observation of the patient and his wound is mandatory.

SELECTION OF PROPER CHEMOTHERAPY AGENT

Whenever possible, this selection should be made on the basis of data resulting from smears, cultures, and sensitivity tests and should be limited to two agents instead of multiple antibiotics. Treatment of serious mixed infections produced by a variety of gram-positive and gram-negative aerobic and anaerobic bacteria usually requires two antibacterial agents for treatment. Aqueous penicillin G and one of the "broad spectrum" antibiotics, such as tetracycline, oxytetracycline, gentamicin, Keflin, or carbenacillin, may be selected. There is some laboratory evidence that antagonism may occur between two or more antibiotics which may decrease their effectiveness, but fortunately there is no significant evidence of this antagonism existing *in vivo*. Repeat cultures and sensitivity tests at weekly intervals in severe prolonged infections are important because of the possibility of acquired bacterial resistance or the development of secondary infections.

Adequate dosage of the antibiotic agents must be employed to obtain sufficient blood and intracellular fluid levels for a period of time long enough to permit the natural defense mechanism of the body to dispose the inhibited but often still viable bacteria. The majority of antibiotic agents exert only a bacteriostatic effect which is greatest on actively growing and reproducing bacteria. Antibiotic treatment should be started as promptly as possible after injury. Late treatment usually results in a more limited or delayed effect, and complications are more numerous. Local application of chemotherapeutic agents to wounds is seldom indicated. Intravenous administration of antibiotics is recommended during traumatic shock to guarantee adequate blood, fluid, and tissue concentrations.

TIMING OF SURGICAL INTERVENTION

The principles of operative treatment for traumatic injuries have not been changed significantly by modern chemotherapy. An attempt should be made to begin antibiotic therapy preoperatively, but the operation should not be delayed.

SUPPORTIVE TREATMENT

Local and general physiologic derangements may be overlooked in the severely traumatized patient. They must be corrected if the full therapeutic effect of antibacterial therapy is to be obtained. Adequate replacement of fluids, electrolytes, and blood, as well as the general care of the patient is essential in treating surgical infections.

UNTOWARD REACTIONS OF ANTIBIOTIC AGENTS

These reactions may be toxic, related to the amount of drug given, or sensitivity reactions due to idiosyncrasy sensitization of the patient; or they may be secondary inflammation or ulcerations produced by superimposed infections. Each antibacterial agent has been shown to be capable of producing one or more of these reactions. Sensitization is a greater problem in certain antibiotics, such as penicillin, than in others. Certain antibiotics such as chloramphenicol and sulfonamides are capable of producing severe depression of the bone marrow probably on the basis of idiosyncrasy. The choice of antibiotic agent employed is more and more dictated by the relative safety of the drug as well as the sensitivity pattern of the offending microorganism. Secondary or superimposed infections usually occur by suppression of susceptible microbial strains and the overgrowth of those resistant to the antibiotic being administered. An example of this type of superimposed infection is the development of staphylococcal enterocolitis following antibiotic therapy. More recently the problem of Candida overgrowth in the gastrointestinal and genitourinary tracts following long-term antibiotic therapy has become more prominent particularly in burn patients.

CLASSIFICATION OF WOUND INFECTION

Traumatic soft tissue injuries may be contaminated and infected by a variety of bacteria resulting in aerobic, anaerobic, gram-negative, gram-positive, or mixed infections. When wound sepsis occurs it may be classified clinically, according to its pathophysiologic type, or bacteriologically according to its microbial etiology. The following is a brief clinical classification of infections developing in these wounds:

CLINICAL CLASSIFICATION

    a. Cellulitis
    b. Suppuration and abscess
    c. Lymphangitis and lymphadenitis
    d. Septic thrombophlebitis
    e. Necrosis and gangrene
    f. Toxemia
    g. Bacteremia
    h. Septicemia

The majority of wound infections start as a cellulitis with hyperemia, edema, pain, and interference with function. Suppuration often follows as a result of local liquefaction of tissue and the formation of pus with the production of an abscess. If the infections spread, they do so by direct, lymphatic, venous, or more rarely by arterial spread. Direct extension is the most common route by way of subcutaneous tissue, muscles, tissue planes, or tendon sheaths.

ETIOLOGIC CLASSIFICATION

Another useful classification of wound sepsis is on an etiologic basis as follows:

Staphylococcal Infections: The treatment of established staphylococcal infections consists of rest, heat, elevation of the infected area, adequate surgical drainage when pus is formed, and antibiotic therapy. An infected wound should be reopened with hemostats at the point of maximum pain, swelling, or fluctuation followed by removal of all skin sutures. The wound should be loosely packed open to keep the edges separated. The packing should be removed within 48 to 72 hours and replaced as indicated. Antibiotic therapy must begin promptly. Aqueous penicillin G should be administered in doses of approximately 3 million units per 24 hours. Erythromycin in doses of 200 mg. every 6 hours orally is likewise effective. The more specific antistaphylococcal antibiotics such as staphcillin and lincomycin, as well as effective broad spectrum antibiotics, such as gentamicin, may be used as indicated. Sodium oxycillin may be given orally in doses of 3 to 4 gm. a day, or methicillin in parenteral doses of 4 to 6 gm. a day.

Streptococcal Infections: Although most frequently produced by the aerobic *Streptococcus hemolyticus,* some infections are caused by the nonhemolytic *Streptococcus viridans, Streptococcus anaerobius,* and microphilic *Streptococcus.* Lesions caused by the aerobic *Streptococcus hemolyticus* characteristically are invasive and run a rapid course initially.

The treatment of hemolytic streptococcal infections consists primarily of controlling their invasive characteristics by antibiotic therapy, rest, and warm applications followed by surgical drainage if abscesses or cutaneous gangrene develop. Penicillin is the agent of choice in doses of approximately 3 million units per 24 hours. Operative treatment should be delayed until the invasive qualities of the infection have been controlled. After operation, treatment includes rest, elevation of the part if possible, and application of moist compresses to the open wounds.

Gram-Negative Bacillary Infections: *Escherichia coli, Pseudomonas aeruginosa,* and *Proteus vulgaris* are examples of organisms capable of causing wound infections in a posttraumatic period. The presence of necrotic tissue, general debility, and so forth, may cause relatively nonvirulent gram-negative bacteria to develop wound infections. A relatively long incubation period is also characteristic of posttraumatic wound infection by these bacilli. Treatment of these gram-negative infections is dependent upon incision and drainage of abscesses, excision of necrotic tissue, and antibiotic therapy based on sensitivity tests when possible. Chloramphenicol is particularly useful in these infections, but the untoward reactions from this drug have limited its use. More recently gentamicin and carbenacillin have been used effectively against these gram-negative infections, particularly those caused by the *Pseudomonas aeruginosa.*

Mixed or Synergistic Infections: A large and miscellaneous group of infections with a polymicrobial etiology are found in association with injuries involving the gastrointestinal, respiratory, and genitourinary tracts. The bacterial toxins and enzymes usually cause a necrotizing and suppurative infection. Examples of mixed infections include human bite infections, peritonitis, empyema, and nonclostridial cellulitis.

Human bite infections are particularly dangerous because of the virulent organisms usually contaminating the mouth. A mixture of bacteria consisting of aerobic and anaerobic streptococci, bacterium melinogenicum, spirochetes, or staphylococci are often found. When infections become established, radical decompression of infected areas and tissue planes by incision is extremely important along with intensive antibiotic therapy.

Crepitant (nonclostridial) cellulitis is a mixed infection which is usually seen as a complication of wounds of the peritoneum, abdominal wall, buttock, hip, thorax, or neck, which have been contaminated by discharges from the intestinal, genitourinary, or respiratory tracts. Proper surgical decompression of all involved areas by multiple incisions is imperative. Aqueous penicillin in doses of 1 million units every 4 to 6 hours is recommended along with broad spectrum antibiotics. Supportive therapy in this form of infection may also be lifesaving.

CLOSTRIDIAL INFECTIONS

CLOSTRIDIAL MYOSITIS

Unfortunately, clostridial myositis is often recognized by the clinical appearance of the patient and his infection in the more obvious, far advanced, and often irreversible stages of disease. Casts, splints, or large dressings necessary for the treatment of major injuries obscure the area of the wound and make the observation and interpretation of local signs difficult. For these reasons, the dressings should be removed promptly and the wound inspected directly if there is the slightest suspicion of this infection. The most important causative microorganism is *Cl. perfringens* (Welchii). It may occur alone or in combination with other clostridia.

Clinical Manifestations: A variable interval exists between injury and the development of the lesion, sometimes a period as short as 6 hours, particularly in wounds associated with gross devitalization and contamination of muscle. The average incubation period is 48 hours. Pain is the earliest and most important symptom, being secondary to the rapid infiltration of the infected muscle by edema and gas.

A rapid and feeble pulse usually follows the onset of pain and is characteristically out of proportion to the elevation of the temperature. Early in the course of infection the blood pressure is normal or slightly elevated. Later it may decrease significantly, falling to shock level.

Temperature elevation in the early stages of the infection may vary considerably. Fever is not a reliable index of the severity and extent of the infectious process, but a low or subnormal temperature associated with a markedly rapid pulse may indicate a grave prognosis. The general appearance of the patient usually includes a peculiar grey pallor, weakness, and profuse sweating. The mental state is often one of apathy and indifference. Stupor, delirium, prostration, and coma are late symptoms indicative of an overwhelming infection.

Early in the course of infection the overlying skin is either white, shiny, and tense or essentially normal in appearance. A dirty-brown watery discharge with peculiar foul odor usually escapes from the wound. As the swelling increases, the overlying skin becomes dusky or bronze in appearance. In far advanced cases further discoloration occurs and vesicles filled with dark-red fluid characteristically appear on the cutaneous surface. Crepitation is a relatively late sign.

Laboratory and X-ray Diagnosis: Blood counts usually reveal a marked reduction in red blood cells, hematocrit, or hemoglobin levels. The leukocyte count is seldom elevated above 12,000 to 15,000. In general, no satisfactory laboratory tests exist for the early diagnosis of gas gangrene. For this reason immediate surgical exploration of any wound suspected of harboring clostridial myositis is advisable. Microscopic examination of the watery discharge usually reveals numerous red blood cells and many large gram-postive bacteria with squared ends, but without spores. In contrast to pyogenic infections, few pus cells are seen. *Clostridium perfringens* and other clostridia usually appear as large gram-positive bacilli with squared ends without evidence of sporulation when the exudate is prepared with Gram's stain.

X-rays taken at intervals of 2 to 4 hours may aid in the diagnosis by differentiating gas in the soft tissues produced by clostridial invasion from that due to mechanical or chemical causes. If the visible gas increases in amount or presents a linear spread along the muscle and fascial planes, an early diagnosis of gas gangrene can be made.

Treatment: Early and adequate operation is the most effective and primary means of treating clostridial myositis. If the diagnosis is made early, while the gangrene is relatively localized, radical decompression of the involved fascial compartments by free longitudinal incisions and excision of infected muscle usually arrest the process and eliminate the need for amputation. If the diagnosis is reached when the process is extensive and has caused irreversible gangrenous changes open amputation of the guillotine type becomes necessary.

Tetracyclines are the drugs of choice in treating this condition with chlortetracycline (Aureomycin) and oxytetracycline (Terramycin) being preferable. Doses of 500 mg. every 6 hours before and after operative treatment are advisable. The intravenous route is usually preferred. Chloramphenicol is also effective. Penicillin is of value only when given in large doses of 3 million units every 3 hours intravenously. Supportive therapy, including blood transfusions, maintenance of fluid and electrolyte balance, adequate immobilization of the infected injured parts, oxygen therapy, and relief of pain, are of great value. In cases of severe toxemia with septic shock, the intravenous administration of steroids should be considered. All secondary operations designed to facilitate healing or restore function of the wounded extremity should be postponed until the infection has been brought under complete control.

The use of polyvalent gas gangrene antitoxin remains controversial. Fifty thousand units given every 4 to 6 hours for 24 to 48 hours before and after operation seems to have been helpful in some cases in controlling the severe toxemia of gas gangrene. Many surgeons, however, continue to doubt the efficacy of gas gangrene antitoxin.

CLOSTRIDIAL CELLULITIS

Clostridial cellulitis is a septic crepitant process involving the epifascial, retroperitoneal, or other connective tissues. Its incubation period is usually 3 to 4 days and its onset is ordinarily more gradual than gas gangrene. Systemic effects are less than with clostridial myositis. However, clostridial cellulitis is not a condition to be regarded lightly. The spread of infection in the tissue spaces may be rapid and extensive, necessitating prompt radical surgical drainage.

Prevention of clostridial myositis and clostridial cellulitis depends primarily on thorough and complete debridement of wounds. Dead and devitalized tissue and foreign bodies must be removed at the time of initial surgery. All wounds in which there has been severe trauma to the soft tissue and wounds from high velocity missiles should be thoroughly debrided, packed open, and frequently inspected. Delayed suturing can be accomplished 4 to 7 days later if the wound has remained clean. The use of gas gangrene antitoxin has not proved of value in the prophylaxis of these infections.

Treatment: The debridement of the wound involved with the anaerobic cellulitis is the most important step in the management of these patients. All devitalized tissue must be excised. When the infection extends along fascial planes above the traumatized area of the wound, long incisions must be made to open these areas and excise the necrotic fascia. Following debridement, the wounds may be irrigated with oxidizing solution in the form of potassium permanganate or hydrogen peroxide. Zinc peroxide cream or ointment when properly prepared may also be of benefit in treating this condition. Intensive systemic antibiotic and supportive therapy similar to that listed for clostridial myositis should also be employed for this serious infection.

TETANUS

Established tetanus is a clinical emergency. Its treatment consists primarily of supportive and symptomatic measures which prevent the complications (usually respiratory) that cause death.

Serotherapy: Considerable controversy has arisen over the effectiveness of serotherapy in the treatment of established tetanus. Protective antibody levels can be obtained with the injection of tetanus antitoxin, but whether or not these protective levels are of benefit to a patient who has fixation of tetanus toxin in the central nervous system remains debatable. The administration of 3000 to 6000 units of human tetanus immune globulin (IM) establishes protective serum levels for up to 14 weeks after injection. Intravenous administration is not recommended.

Surgical Excision of Wound: If a primary wound is present and can be surgically excised or extensively debrided with removal of all foreign material and necrotic tissue, injection of the area with antisera one hour prior to surgical incision is recommended.

Sedation: Sodium pentothal has been our drug of choice for general sedation of the patient to control convulsive seizures. It has been administered in dilute solution (0.5 to 1.0 gm. per 1000 cc.) in a continuous, slow, intravenous drip. The dosage is adjusted to produce sleep, from which the patient can be aroused, by moderate external stimuli, to obey commands. Should a convulsive seizure occur, a 2.5 per cent solution of Pentothal is injected intravenously immediately. A syringe with this more concentrated Pentothal solution should be connected by a stopcock to the continuous intravenous drip tubing.

Muscle Relaxant Drugs: Some clinicians have been enthusiastic about the use of these drugs to control convulsive seizures, but in our experience they have been more difficult to manage and have not prevented death from respiratory arrest. Drugs most commonly suggested are Robaxin, Tolserol, d-tubocurarine, and succinylcholine.

Tracheostomy: Early tracheostomy employing a cuffed tracheostomy tube may be of benefit in treating severe cases of tetanus. Tracheostomy allows a constant open route for suctioning and prevention of aspiration. It also decreases the anatomic dead space and maintains a route for resuscitation with positive pressure breathing.

Mechanical Respirators: The use of an intermittent positive pressure breathing apparatus may be helpful for insuring adequate ventilation in the presence of heavy sedation.

Constant Nursing Attendants: A special nurse or physician should be at the patient's bedside at all times. This is extremely important so that convulsive seizures and episodes of respiratory arrest can be immediately recognized and treated by the institution of adequate therapeutic regimen as previously discussed.

External Stimuli: The patient should be kept in a darkened, quiet room, and all forms of stimulation should be kept to a minimum. Loud sounds or sudden stimulation of any type may excite seizures and cause respiratory arrest.

Adequate Fluid, Electrolyte, and Calorie Intake: Only a limited number of calories can usually be administered to a patient through the continuous intravenous drip containing dilute solution of sodium pentothal.

Chemotherapy: Although antibiotic therapy probably is of no beneficial value once tetanus infection has become established, it is recommended during the course of tetanus to minimize or control the development of other wound infections by secondary invading bacteria or respiratory infections including pneumonia.

Steroid Therapy: Although not used routinely, steroid therapy has been employed in a few severe cases of tetanus in which the prolonged course of the disease seemed to threaten adrenal exhaustion.

Hyperbaric Oxygen: This form of therapy must be considered experimental at the present time and should not be recommended for general use until more experience has been gained.

Chapter 5

Anesthesia

Regardless of the urgency of the situation, the principles of good anesthetic management in the injured patient deserve emphasis. The few moments needed to prepare the patient for anesthesia and operation may save hours of anguish for the physician, the patient, and the relatives.

PREANESTHETIC EVALUATION

HISTORY

The anesthesiologist should personally review the history of the circumstances of the injury and the management of the patient after injury. He should give particular attention to drug administration, the nature and time of the last ingestion of food or fluid, allergies, and any history of chronic illness.

Consider a patient having an emergency operation as having a full stomach.

The anesthesiologist should speak directly with the physician responsible for the patient so that they may institute any additional studies or treatment that may be necessary while the operating room is being prepared.

PHYSICAL EXAMINATION

First, determine the effectiveness of respiration and assure patency of the airway. Obstruction by blood, vomitus, foreign bodies, or soft tissue must be removed. A nasal or oral pharyngeal airway, a nasal or oral endotracheal tube (Fig. 5–1), or a tracheostomy may be necessary to maintain a good airway.

An unconscious patient has respiratory obstruction until proved otherwise.

Figure 5–1 Technique for establishing a safe airway rapidly by endotracheal intubation. The patient's neck is flexed and his head is extended and supported, in order to bring the mouth, larynx, and trachea in line. A laryngoscope is introduced, and the vocal cords and the glottic opening are visualized. A cuffed endotracheal tube is passed alongside the laryngoscope to 3 or 4 cm beyond the glottis. When the laryngoscope is removed, the cuff of the tube is inflated to seal the trachea. (Modified after Netter, in CIBA Clinical Symposia, Vol. 22, No. 3, 1970.)

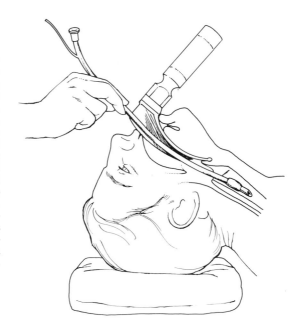

Second, determine by means of inspection and auscultation the ability of the patient to breathe satisfactorily and the adequacy of ventilation of *both* lungs. If ventilation is inadequate, assist it by whatever means is available, such as bag and mask, respirator, or mouth-to-mouth resuscitation.

Administer oxygen to all patients with cyanosis or hypotension.

Next, assess the status of the cardiovascular system. Note repeatedly the rate and quality of the pulse, skin color and temperature, capillary perfusion, arterial and venous pressures, and urinary output. Adequate excretion of urine, providing the urinary tract is anatomically intact, is a good measure of adequate circulating blood volume and tissue perfusion.

A single observation of blood pressure, pulse rate, respiratory depth and rate, central venous pressure, and urine output has little meaning.

Finally, discuss the nature and the extent of the injury or injuries and the proposed operation with the surgeon.

PREANESTHETIC MEDICATION

Preanesthetic medication is given for two reasons: (1) to relieve pain and (2) to inhibit harmful reflexes. Increments of diluted narcotics may be given intravenously to achieve the desired effect, but it must be remembered that the less adequate the circulation, the longer it takes to attain the maximum effect.

DOSAGE IN ADULTS

Morphine: Dilute to 1 mg/ml in sterile saline solution. Give intravenously in 1-mg increments to obtain the desired effect, waiting between doses to observe the effect.

Meperidine (Demerol): Dilute to 5 mg/ml. Give intravenously in 5-mg increments.

DOSAGE IN CHILDREN

Morphine: Dilute to 1 mg/ml. Give intravenously in 1-mg increments. Estimate the dose at 1 mg per 10 pounds of body weight, up to 100 pounds.

Meperidine: Dilute to 5 mg/ml. Give intravenously in 5-mg increments. Estimate the dose at 10 mg per 10 pounds of body weight, up to 100 pounds.

A *belladonna derivative* such as atropine (0.2 mg) or scopolamine (0.2 mg) may be given intravenously to block reflex bradycardia and reduce salivary and bronchial secretions.

Barbiturates are contraindicated because they give no pain relief and they remove cortical control, resulting in an uncooperative patient.

Give no intramuscular injections or depressants to the patient in shock.

GENERAL ANESTHESIA

Choice of the anesthetic technique and agent depends upon each particular set of circumstances and the skill of the individual administering the anesthesia. As a general rule, there are no safe techniques or agents, only safe individuals using these techniques and agents.

The anesthesiologist should use the agent and technique with which he is most familiar.

Consider a patient undergoing an emergency operation as having a full stomach that cannot be emptied by the use of a nasogastric tube. The induction of vomiting by means of the gag reflex or by drugs may be more harmful to the patient than beneficial. One of several techniques may be selected to establish a safe airway in the patient who has a full stomach. The throat may be anesthetized topically and an endotracheal tube with a cuff inserted while the patient is awake (Fig. 5–1).

Topical anesthetics require the same precautions as other anesthetics.

Another method of establishing a safe airway is to preoxygenate the patient, followed by a rapid induction and complete muscular paralysis, followed by insertion of a cuffed endotracheal tube (Fig. 5–1). Or one may introduce a cuffed tube through a tracheostomy accomplished under local anesthesia. (See Chapter 11.)

Assure adequate suction for catheter aspiration of the pharynx and trachea before starting.

Turning on the motor of a suction machine does not necessarily indicate adequate suction at the tip of the catheter.

In general, the smallest effective doses of agents for general anesthesia should be used at all times and the patient kept in as near a physiologic balance as possible.

All anesthetics are depressants. The severely injured and severely ill require but a fraction of the dose of a depressant ordinarily used in an uninjured patient of the same size and age.

REGIONAL ANESTHESIA

The four regional anesthetic techniques described in the following pages are useful for operations on the head, the upper extremity, the trunk, and the lower extremity.

Aside from needing to know the pharmacology of the drugs used, it is important for the anesthesiologist to make the proper psychological approach to the patient who is about to have an operation under regional anesthesia. The patient must be made to understand that he will retain some feeling. He should feel no pain but he may retain the sensations of touch and pressure. Mild sedatives such as a small intravenous dose of a barbiturate or narcotic may be used to enhance the effectiveness of regional anesthesia in a good-risk patient. Allow an adequate time interval between completion of the regional block and the start of the operation. Thirty minutes is a desirable time interlude during which preparation for the operation can be carried out.

As with general anesthesia, all patients under the major regional blocks described below should be monitored. Before any regional technique is undertaken, apply a blood pressure cuff and start an intravenous infusion of 5% dextrose in electrolyte solution.

Local anesthesia is most dangerous in the patient not being monitored. Patients under spinal or local anesthesia may require and should have oxygen.

AXILLARY BLOCK

Indications: Operations upon the hand and arm up to (but not including) the elbow.

Technique: With the patient supine, place the elbow and shoulder at a 90 degree angle with external rotation at the shoulder. Position a pillow under the hand and forearm for comfort. After suitable skin preparation and draping, stand at the side of the patient and palpate the axillary artery approximately 3 cm proximal to the point of insertion of the pectoralis major muscle. Place both the left index and middle fingers 2 cm apart along the course of the artery. Make a skin wheal between the fingers with a 25 gauge 2-cm needle attached to a ring syringe in the right hand. Advance the needle slowly until you elicit paresthesia or until you feel the needle penetrate the axillary fascia (Fig. 5–2). If paresthesias are evoked, withdraw the needle 1 to 2 mm. Aspirate with the bevel of the needle in each of at least three quadrants before injection. Deposit up to a total of 25 ml of local anesthetic solution above and below the artery. If the needle penetrates the axillary artery or veins, withdraw the needle point 2 to 3 mm, aspirate again and inject the solution.

Choice of Drugs

1. Use 1.5% solution of lidocaine (Xylocaine) with epinephrine 1:200,000. Duration—2 to 3 hours. This formulation is available in a 30-ml single-dose ampule or may be prepared by mixing a 1% multiple-dose vial containing no epinephrine with a 2% multiple-dose vial with epinephrine 1:100,000, of equal volume.

2. Use 1.5% solution of lidocaine with 1:25,000 phenylephrine (Neo-Synephrine). Duration—2 to 3 hours. Prepare this formulation by adding phenylephrine 1 mg/25 ml to the 20-ml single-dose ampule of 1.5% lidocaine without epinephrine, or to a mixture of equal parts of a 1% multiple-dose vial and a 2% multiple-dose vial, both without epinephrine.

3. Use either 1 or 2 with 0.15% tetracaine (Pontocaine). Duration—5 to 7 hours.

Precautions

1. Beware of a history of reaction to local anesthetic.

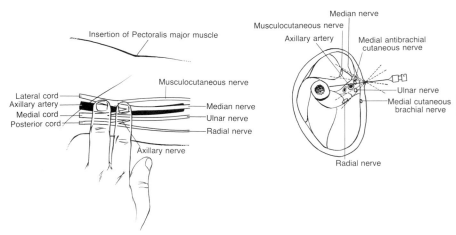

Figure 5–2 Technique for axillary block. Place the index and middle fingers along the axillary artery at a point 3 cm proximal to the insertion of the pectoralis major muscle on the humerus. Make a skin wheal between these fingers. Advance the needle until the point is felt to penetrate the axillary fascia—or until the patient describes paresthesia. Aspirate and inject 25 ml of the anesthetic above and below the artery. (Modified from Moore, D. C.: *Regional Block*, 3rd Edition. Springfield, Illinois, Charles C Thomas, 1961.)

2. The aforementioned dosages are for a healthy young adult. Use one-half the dose in a 40-kilogram child; one-fourth in a 20-kilogram child. Cachetic patients and older patients require less than the 25 ml mentioned.

3. Omit epinephrine in patients with hypertension, heart disease, and diseases of hypermetabolism; phenylephrine is safer.

4. Limit the total dose to 25 ml of 1.5% lidocaine.

INTERCOSTAL BLOCK

Indications: Superficial wounds of the abdomen, flank, and lower thoracic areas.

Technique: Position the patient on his back with pillows under the hip and shoulder of the side to be blocked, or place him on his side so that the side to be blocked is up. Internally rotate and abduct the shoulder so that the scapula will slide forward and upward, allowing the upper nerves to be blocked. After the skin preparation and draping, stand at the patient's back and palpate each rib which corresponds to the nerves to be blocked, starting with the twelfth. Block the nerves at the posterior axillary line. Placing the left index and middle fingers in the intercostal spaces straddling the rib, use a 25 or 22 gauge, 2- to 3-cm needle attached to a ring syringe in the right hand to make a skin wheal. Slowly advance the needle until the rib is contacted with the needle. Walk the needle inferiorly until it slides past the rib not more than 0.5 cm. After aspiration, inject 2 to 3 ml of solution turning the bevel of the needle in each of at least three quadrants. It is essential that the needle be absolutely perpendicular to the rib in its final placement. Since there is an overlap of innervation of intercostal nerves, block one nerve above and one nerve below the site of operation.

Choice of Drugs: Same as axillary block.

Precautions

1. Same as axillary block.

2. Advance the needle no more than 0.5 cm from the external surface of the rib.

3. Signs and symptoms of pneumothorax may appear as late as 8 to 10 hours after the block.

4. Limit the total dose to 25 ml of 1.5% lidocaine (Xylocaine).

SCALP BLOCK

Indications: Injuries of the scalp from the eyebrows to the external occipital protuberance.

Technique: Position the patient sitting or supine. Select a point in the midline just above the eyebrows and a second point just above the external occipital protuberance. After preparing the skin, make a skin wheal at each site. Introduce a 22 gauge 15-cm needle, attached to a ring syringe, into the subcutaneous tissues of the occipital area. Advance the needle to a point just above the right ear. The index finger of the left hand keeps pressure at the needle point which forces the needle to follow the

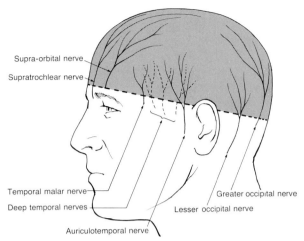

Supra-orbital nerve
Supratrochlear nerve
Temporal malar nerve
Deep temporal nerves
Auriculotemporal nerve
Greater occipital nerve
Lesser occipital nerve

Figure 5–3 Technique for scalp block. Infiltrate the anesthetic solution beneath the skin along the dotted line. The shaded area shows the area of anesthesia that results. (Modified from Adriani: *Labat's Regional Anesthesia*, 3rd Edition. Philadelphia, W. B. Saunders Company, 1967.)

curve of the skull. Inject 10 to 15 ml of local anesthetic solution as the needle is withdrawn. You need not aspirate providing you keep the needle point moving. Direct the needle to a point just above the left ear and repeat the procedure. Utilizing the skin wheal in the midline in the front of the head, place the needle toward the right ear and toward the left ear as described. A total of 40 to 60 ml of drug is necessary for a ring block completely around the head (Fig. 5–3).

Choice of Drugs

1. Use 0.5% lidocaine solution with 1:200,000 epinephrine. Duration — 1 to 2 hours. Available in multiple-dose vial.

2. Use 0.5% lidocaine solution with 1:25,000 phenylephrine. Duration — 1 to 2 hours. Prepare by adding phenylephrine 1 mg/25 ml to the multiple-dose vial without epinephrine.

3. Use either 1 or 2 with 0.1% tetracaine. Duration — 2 to 4 hours.

Precautions

1. Same as axillary block.

2. Limit the total dose to 60 ml of 0.5% lidocaine.

UNILATERAL SPINAL

Unilateral spinal block has the virtue of limiting the effect of the anesthetic on the autonomic, sensory, and motor nerves to one hind quarter.

Indications: Injury to leg, buttock, or groin.

Technique: Place the patient in the lateral position, injured side down, with the neck, back, hip, and knees flexed. Elevate the head of the operating table so that the cephalad spine is tilted 5 degrees above the horizontal. After preparing the skin and draping the field, tap the subarachnoid space at the level of L3–4, L4–5, or L5–S1 with a 22 gauge 8- to 10-cm needle. Rotate the needle bevel so that it points toward the injured side. Place the heel of the left hand against the patient's back, grasping the hub of the needle between the thumb and the index finger. Attach the syringe with the right hand and inject the solution over a period of two to three minutes by the clock. Do not aspirate once the injection has begun. Remove the needle and keep the patient in the lateral position for 20 minutes. During this time, check the blood pressure, pulse and respirations every half minute for the first two minutes, every one minute for the next 10 minutes, and then every five minutes until the end of the operation. After 20 minutes, roll the patient gently to the supine position. If movement by the patient is limited and the change in the position is done carefully, the effects of the anesthetic will be limited to one side. Check the level of analgesia periodically during the 20-minute waiting period and for five minutes after placing the patient in the supine position.

Always check the blood pressure immediately after moving a patient under spinal anesthesia.

Choice of Drugs

1. Use 0.3% solution (3 mg/ml) tetracaine (Pontocaine) premixed with dextrose 6%. Duration—1 to 2 hours. The average adult will require 8 to 10 mg of tetracaine.

2. Use 2% solution (10 mg/ml) tetracaine added to dextrose 10% in equal volume. Duration—1 to 2 hours.

3. Use 1:1000 solution (1 mg/ml), epinephrine, adding 0.1 ml to each 3 ml of spinal drugs. Duration—2 to 4 hours.

4. Use 1% solution (10 mg/ml) phenylephrine, adding 0.1 ml to each 3 ml of spinal drugs. Duration—2 to 4 hours.

Precautions

1. The eventual level of anesthesia will depend upon (a) volume of solution injected, (b) site of lumbar puncture, (c) rate of injection, (d) dosage of drug, (e) length of the dural sac, (f) diameter of the spinal cord, and (g) curves of the vertebral column.

2. Spinal anesthesia should not be used in the presence of: (a) shock, (b) significant blood loss, (c) central nervous system diseases, (d) diseases that have central nervous system sequelae, e.g., mumps.

3. The anesthesiologist must be prepared to treat: (a) hypotension. The hypotension of spinal anesthesia by itself is best treated by (1) anticipating the drop in pressure and (2) infusing a dilute solution of vasopressor intravenously, e.g., 5 mg phenylephrine in 1000 ml 5% dextrose in water. (b) nausea and vomiting, (c) respiratory depression or arrest, (d) cardiac failure.

REGIONAL TECHNIQUES FOR OTHER SITES

Face and Neck: Blocks of individual nerves may be accomplished but infiltration of the wound is usually preferable.

Fractures: In the presence of severe injuries, injection of a local anesthetic into a fracture site is acceptable as a compromise.

POSTANESTHETIC CARE

Since many injuries occur at night when recovery rooms are not staffed, the anesthesiologist has responsibility to stay with the patient until his protective reflexes have returned or to see that some other competent person stays with the patient. The dangers of vomiting, aspiration, hypotension, and hypoxia are as real when the patient emerges from an anesthetic as during induction.

The most dangerous times in the anesthetic experience are the induction and recovery periods.

Local anesthesia and block anesthesia require careful observation of the patient after operation, just like general anesthesia.

Chapter 6

Thermal, Electrical, Chemical and Cold Injuries

THERMAL BURNS

A major thermal burn is a catastrophic injury—medically, financially, and psychologically. Since providing adequate medical care for patients with major burn injuries can prove taxing to hospital facilities, most major burn injuries are best treated in larger hospitals and, more specifically, in burn units especially staffed and equipped for the management of burns.

CAUSES OF BURN INJURIES

Scald burns are most common in children under 3 years of age. Most burns in the 3- to 15-year age group are flame injuries stemming from the misuse of matches and fire. Burn injuries in adults usually result from clothes catching fire. Smoking in bed contributes a significant share of burn injuries among the aged and the infirm. Burns among military personnel are frequent, resulting from occupational hazards including aircraft accidents, explosions, flame throwers, white phosphorus, and accidents involving fuel for vehicles and aircraft. Chemical and electrical injuries commonly result from industral accidents.

PATHOPHYSIOLOGY OF THE BURN INJURY

Major burn injuries induce alterations in the normal physiology primarily as a result of the three following factors: (1) disruption of the normal protective functions of the skin, (2) injury to the vascular tree and blood elements, and (3) the general metabolic effects of major trauma. The magnitude of the changes seen in these three parameters in patients with major burns probably exceeds that seen in any other form of injury.

SKIN FUNCTION

The primary protective functions of the skin under normal conditions stem from its ability to act as a barrier against invasive infection by microorganisms and its ability to impede the loss of water and heat from underlying tissues. Both of these functions are largely lost after a full-thickness injury of the skin occurs as in a third-degree burn. Alterations also occur in partial-thickness injuries of the skin, but to a lesser extent. Invasive infections of the third-degree eschar is the leading cause of death in patients with major burn injuries.

The magnitude of the insensible water losses occurring through burned tissue has only recently begun to be appreciated to its full extent. Evaporative water losses in major burns have been measured as varying from 100 to 300 ml per hour per square meter of body surface area. Thus it can be seen that larger burns may require from 2.5 to 6 liters or more of fluid per day to replace evaporative water losses. Closely associated with the large evaporative water losses occurring in major burns are the tremendous energy expenditures. Each gram of water evaporated from the burn surface removes approximately 0.580 of a kilocalorie of heat from the body. The metabolic rate must be correspondingly increased to maintain body temperature.

VASCULAR INJURIES

Thermal injury to the vascular tree and blood elements results in loss of vascular integrity and destruction of red cell mass. Injury to the capillaries causes abnormal capillary permeability which allows protein-rich fluid to escape into tissue spaces. It has also been demonstrated that capillary permeability increases not only in areas of direct burn injury but also in other areas of the body. The rate of fluid loss resulting from a burn is greatest during the first few hours and diminishes progressively over the following 48 hours. This fluid is manifested clinically as a state of hypovolemia coupled with edema.

METABOLIC EFFECTS

The general metabolic effects of a major burn are those associated with any form of major stress or trauma. These include a markedly negative nitrogen balance, depletion of the body fat stores, increased potassium losses, and increased urinary excretion of adrenal corticoids and catecholamines. Adrenocortical exhaustion does occur in patients with major burns, but is relatively uncommon.

ESTIMATION OF THE SEVERITY OF THE BURN

The severity of any burn injury and implied prognosis are best evaluated by considering the following factors: (1) extent of burn, (2) depth of burn, (3) age of the patient, (4) location of the burn, (5) previous state of health, and (6) associated injuries.

EXTENT OF BURNS

The extent of burn is expressed as the percentage of the total body surface area involved by the burn. A good rapid method for the estimation of the extent of burn is the **Rule of Nines.** According to the Rule of Nines, the body surface is divided into regions, each of which represents 9 per cent or a multiple of 9 per cent of the body surface (Fig. 6–1). A more accurate method for the determination of the extent of burn, and one which makes allowance for the varying surface area of different anatomic areas in children, is the **Lund and Browder chart** (Fig. 6–2).

Based on extent and depth, burn injuries are categorized as minor, moderate, or critical. **Minor burns** include partial-thickness burns of less than 10 per cent of the body surface area and full-thickness burns of less than 2 per cent of the body surface. Burns of this limited magnitude do not require intravenous fluids and can ordinarily be managed on an outpatient basis.

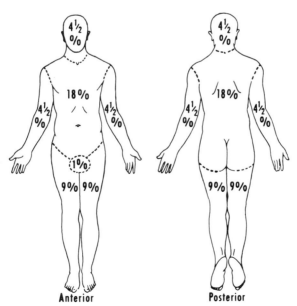

Figure 6–1 Schematic outline of the Rule of Nines. This formula provides an easy and fairly accurate method of determining the percentage of the body surface area burned.

*Adapted from Lund and Browder.

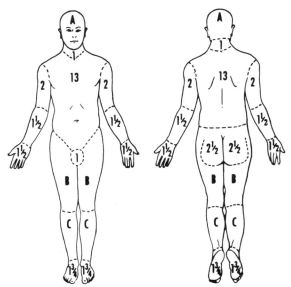

Relative Percentage of Areas Affected by Growth

			Age in Years			
	0	1	5	10	15	Adult
A—½ of head	9½	8½	6½	5½	4½	3½
B—½ of one thigh	2¾	3¼	4	4¼	4½	4¾
C—½ of one leg	2½	2½	2¾	3	3¼	3½

Figure 6–2   The Lund and Browder chart, a more accurate method for determining the extent of a burn. Such a chart should be included on every hospital record of a burned patient.

Moderate burns are either second-degree burns which cover less than 30 per cent of the body surface or third-degree burns which cover less than 10 per cent of the body surface area. Burns in this category usually can be managed in community hospitals.

Critical burns are second-degree burns which cover more than 30 per cent of the body surface area, third-degree burns of more than 10 per cent of the body surface area, or significant burns which are present on the face, hands, or feet. Burns complicated by a respiratory tract injury, fractures, or major soft tissue injury as well as electrical injury are also best placed in this category. These burns should be managed in specialized treatment centers. This classification is of the utmost importance in establishing a triage of burns in mass casualty situations.

DEPTH OF BURN

The depth of any given burn is ordinarily categorized as first-, second-, or third-degree. First- and second-degree burns are frequently referred to as **partial-thickness burns,** while third-degree burns constitute **full-thickness** skin injury. **First-degree burns** are frequently seen after brief flash burns, contact with hot liquids, or prolonged exposure to sunlight. They are characterized by a simple erythematous flush. The burns are dry and quite painful and sensitive to touch. Blisters when present are minute.

Second-degree burns commonly result from brief exposure to hot liquids and flash explosions. Examination of a second-degree burn reveals marked erythema, blisters, a moist surface, pain, and sensitivity to light touch and pin prick. The deeper dermal elements remain viable and second-degree burns heal spontaneously if significant infection does not supervene.

Third-degree burns are usually caused by flames or contact with hot objects. The surface of the third-degree burn presents a dry and whitish or charred appearance. Third-degree burns are rarely significantly painful because of destruction of the nerve endings within the skin. For the same reason, sensitivity to light touch and pin prick is absent. Third-degree or full-thickness burns imply full-thickness destruction of the skin and spontaneous healing will not occur. For diagnosis of burn depth refer to Table 6-1.

AGE OF PATIENT

The age of the patients is also an important factor in determining the severity of a given burn. In general, children less than 5 years of age and adults more than 30 years of age tolerate burns relatively poorly.

LOCATION OF BURN AND COMPLICATIONS

The location of the burn is important in assessing severity of burn injury. Obviously, burns of the head and neck are more frequently associated with respiratory tract complications and a higher mortality. Mortal-

TABLE 6-1   DIAGNOSIS OF BURN DEPTH

	Second-degree	*Third-degree*
Etiology	Scald, flash	Flame
Appearance	Pink, red	Pearly white or charred, thrombosed subcutaneous vessels visible
Physical characteristics	Moist surface, blisters, painful, sensitive to light touch and pin prick	Dry, anesthetic

ity in burned patients is also adversely affected by the presence of significant cardiac, pulmonary, renal, or other chronic disease.

FIRST AID AND TREATMENT OF MINOR BURNS

One of the best first-aid measures for burns is the **application of cold.** If a patient is seen in the emergency department with a burn of the face, wet towels soaked in ice water should be placed over the face to bring about immediate pain relief. If other burned areas are causing stinging pain, they should be covered with moist cold towels. As in any case of major trauma, a patent airway must be maintained by any means available. It may be necessary to give the patient a dose of morphine intravenously. Burned patients are frightened and need to be reassured.

Chemical burns caused by acid or alkali should be washed immediately with large quantities of water to remove the injurious agent. Looking for a specific antidote may be a waste of time. The clothing should be removed and if a large quantity of chemical burning agent has come in contact with the skin, the patient should get under a shower or in a bathtub.

The burn wound should be cleansed initially and debrided and then covered with a dry sterile dressing. Dressing changes should be performed at 3- to 5-day intervals. At each dressing change, the burn wound should be cleansed and irrigated. These procedures should be continued until the burn wound has healed completely or until an area suitable for grafting is obtained in case of full-thickness burns. Dressings are necessary in the management of most minor burns to protect the burn wound and to prevent contamination. Patient comfort is also enhanced by using dressings.

TRANSPORTING THE BURNED PATIENT

The real problems in transporting a burned patient become evident when a burned patient must be transported from a local physician's office or small community hospital to a larger facility some distance away. (Burns of less than 20 per cent of the body surface can usually be handled in any small hospital unless critical areas — such as the hands and face — are involved. More extensive burns require the specialized facility of a large well-equipped institution.) Moving a patient with moderately severe burns over a long distance requires thought and preparation. The referring physician should call the receiving hospital and make arrangements for admission, describing the type of transportation, the approximate time of arrival, who will accompany the burned victim, and medical details of the injury.

The best time for transporting a seriously burned patient is during the first 48 hours after injury. Fluid losses can usually be anticipated during this time, and if fluids are replaced by appropriate therapy as they are lost, the patient usually remains in relatively good condition for the first 24 hours.

Since moving a patient over a long distance usually intensifies injury, the patient should be prepared for transportation. It is the referring physician's responsibility to see that the patient arrives at his destination in good condition. Since all patients are more comfortable after their burn wounds are dressed, a large bulky dressing should be applied prior to transport. If the transportation will require more than one hour, intravenous fluids should be started so that resuscitative therapy can be given before and during transport. The patient should be given nothing by mouth. If movement to the receiving facility will require 3 or more hours, a urinary catheter should be inserted. Occasionally a tracheostomy is necessary when there has been marked inhalation of smoke or when there is appreciable edema of the neck that might interfere with respiration. It is always wise to send a detailed and accurate history of the accident, as well as an explanation of the type and time of medication administered.

IMMEDIATE HOSPITAL CARE

As in all patients who have sustained major trauma, an initial rapid assessment of the patient's general condition should be made when the patient is first seen. A factor of prime importance is airway patency. If respiratory difficulty is apparent or seems imminent, endotracheal intubation or tracheostomy should be performed. Major associated injuries such as fractures and deep lacerations should be noted and cared for appropriately. At this point, a brief initial history and physical examination should also be obtained and recorded. An estimate of the extent of burn should also be made at this time.

Intravenous fluid therapy should then be instituted. Intravenous fluids should always be administered through a large-bore indwelling venous cannula. Reliance for any prolonged length of time on intravenous needles for fluid administration is dangerous because of the frequency with which needles dislodge. When a cutdown is done, initial blood samples for laboratory analysis should be obtained. The tests should include cross matching, hematocrit, blood urea nitrogen, and any other specific determinations that appear necessary. Infusion of lactated Ringer's solution or a suitable colloid should then be initiated through the intravenous cannula.

If **narcotics** are necessary to relieve pain, they should be administered intravenously. In instances of poor tissue perfusion, subcutaneously administered narcotics will be poorly absorbed and ineffective. In addition, because the initial doses may not produce the desired effect, more of the narcotic is frequently administered. When circulation improves, the previously administered dose of narcotics may be absorbed rapidly and result in a toxic overdosage. It is wise when performing the initial cutdown to place the catheter in a position suitable for measuring central venous pressure to provide an additional parameter for monitoring the patient's response to therapy.

An **indwelling catheter** should be placed in all patients with major burns. The most reliable method for monitoring fluid replacement in patients with major burns is the hourly measurement of urinary output. Ordinarily the catheter can be removed within 48 to 72 hours.

A budget or over-all plan of intravenous fluid and colloid administration should be settled on at this point. Numerous methods of determining the approximate amounts of fluid and colloid necessary in the treatment of the shock phase of major burns are available. No mathematical formula exists which is suitable for all patients under all conditions. Consequently, the response of the patient to the resuscitative therapy must be constantly monitored and the dosage and rate adjusted.

Of the methods of fluid estimation currently available, the most popular is the **Brooke formula.** It estimates the following requirements during the first 24 hours after burning:

> colloid (dextran, Plasmanate, or plasma) — 0.5 ml/kg/per cent
> of body surface burned
> electrolyte solution (lactated Ringer's) — 1.5 ml/kg/per cent of
> body surface burned
> water requirement (given as dextrose and water) — 2000 ml
> for adults; children correspondingly less

Approximately one-half of the fluid calculated by this formula should then be administered within the first 8 hours following injury, and the remaining one-half during the next 16 hours. During the second 24-hour period after a burn is sustained, usually about one-half of the aforementioned amounts of fluids will be required. A useful rough guide to the daily water requirements in infants and children is as follows:

0 to 2 years	120ml/kg
2 to 5 years	100 ml/kg
5 to 8 years	80 ml/kg
8 to 12 years	50 ml/kg

It must be remembered that the ratio of fluid requirement to body surface area burned is not linear. Consequently, burns of greater than 50 per cent of the body surface area should be calculated as 50 per cent burns. Other factors that must be considered in altering the fluid budget are the age of the patient (children and elderly patients tolerate rapid fluid infusions poorly) and the presence of cardiac, pulmonary, or renal diseases.

The adequacy of therapy is best monitored by hourly evaluation of pulse, urinary output, and central venous pressure. Serial hematocrit determinations are also of value. The rate of fluid infusion should be adjusted to maintain a urinary output of from 30 to 60 ml per hour. If the output should fall outside these limits, the rate of fluid infusion must be adjusted accordingly. In infants and children, a urinary output of 10 to 20 ml per hour is usually considered adequate. Ideally, the central venous pressure should remain between 6 and 12 cm of water, and the hematocrit should be maintained within normal limits. A rapidly rising hematocrit indicates an inadequate rate of fluid administration. After the first 48 hours, most patients can be maintained on oral fluids and feeding.

Tetanus prophylaxis must always be given in patients with burn injuries, even though the injury is minor. If the patient has no record of previous immunization, tetanus immune globulin (human) must be utilized. If previously immunized, the patient should be given a booster dose of tetanus toxoid.

Prophylactic antibiotic therapy is probably not necessary. Prophylactic antibiotics were frequently used in previous years primarily to prevent the occurrence of streptococcal burn wound infection. If, however, one of the currently available topical chemotherapeutic agents is utilized in the treatment of the burn wounds, prophylactic antibiotics are probably superfluous.

After the initial shock phase has been successfully treated, meticulous attention must be paid to the patient's **nutritional status** until the wounds have healed completely. Reference has already been made to the fact that burned patients have a tremendously increased requirement for calories and protein. A daily protein intake 2 to 3 gm/kg of body weight is desirable. The caloric intake should be 50 to 75 calories/kg/day. In addition, routine vitamin supplements are recommended as follows: ascorbic acid 1500 mg, riboflavin 50 mg, and nicotinamide 500 mg.

Blood volume must also be maintained during the phase of wound management and wound closure. Frequent hematocrit determinations should be made and sufficient blood given to maintain it at about 40.

GENERAL SUPPORTIVE MEASURES

BODY POSITION

Patients with extensive burns should be positioned in bed for maximum comfort. For patients with burns of the head and neck the head of the bed should be elevated to minimize dependent edema and the increased possibility of airway obstruction. Patients with circumferential burns of the trunk and legs can usually be handled best on a turning frame or circoelectric bed.

ESCHAR

One of the most underestimated complications of full-thickness burns is the constricting effect of a circumferential eschar on an extremity and, sometimes, on the chest. In the arms and legs, the edema which forms rapidly beneath the unyielding eschar produces pressure sufficient to occlude first the venous circulation and then the arterial circulation, resulting in ischemic necrosis. Circulatory embarrassment can be recognized by early congestion with poor capillary flow in the nail beds. Later, pain and pallor are prominent. The treatment is incising the eschar, without anesthesia, down to the fascia.

PHYSICAL THERAPY

Physical therapy should be begun as soon as the initial phase of edema has started to abate. This is particularly important in the management of deep burns of the hands. In the case of burns of the feet, a foot board should be used at all times to prevent foot drop. Meticulous attention to these details can obviate the development of severe limitation of joint function in almost all instances. Once fibrosis and calcification of tissue in and about the joints with subsequent limitation in the range of motion has developed, treatment is extremely difficult. If these complications are not prevented, permanent and severe disability usually results.

EMOTIONAL CARE

A frequently neglected aspect of the management of patients with critical burns is the psychologic one. Patients suffering major burns understandably experience severe emotional difficulties. Initially, the fear of death, disability, and disfigurement is usually present. Frequent reassurance and honest appraisal of the patient's course is helpful in allaying the patient's fears. In the recovery phase, a period of severe depression is common as the patient contemplates the difficulties to be encountered in attempting to return to a normal life. Adequate physical and occupational therapy during the period of hospitalization does much to restore the patient's confidence in his abilities. Psychiatric counseling as well as consultation with vocational rehabilitation agencies is often helpful in minimizing the problems of adjustment.

MANAGEMENT OF THE BURN WOUND

WOUND CLEANSING

The initial management of the burn wound is devoted primarily toward obtaining as clean a wound as possible. After resuscitative therapy has been instituted, adherent clothing, dirt, and foreign material should be removed. The wound should be cleansed with an antibacterial detergent in warm sterile water or saline. Although strict asepsis in the initial cleansing and debridement of the wound is impossible, sterile techniques should be adhered to as much as is practical. Loose, devitalized tissue and blisters should be debrided. If the burned patient is to be transported to another facility, it is wise to apply dry occlusive dressings after the initial cleansing and debridement. The use of the closed method of wound management facilitates the transportation and handling of the patient and minimizes further contamination of the burn wound.

TOPICAL GERMICIDAL AGENTS

The development of methods of effective topical wound management has recently provided one of the major advances in the management of extensive burns. A number of topical germicidal agents are currently available which appear to be highly effective in the prevention of invasive burn wound sepsis. These agents include Sulfamylon, silver nitrate, and gentamicin. Many other agents are currently under intensive investigation and may prove equally effective.

Currently, the most widely used topical agent is **Sulfamylon.** After the initial cleansing and debridement, Sulfamylon is applied to the entire burn wound. Thereafter, the patient is placed in a Hubbard tank once daily, the Sulfamylon washed off and then reapplied. Complications secondary to the use of Sulfamylon have been limited, but include sensitivity reactions and the development of metabolic acidosis. Sulfamylon is a carbonic anhydrase inhibitor, and significant amounts are absorbed through the burn wound. This occasionally leads to a metabolic acidosis. Hyperventilation is frequently an early warning sign of the development of metabolic acidosis. Reversal of the chain of events occurs rapidly after removal of the Sulfamylon and treatment with intravenous sodium bicarbonate solution.

GRAFTING

Separation of the burn wound eschar usually begins approximately three weeks after the initial injury. **Debridement** under general anesthesia may be necessary to hasten this process. As soon as suitable areas of granulation have developed, grafting should be initiated.

Preferred **donor sites** are the back, abdomen, upper thighs, chest, upper arms, buttocks, and legs. The electric or air-driven dermatome is useful for the rapid removal of large amounts of split-thickness autograft. An attempt should be made to remove split-thickness grafts at a thickness of approximately 0.010 of an inch. If repeated crops of autografts are to be obtained from the same donor sites, as is frequently the case on a major burn, the grafts removed must be thinner.

After removal of the split-thickness graft, the donor site is covered with a single layer of dry, fine-mesh gauze, and a warm moist pad is applied to obtain hemostasis. After hemostasis has been obtained, the pad is removed with the gauze left in place. Blood and serum form a coagulum in the gauze which creates an effective barrier against infection. The gauze will peel away spontaneously as epithelial regeneration occurs beneath.

The removed grafts are then applied to the granulating surfaces. Preferably, the grafted site is left exposed and no sutures or dressings are used. The skin grafts rapidly become adherent to the underlying wound. In dependent areas and in areas of circumferential wounds, dressings are usually necessary for approximately 72 hours to prevent dislodgment of the graft.

After the wound has healed, any remaining small open areas of granulating tissue should be kept scrupulously clean. This can be accomplished in the ambulatory patient by daily shower baths and by washing with a mild detergent soap. Dry, fine-mesh gauze patches should then be applied to the open granulating areas. In the nonambulatory patient, daily soaks in the Hubbard tank and cleansing should be continued.

SPECIAL TYPES OF BURNS

Although the general principles remain the same, certain types of burns require modification of the treatment techniques which have been discussed in the preceding section. Included in these special types of burns are electrical injuries and chemical injuries.

ELECTRICAL INJURIES

Electrical injuries differ from thermal burns primarily in the extent of injured tissue present. Electrical injuries characteristically result in necrosis of a relatively large volume of tissue underlying the cutaneous wound. In contrast to simple thermal burns, although the surface extent of the burn may be limited, destruction of tissue usually extends for a significant depth into the soft tissues and bone underlying the cutaneous injury.

The volume of **fluid required** for resuscitation of a patient who has suffered an electrical injury over a given percentage of the body surface area usually exceeds significantly that which would be predicted from merely viewing the surface area involved by the burn. The incidence of **acute renal tubular necrosis** is much higher in patients who have sustained electrical injuries than in the usual thermal burn.

Because of the extent of the injury, **early excision** of electrical injury is advisable. After the patient has been properly resuscitated, the burn eschar and all underlying nonviable tissue should be excised. The dressing should be changed and subsequent excisions repeated until all nonviable tissue has been removed. Split-thickness skin grafting is then accomplished.

CHEMICAL BURNS

Chemical burns resulting from contact with acid or alkali are commonly the result of industrial accidents. Strong acids develop an intense exothermic reaction, precipitate intra- and extracellular protein, and cause cellular dehydration and necrosis. Strong bases such as potassium and sodium hydroxide likewise result in strongly exothermic reactions. They are also associated with hygroscopic cellular dehydration, saponification of fat, and protein denaturation. Initial treatment should be directed toward copious irrigation of the affected area with water. After dilution has been accomplished, strong acids should be neutralized with a weak base such as sodium bicarbonate; strong bases should be neutralized with a weak acid such as dilute acetic acid. Neutralization should never be attempted prior to irrigation because of the sudden and intense increase in the exothermic reaction which results. After these initial methods of treatment, the burn wound should be cared for in the same manner as a simple thermal burn.

Phosphorus burns are rarely seen in civilian practice but are quite common as a military injury. Initial treatment should consist of irrigation with copper sulfate solution. Copper sulfate prevents the oxidation of organic phosphorus and inactivates it. It also causes a black discoloration of the phosphorus particles and allows them to be located more easily and removed. Thereafter, the tissue injury is managed in a method similar to the usual thermal burn.

COLD INJURIES

Frostbite is a serious injury with potentially disastrous consequences which are often not immediately apparent.

CLASSIFICATION

Since the following classification can be made only in retrospect it has limited value in prognosis and treatment of frostbite.

First-Degree: Erythema, swelling, burning and tingling without bleb formation.

Second-Degree: Edema, bleb formation, paresthesia, anesthesia, and marked hyperemia after warming.

Third-Degree: Early edema and necrosis of the skin but without loss of a part.

Fourth-Degree: Early pallor and lack of edema of the skin with total necrosis and loss of a part.

EARLY TREATMENT

1. **Rewarm the body** to normal temperature.
2. **Anticipate shock** and treat it.

3. **Rapidly thaw** the injured parts by immersion in water at 40° to 42° C (104°–107° F) until distal vascular bed shows flushing. Use whirlpool bath, if available, with antiseptic soap.

4. **Relieve pain** with analgesics. The intravenous or intra-arterial use of 25 mg tolazoline hydrochloride (Priscoline) may aid in the relief of pain.

5. **Give toxoid or human immune globulin** for tetanus prophylaxis.

6. **Confine the patient to bed in a hospital** until edema subsides and blebs dry.

7. **Treat the injured parts openly with asepsis:** (a) place sterile gauze between toes; (b) use sterile sheets; (c) preserve blebs; (d) give a whirlpool bath at body temperature with antiseptic soap for 20 minutes, twice a day; and (e) have the patient move every joint at every part every waking hour.

OTHER TREATMENT

Low molecular weight dextran has shown encouraging results clinically and in the laboratory.

Some have reported benefit from **sympathectomy** within 24 hours; further experience will determine its place.

Heparin, although used extensively, has shown equivocal results.

PROGNOSIS

Favorable signs: A prompt return of sensation and the appearance of large, light pink blebs extending to the digit tips.

Unfavorable signs: The absence of edema, the presence of purple blebs, and cold and cyanotic digits distal to the blebs.

Chapter 7

Bites

HUMAN BITES

TYPES OF INJURIES

Injuries resulting from contact with human teeth may vary from superficial abrasions and small puncture wounds to deep lacerated wounds or complete avulsion of a part, for example, a nose, a lip or an ear.

Hitting teeth with a fist may injure the extensor aponeurosis and metacarpophalangeal joint of the fingers as well as the overlying skin.

The degree of contamination with mouth organisms depends upon the depth of the wound and the tissues exposed. Badly crushed tissue is likely to become necrotic and thus add to the hazard of infection.

TREATMENT

The following series of steps constitute suggested treatment for human bites.

1. The skin about the wound is shaved and scrubbed with soap and water; then the depth of the wound is flushed with copious amounts of sterile physiologic salt solution. Detergent substances with an antibacterial agent, such as hexachlorophene, are excellent for skin cleansing, but are too irritating to be used on or near mucous membranes. They should not be used on large open wounds where absorption might be a critical factor. While the wound is being washed, any damaged tissues and foreign bodies are carefully removed.

2. Anesthesia, if required, may be either local or general. A local field or nerve block is usually preferable about the lips and cheeks, where equipment for general anesthesia is inconvenient and may add to the risk of contamination. Most surgeons who treat hand injuries prefer general

73

anesthesia, but nerve block at the wrist or axilla is simple and satisfactory for the experienced physician.

3. A tooth wound which is treated promptly may be closed immediately. Most deep wounds and all those which are not treated soon after injury, should first be cleansed thoroughly and then loosely sutured after the threat of infection has passed. As a compromise procedure, the wound edges may be approximated loosely with sterile tape strips which can be removed easily and quickly if marked edema or frank infection becomes apparent. Exposed tendons are not to be repaired initially. If the wound is on the dorsum of the hand, the fingers are splinted in moderate extension. If the wound is a true bite, penetrating deeply into the palmar surface, the hand is dressed with the fingers in the "physiologic position" of midflexion.

4. Tissues of the lip, nose, cheek, ear, or finger should be debrided conservatively, sparing all that might recover.

5. If in doubt, do not close the wound. Wounds that are not sutured are treated with daily dressing change and flushing with saline. Moist saline dressings may be used. If infection is not apparent after four days of observation, the wound may be closed with a few, loosely-tied sutures.

6. Aerobic and anaerobic cultures are to be taken at the time of first treatment. Penicillin may be started because most mouth organisms are sensitive to it. If any gram negative or anaerobic organisms that are not sensitive to penicillin are found, an appropriate antibiotic should be added while treatment with penicillin is continued.

7. If the wound is observed late and the tissues are already edematous or covered with exudate, the wound is to be treated open with warm saline compresses or sodium hypochlorite dressings, and systemic antibiotics. When edema subsides and necrotic tissue has separated, the wound may be closed.

8. Tetanus prophylaxis is indicated.

9. Thermal or chemical cautery is contraindicated.

ANIMAL BITES

PREVENTION

It is estimated that each year at least one million people are bitten by domestic pets—chiefly cats and dogs. Since a high percentage of the victims are children, the following rules are pertinent:

1. Infants should not handle pets.

2. All children should be instructed concerning handling of pets.

3. Strange or sick animals should be avoided.

4. Mature, male animals are said to be the safest pets.

5. Laws pertaining to the use of leashes, muzzles, and other restrictions should be followed.

TREATMENT

Despite the often quoted cliché: "clean as a hound's tooth" most animal bites carry the same potential for infection as do human bites, with the added threat of rabies.

Irrigation and debridement of the wound is to be carried out promptly and completely. This reduces the threat of rabies as well as pyogenic infection.

The traditional chemical or thermal cauterization is no longer recommended.

RABIES

In most parts of North America the incidence of rabies has been reduced to the point where no more than one death per annum has been reported as due to rabies. The incidence of rabies is greater in wild animals than in domestic pets. Significant pockets of rabies may exist among skunks, foxes, and bats. Although these animals do not often attack humans, they may do so. They are far more likely to contaminate domestic animals.

If a cat or dog bites a human, an accurate description of the biting incident is essential. The normal animal will not usually attack a human viciously. When such an attack occurs, it raises the question of the animal being sick or possibly rabid. This is no more a reliable criterion, however, than the generalization that dog- and cat-bites are usually provoked by rough play.

The animal should be confined under observation for from 7 to 10 days, and any sign of illness should be reported to the local Department of Health. If the animal dies, the head should be packed in ice and transported to the nearest qualified laboratory for examination. If the animal involved is wild, it should be captured and observed or killed. If killed, its brain should be examined for evidence of rabies.

Since the incidence of rabies varies greatly in different parts of the country, and since the local physician may or may not be conversant with the regional situation, he may be well advised to consult the local Department of Health relative to the incidence of the disease in the area and the rules regarding prophylaxis and treatment.

POSTEXPOSURE PROPHYLAXIS

In the past many physicians concluded that the Pasteur treatment was more hazardous than the disease it was expected to prevent. This fear is less justified today since better and less toxic vaccines and sera are presently available.

Active Immunization.   Duck embryo vaccine (DEV) and nervous tissue vaccine (NTV) have proved to be about equally effective in preventing rabies among exposed individuals, but since fewer neurotoxic reactions have occurred with DEV, it is the choice of the Public Health Service Advisory Committee on Immunization Practices. For at least 14 days a daily injection, in the dosage recommended by the manufacturer, is given subcutaneously in the abdomen, lower back, and lateral aspect of the thighs, in rotation. Additional booster doses are given 10 and 20 days after the completion of the initial course.

The antigenicity of the vaccines must be considered, and for individuals with a history of hypersensitivity to avian or rabbit tissue, readily available antihistamines and epinephrine should be on hand. If meningeal or neuroparalytic reactions occur, treatment is discontinued. Corticosteroids have been recommended, but are of doubtful value.

Passive Immunization. Hyperimmune serum, in combination with vaccine, provides the best postexposure prophylaxis, but the usefulness of serum is limited by the fact that most of the material available is of equine origin. An allergic response may be expected in at least 20 per cent of those receiving it. When hyperimmune serum is employed, part of the dose is injected into and about the wound.

PREEXPOSURE PROPHYLAXIS

The relatively low frequency of reactions to DEV has made it practical to offer active immunization to individuals in high risk occupations, such as mailmen, veterinarians, and those stationed in areas where rabies is a constant threat. Two 1.0 ml. injections of DEV are given subcutaneously in the deltoid areas 1 month apart, followed by a third dose 7 months later. Those receiving such immunizing injections are advised to have a serum test for neutralizing antibodies 3 to 4 weeks after the last injection. Additional booster doses may be necessary if the antibody titer is inadequate and may be indicated following exposure to known rabies.

SNAKE BITES

Although there are several thousand snake bites recorded in the United States each year, only about 20 deaths due to snake bites are recorded during the same interval. The pit vipers are the major source of such lethal episodes (Fig. 7-1). Ninety per cent of the bites are on extremities. About 55 per cent of the victims are under 20, and 35 per cent are under 10 years of age.

Bites of nonpoisonous snakes produce a "V" of small punctures, while poisonous bites leave one or two distinct penetration marks on the skin (Fig. 7-2). Excruciating pain is the most significant symptom of the poisonous bite. The area usually swells and discolors rapidly.

Venenation does not always accompany a bite by a poisonous snake.

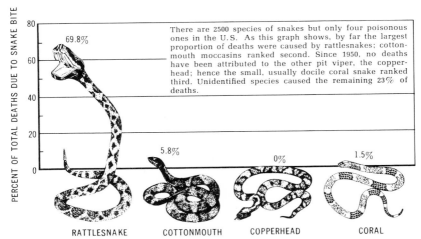

There are 2500 species of snakes but only four poisonous ones in the U.S. As this graph shows, by far the largest proportion of deaths were caused by rattlesnakes; cottonmouth moccasins ranked second. Since 1950, no deaths have been attributed to the other pit viper, the copperhead; hence the small, usually docile coral snake ranked third. Unidentified species caused the remaining 23% of deaths.

Figure 7-1 Line-up of killers: deaths attributable to each species. (From Consultant. July-August, 1963. Smith, Kline and French Laboratories.)

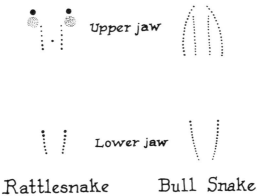

Rattlesnake   Bull Snake

Figure 7-2 Bite marking made by poisonous snake compared with nonpoisonous snake (natural size for average size mature snake). On the left are the bite markings (upper and lower jaw) made by the fangs and teeth of the western diamondback rattlesnake. The two large black dots represent the puncture wounds made by the fangs. The stippled areas under the fang marks represent the areas where the venom is deposited under the skin; because of the curvature of the fangs and their tendency to fold at the termination of the strike, the deposit of venom will be slightly below the puncture wound made by the fangs. This indicates that the cruciate incision made to evacuate venom should actually be centered over this deposit, although cutting through the fang marks. The parallel rows of dots below and medial to the fang marks are marks made by the teeth of the upper jaw. They, as well as the lower jaw teeth markings shown below, may not be visible, particularly if the strike was made through clothing. On the right are upper and lower jaw markings made by the nonpoisonous bull snake. Seldom will the entire pattern be visible. (After Pope and Perkins. Arch. Surg., 49:331, 1944.)

If no local symptoms develop within a matter of minutes, then the customary treatment for a nonpoisonous snake bite is followed.

TREATMENT

1. A **tourniquet** is applied proximal to the wound, only tight enough to impede the superficial lymphatic and venous flow. If swelling appears above the tourniquet, then it should be reapplied proximal to the swelling.

2. The fang marks are **excised** and **suction** is applied by employing an inverted syringe barrel which is attached to wall suction or another source. The suction is applied as continuously as possible; if discontinued for several hours, it is not usually reinstituted.

3. After suction is discontinued, **cracked ice,** if available, is applied to the wound in order to slow the absorption of venom. This suggestion, however, does not imply approval of cryotherapy, which was formerly advocated but is now regarded as unproductive and probably hazardous.

4. While **peroral alcohol** has been a popular remedy for snake bite, it is no longer regarded as a valid part of therapy.

5. The patient is placed at **rest** to reduce the flow of blood and lymph from the limb.

6. **Tetanus prophylaxis** and a broad spectrum antibiotic are employed upon the assumption that snake saliva may be contaminated both with anaerobic and aerobic organisms. If mouth suction has been employed as an emergency measure (other methods are preferred whenever available), there is also possible contamination from this source. On the other hand, it is possible that the person who applied the mouth suction may be poisoned with venom, especially if some ulceration of the oral cavity is present. Such instances have been reported.

7. **Hospitalization** is in order to permit close observation with adequate laboratory facilities. A physiologic solution of electrolyte in water is started intravenously in anticipation of possible shock and to provide a convenient vehicle for specific therapy. A tracheostomy set should be available.

8. **Antivenin.** Crotaline Antivenin Polyvalent, USP, which is commercially available throughout North America, is effective against the venom of the more common poisonous snakes, with the exception of the coral snake. Fortunately, this snake is seldom involved. The individual should be skin tested for sensitivity even though this material is not prepared in horse serum. There may be theoretical advantage in the use of a monovalent antivenin, if it is available and if the snake has been accurately identified. Valuable information may be obtained from the nearest poison-control center. Investigation under way in this field may change the recommended management.

If the patient has only a superficial abrasion or tooth mark with no local or systemic reaction, the area is carefully cleansed, tourniquet and ice are applied, and the patient is observed. Some experts believe that antivenin is not indicated if the local edema and erythema about the fang marks is not more than five inches in diameter. When, however, the patient is obviously ill and the reaction is spreading rapidly, antivenin should be administered promptly, giving one-half the vial in the region of the bite and the other half in one of the large muscles of the bitten extremity; a second vial is given intravenously in the liter of electrolyte in water already started. Whether the initial dose is to be repeated on subsequent days will depend upon the systemic response and the extent of local reaction. Failure to respond may be an indication for increasing the dosage.

Pain is severe in the early stages of venenation and usually lessens with effective treatment.

During the stage of neuron involvement and possible respiratory paralysis, **tracheostomy** and assisted respiration may be indicated.

Adrenal support with steroid therapy may be required because of allergic response either to the venom or the antivenin. In desperate cases it may be indicated from the onset.

If shock persists with renal shutdown, **dialysis** may be necessary.

Severe hemorrhage due to venom-induced hypoprothrombinemia may necessitate *blood transfusions* and administration of *vitamin K*. Adequate **fluid** and **electrolytes** are to be given throughout the illness.

INSECT BITES

Each year millions of individuals suffer the consequences of insect bites, most of which involve only erythema, induration, and pruritus. Among the varieties of arthropods which produce annoying bites are: horse flies, stable flies, deer flies, black flies, tsetse flies, mosquitoes, fleas, midges, lice, chiggers, ticks, bed bugs, bees, wasps, hornets and yellow jackets, spiders, and scorpions, most of which are found in North America.

Some produce minimal local effect, but transmit to the host (as in the case of the mosquito, tick, and tsetse fly) a serious systemic disease or infection such as malaria, yellow fever, filariasis, onchocerciasis, encephalitis, trypanosomiasis, leishmaniasis, plague, tularemia, epidemic and marine typhus, scrub typhus, Rocky Mountain spotted fever, Q-fever, and several rickettsial variants. Some of these are endemic in restricted areas, but with a highly mobile population they may appear almost anywhere.

On the other hand, some of the biting arthropods may cause very severe local tissue destruction, with or without severe systemic symptoms. Some like the bee, hornet, spider, and scorpion, inject a toxic substance and leave a part of the stinging apparatus in the tissues of the host. Or, in the case of ticks, the biting mouth parts may be retained within the tissues and produce a granuloma. The injected material may cause only mild malaise or may be neurotoxic and rapidly lethal. It may cause very severe local tissue destruction, or it may evoke a mild or severe allergic response. In general, **venom sacs** retained in the tissues should be removed surgically, since their retention leads to more local destruction or absorption of the toxic material they contain.

While an atopic history has been given in a high percentage of individuals who have serious or fatal reactions from the stings of *Hymenoptera* (bees, wasps, yellow jackets, and hornets), many have no known history of allergic response prior to the bite or sting. It has been noted that a known, severe reaction to an insect sting in the past may well predict a more serious reaction to a similar sting later, irrespective of any history of allergy. It has been estimated that at least 20 fatalities occur each year due to insect bites or stings, and that one-third of these occur within an hour after exposure.

TREATMENT

These facts point up the importance of employing *antihistaminic* and suppressive corticosteroid therapy as soon as possible after the insult, as well as instructing the individual to avoid contact with such insects in the future. Some allergists advise previously exposed individuals (the majority being children) to carry an **emergency insect sting kit** including a tourniquet, a sterile syringe containing epinephrine HCl (1:1000), an antihistaminic, and a tablet of ephedrine sulfate. Some advise using whole **bee extract** to immunize children who are obviously sensitive to bee stings.

Although presently available **insect repellents** have not been proven to be completely effective, it seems pertinent to suggest that a container of aerosol insecticide spray be carried in the glove compartment of automobiles to discourage any errant stinging insect that finds its way inside the vehicle.

When the victim of the insect sting is brought to the emergency department in obvious shock, or unconscious, an intravenous "cocktail" of hydrocortisone (100 mgms in 500 ml of 5 per cent dextrose in water), aminophylline, and an antihistamine may be helpful if administered immediately.

SPIDER BITES

The **black widow spider** (*Latrodectus mactans*) has been accorded impressive attention in both professional and lay press, and several deaths have been attributed to its neurotoxic bites. It is identified by a red hourglass marking on the abdomen and a shiny black "shoe button" body. Bites have been followed by abdominal rigidity, pain and muscle stiffness in the trunk and extremities, shock, pareses, urinary retention, convulsions, and respiratory difficulty. Supportive intravenous therapy and corticosteroids seem to offer the best chance of improvement. Intravenous calcium gluconate often produces marked improvement.

The **brown recluse spider** (*Loxosceles reclusa*) has been reported in at least 13 states and may actually be more dangerous than its more publicized cousin, the black widow spider.

Although in the case of the black widow spider, the venom is a product exclusively of the female, in the brown recluse spider, the male can also produce venom but apparently in lesser amounts than the female. Both spiders have the unfriendly habit of hiding in dark crevices of man-made structures, particularly outhouses, from which vantage point they attack surreptitiously exposed regions of the unsuspecting victim's body. While the bite of the black widow may be difficult to find when toxic symptoms appear, the brown recluse deposits a tissue toxin that produces a local reaction which proceeds within a matter of hours to necrosis, accompanied by increasing systemic symptoms. Large doses of **methyl prednisolone** have been recommended (intramuscularly and intravenously) to lessen the tissue necrosis and toxic symptoms.

Surgeons with extensive experience in treating brown-recluse-spider bites have expressed doubt that steroid treatment alone will suffice. Initially the sting from the bite may seem minimal, but shortly thereafter the victim begins to experience severe pain at the site and seeks medical attention. Soon a small area of necrosis appears which spreads gradually, increasing daily. Without excision the involved and necrotic skin must eventually slough. Observations have led to the conclusion that the most satisfactory treatment is to excise the involved skin as soon as a diagnosis of brown-spider bite can be established. If done early enough, healing will take place without further operation. If delayed until later, the area usually requires skin grafting 5 to 10 days following the excision.

From the standpoint of differential diagnosis, two other lesions should be mentioned: (1) blisters or blebs on the skin surface produced by vesicant fluid secreted by the "blister beetle," and (2) the grid-like pattern of rows of painful papules or vesicles which result from contact with the "puss caterpillar."

MARINE ANIMAL BITES

There are few, if any, inhabitants of fresh water that are a serious menace to man, other than snakes and microscopic creatures such as the *Schistosoma haematobium*, which gains access through small apertures like the urethra. The usually friendly catfish may inflict wounds with its dorsal and pectoral spine.

Sharks are probably the most important of the salt water creatures which attack humans. Of the large family of sharks, about 20 species are said to attack man, and the wounds they create are massive and always life-threatening. Occasionally a barracuda, giant grouper, or moray eel will inflict a massive injury.

The most compelling problem for the victim of a shark attack is to get free of the attacker and out of the water and under the care of someone able to give prompt and effective treatment for massive blood loss. From that point on the mutilating and usually lethal injuries produced by the shark are not unlike those experienced with massive trauma of any other variety.

Most other injuries caused by marine creatures are due to stings from the jellyfish, Portuguese man-o-war, octopus, fire coral, stinging bristle worm, sea urchin, stingrays, and catfish. The last two account for the greatest number of injuries, which are usually caused by brushing against or stepping on the venom-containing apparatus. Usually one of the tentacles, spines, "teeth," or other venom-secreting organs is imbedded in the skin or subcutaneous tissue. These should be removed, if practical.

TREATMENT

There is no specific antivenin for the toxic secretions of any of the marine animals. The treatment as outlined below is the same as for bites or stings for which no specific antagonist to the toxic agent is available:

1. Cleanse the skin surface.
2. Remove foreign material.
3. Apply sodium bicarbonate topically.
4. Place proximal tourniquet, not too tightly.
5. Apply ice, to delay absorption.
6. Elevate affected part and see that patient has bed rest.
7. Treat for shock and blood loss.
8. Give tetanus and antibiotic prophylaxis.
9. Administer antihistaminic and steroids as needed.
10. Provide respiratory and cardiac support when indicated.

Chapter 8

Head

Most patients with head injuries are treated initially by persons who are not specialists and who are relatively inexperienced in the management of neurosurgical problems. Those who survive the initial period following injury will probably receive skilled care later. However, it is not generally recognized that ultimate mortality and morbidity are highly dependent on the quality of initial care. Lay attendants can become exceedingly proficient in the management of patients with head injuries. Perhaps in no field of medicine is unceasing, dedicated vigilance more important. An understanding of fundamental principles and objectives, a sense of dedication, and considerable optimism are essential to success.

PRIMARY CONSIDERATIONS

RESPIRATORY EXCHANGE

Establishing and maintaining an adequate respiratory exchange are the most important of all considerations in the management of patients with head injuries. Adequate exchange can be accomplished in several ways:

1. The patient may be placed in the lateral decubitus position with face dependent (Fig. 8–1). An unconscious patient should be transported on his side.

2. On a hand litter, the lateral decubitus position cannot be maintained, however, so a prone position with an oropharyngeal tube is used.

3. In the acute stage, an endotracheal tube often is lifesaving and may be preferred to tracheostomy. When a skilled anesthesiologist is present a plastic tube may be left in the trachea for 24 to 48 hours. A safe procedure, however, is the use of tracheostomy and a tube with a cuff.

4. Frequent aspiration of the airway is essential.

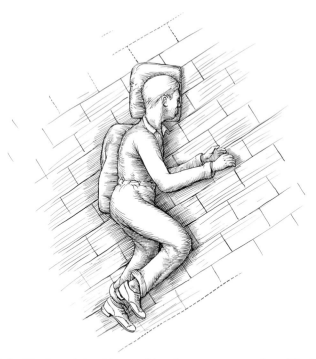

Figure 8–1   The lateral decubitus position for a comatose patient. The head is slightly turned so that the secretions may drool from the dependent corner of the mouth.

5. Oxygen by nasal catheter, endotracheal tube, or tracheostomy is indicated.

6. Intermittent positive pressure apparatus may be necessary to assist respiration or, in some cases, may serve as a respirator to maintain respiration (see Chapter 12, Chest).

Hypoxia of the brain is the most frequent cause of death following head injury. So sensitive is the brain to insufficient oxygen that the maintenance of an adequate airway usually is more important than the arrest of hemorrhage. The signs of progressive cerebral hypoxia are usually indications for immediate surgical correction of the lesion. If cerebral hypoxia or anoxia continues for more than a few minutes, operative correction may be useless, for by that time the brain may be dead.

All who attend the patient with a head injury should understand that cerebral anoxia can develop not only as a result of inadequate respiratory exchange but also from swelling or an expanding mass within the rigid cranial box which reduces the cerebral circulation and, thus, oxygenation of the brain. Patients, conscious and unconscious, who have sustained moderately severe blows to the head should be watched for signs of increasing intracranial pressure.

With a *rapid rise in intracranial pressure*, both early and during the period of compensation, vital signs are as follows:

  a. The pulse becomes slow.
  b. The respiratory rate becomes slow.
  c. The blood pressure rises.
  d. The temperature is elevated.

However, these manifestations may be late in developing. If other signs suggest intracranial hypertension, definitive diagnostic procedures should be instituted promptly.

A further rise in intracranial pressure will lead to the *state of decompensation*. Decompensation is associated with dangerously low cerebral oxygenation due to compression of the cerebral circulation; the vital signs then become reversed:

  a. Consciousness is progressively depressed.
  b. The pulse becomes rapid.
  c. The respiratory rate becomes rapid.
  d. The blood pressure may or may not fall.
  e. The temperature usually remains elevated.

As decompensation develops the pulse may fluctuate in rate. The conscious patient is apt to become drowsy and restless and scream with headache. Usually such signs of increased intracranial pressure require surgical intervention to prevent the death of the patient.

STATE OF CONSCIOUSNESS

The adequacy of oxygenation of the brain is reflected in the reactions or the level of consciousness of the patient. The *level of consciousness is by far the most important measure of the patient's condition.*

Assessing the State of Consciousness. The state of consciousness must be determined and recorded frequently. The following procedures and observations will aid in making this assessment.

  1. Ask the patient to speak.
  2. Determine the response to a command such as "Stick out your tongue."
  3. Note the response to painful stimuli, such as when the skin is pinched or the supraorbital nerve compressed.

      a. Quick, purposeful movements of both extremities are favorable signs.
      b. Slow or delayed, not purposeful or protective, unilateral movements of the extremities are unfavorable signs.

  4. Test the pupils frequently; the size and reactivity of the pupils give an indication of the degree of impaired consciousness.
  5. Watch for bedwetting; bedwetting suggests cerebral compression, and in the aged may be the first sign of a subdural hematoma.
  6. Note any restlessness. Restlessness is more frequently the result of contusion and laceration than of compression from an expanding lesion.

However, restlessness, appearing in a previously quiet patient, may be the first sign of an expanding lesion—compression due to edema or hemorrhage. It may also be produced by a distended bladder or a painful bandage or cast.

7. Record the state of consciousness, along with vital signs, i.e., pulse, blood pressure, respirations, and the size and reactivity of the pupils, every 15 minutes, if possible.

Course of Consciousness. The dynamics of the state of consciousness should be constructed from the history.

1. Initial consciousness followed by unconsciousness suggests increasing compression from swelling or hemorrhage.

2. Continued unconsciousness from the time of injury indicates that unconsciousness probably was due to the initial cerebral trauma, contusion, or laceration. Since one is deprived of the keystone of clinical evaluation (level of consciousness) echoencephalography, angiography, or cranial exploration may be necessary to establish whether or not an expanding lesion is present.

3. If consciousness is quickly regained, the ultimate prognosis should be good.

4. If consciousness and response to stimuli return slowly the prognosis is more guarded.

5. If the conscious patient becomes stuporous, or if more painful stimuli are required to arouse him, he probably has cerebral hypoxia or anoxia due to compression of the brain by either hemorrhage or edema. A dilating pupil is the best guide as to the side of the lesion.

6. If coma is immediate and continuous, it is probably due to laceration and contusion, which as a rule are not helped by surgical operation.

MANAGEMENT

INITIAL TREATMENT

1. Protect wounds with generous sterile dressings.
2. Do not manipulate or disturb foreign bodies.
3. Apply adequate compression with gauze or elastic bandage.
4. Treat shock as in any other injury. Patients with multiple injuries and cranial trauma should not be rushed to the x-ray room for diagnostic purposes unless a depressed fracture or a penetrating wound is suspected. In those situations radiological examination should be made before the wound is closed. Careful observation of vital signs and level of consciousness is more important in the seriously ill patient than an exact roentgenographic diagnosis.
5. Consider the possibility of cervical spine injury.

SIMPLE WOUNDS

In general, the management of simple wounds involving only the tissue of the scalp consists of (1) protecting the patient from further soft tissue injury, hemorrhage, and infection; (2) establishing an accurate diagnosis; (3) performing thorough cleansing and debridement; and (4) making a snug closure.

Control of Bleeding: If cerebral oxygenation is good, hemorrhage often will cease spontaneously. After the scalp area has been shaved, cleansed, and surgically prepared and draped, the wound may be examined with a sterile, gloved finger. Bleeding from the margin is controlled by grasping the galea in a hemostat. If the scalp wound divides the galea, the wound will gape. If the galea is intact the wound may extend down to the galea with the skin edges well approximated.

Leakage: If blood or spinal fluid is dripping from the ear or from the nose, no attempt should be made to pack the orifice. A sterile dressing applied over the ear or nose and changed as indicated is usually adequate until the drainage ceases spontaneously.

Other Considerations: It is rare for a patient to be in *shock* from a head injury or scalp laceration alone. Intracranial clots of surgical significance are rarely found in patients admitted in shock. Opiates should be avoided; even sedatives such as paraldehyde or phenobarbital should be given to the restless patient only when the likelihood of intracranial bleeding has been eliminated. Antibiotic agents are indicated if an open skull fracture exists.

Fluid and electrolyte balance should be maintained. Do not dehydrate or give hypertonic solutions in an attempt to produce dehydration!

Since the level of consciousness is likely to change abruptly, and since vomiting is likely to occur in patients with head injuries, great care is taken to avoid regurgitation and aspiration of stomach contents.

Brain function may be interrupted by severe contusions or lacerations or by reduced blood supply. Hemorrhage or the edema of inflammation will displace normal fluids (the cerebrospinal fluid and the normal blood volume of the brain) from the cranial cavity. Displacement of cerebrospinal fluid produces no clinical symptoms, but reduction of normal blood supply causes profound alterations in cerebral function. Signs of irreversible brain damage due to hypoxia may appear after minutes, hours, days, or weeks. Small, rapidly expanding lesions may kill immediately. A massive hematoma which develops slowly may be tolerated for a long time.

If headache and vomiting persist in a conscious patient, the situation is grave.

APPRAISAL OF CRANIAL NERVES

Cranial nerve function provides useful information which must be recorded at the time of the initial evaluation of the patient and must be reassessed and recorded frequently thereafter. Loss of function, simultaneous with injury, usually indicates destruction or laceration of a nerve, while subsequent loss of function probably is the result of compression or hypoxia secondary to an expanding lesion within the cranial cavity.

1. OLFACTORY NERVE

The presence or absence of loss of smell is of little significance in the acutely injured patient. It may be a permanent and unpleasant complication.

2. OPTIC NERVE

Bilateral blindness is rare; unilateral blindness is not uncommon, and is usually the result of a laceration of the nerve associated with a fracture involving the optic foramen.

3. OPTIC FUNDI

Retinal hemorrhages may develop immediately with injury. Significant diagnostic fundal changes developing after injury are rare. Thus, papilledema and retinal hemorrhage are rare following trauma. In spontaneous hemorrhage from an aneurysm or a stroke, they are common.

4. THIRD CRANIAL NERVE

Note the size of pupils and their reaction to light with a flashlight. Progressive dilatation of a pupil usually indicates an expanding lesion. The degree of dilatation is not commensurate with the size of the lesion but is suggestive of the degree of herniation of the temporal lobe through the incisura. A large lesion may be present without dilatation of the pupil. Any change in pupillary reaction associated with changes in pulse, respiration, and blood pressure may require immediate action! Marked but equal dilatation or constriction, or variation from one to the other, is not unusual in the patient with injury of the brainstem. Dilatation of one pupil, developing after injury, is due in most instances to pressure produced by herniation of the temporal lobe through the incisura. Thus, dilatation of the pupil reflects in some degree the extent of herniation. The fourth and sixth nerves are not so affected in the majority of instances of temporal lobe herniation. The temporal lobe herniation must be reduced at operation.

5. FOURTH AND SIXTH NERVES

Posttraumatic paralysis of the extraocular muscles is rarely the result of intracranial hematoma or swelling. The following diagnostic signs are reliable only when corroborated by other localizing signs:
   a. In cortical lesions, the eyes tend to turn toward the side of the lesion.
   b. In brainstem injury, the eyes tend to turn away from the side of the lesion.

c. Laceration or contusion of one hemisphere or the other may produce conjugate deviation of the eyes, or nystagmus.

6. FIFTH NERVE

Lesions of this nerve are not helpful diagnostically. The trigeminal nerve may be lacerated when the base of the skull is fractured, but usually such a lesion cannot be corrected surgically.

7. SEVENTH NERVE

With **fractures of the base of the skull,** the patient may have complete peripheral facial nerve paralysis, with inability to move any facial muscles and with impaired sense of taste at the tip of the tongue.

Weakness of the facial muscles from a **hemispheral lesion,** a central nerve lesion, is usually only present in the lower part of the face, with the eyelid muscles only slightly affected.

Paralysis of the face developing **after injury** is usually associated with a fracture of the base of the skull, does not reflect the presence of an intracranial clot, and usually disappears spontaneously. This is a peripheral nerve lesion.

8. EIGHTH NERVE

Injury of the acoustic nerve is associated with fracture of the petrous portion of the temporal bone and may be accompanied by bleeding or leakage of cerebrospinal fluid from the ear.

No local treatment is required. The ear canal should not be irrigated nor plugs, such as cotton, inserted into the ear. In comatose patients with normal tympanic membranes, impaired reactions of the eyes to vestibular stimulation with cold water is indicative of brainstem damage. An absence of vestibular induced nystagmus is usually a serious omen.

9. NINTH, TENTH, ELEVENTH, AND TWELFTH NERVES

These nerves may be affected by trauma, but their involvement rarely requires surgical intervention.

ADDITIONAL OBSERVATIONS

If the head is held at a wry angle, if there are bruises on the side of the head and shoulder, or if the extremities do not move when a pin prick is applied, a concomitant spinal cord injury should be suspected (see Chapter 9).

Attendants should check motor function frequently. This can be accomplished by comparing the power of the hand grip on the two sides or by observing the ability of the patient to support the extremities in the air. If the patient is restless the extremities of one side may be moved more than those of the other.

PARALYSIS

Immediate paralysis or weakness involving one entire side of the body results from laceration or contusion of the opposite side of the brain.

A depressed fracture, such as that produced by a golf ball, may produce immediate focal paralysis, and not hemiparesis.

Paralysis due to hemorrhage begins after injury, is usually focal, and may spread to other regions.

CONVULSIONS

Convulsions following head injury may be associated with intracranial hemorrhage. Focal Jacksonian seizures and generalized seizures require special studies to prove or disprove the presence of an expanding or mass lesion. The convulsing patient is subjected to systemic hypoxia because secretions collect in the respiratory tree as the result of an impaired cough reflex and because the spasmodic contractions interfere with respiration. Moreover, at such times the brain requires larger amounts of oxygen than during normal activity.

When a surgical lesion has been ruled out, medical treatment of convulsions should be instituted promptly. A soluble preparation of Dilantin sodium given intravenously in doses of 250 to 300 mg, if necessary at 4- to 6-hour intervals, will usually control the attacks. Intravenous phenobarbital (120 to 200 mg) may be added, but if the attacks persist the patient should be anesthetized by the intravenous administration of Pentothal by an anesthesiologist. Upon recovery from the anesthesia, Dilantin (100 mg) or phenobarbital (100 mg) 3 times a day is usually adequate to prevent further attacks.

DECEREBRATE RIGIDITY

Decerebrate rigidity may occur from contusion of the brainstem and is a serious injury. The patient is unconscious, but painful stimuli produce extensor rigidity of all extremities. Rotation of the head may produce extension of the ipsilateral extremities and flexion of the opposite limbs like the righting reflex of the cat. Grinding of the teeth is seen frequently. The pupils often are small, but may be dilated and fixed. The skin alternates between sweating and a flushed, dry, fixed condition.

RESTLESSNESS

Restlessness or thrashing about in bed is a fairly common symptom of brain injury and cerebral hypoxia. Its development in a previously quiet patient may be the first clinical expression of an expanding intracranial lesion.

Restlessness often can be controlled by correction of the cause. Cerebral anoxia is a frequent cause, and primary attention should be given to this. On the other hand, a distended urinary bladder or painful bandages or casts may induce restlessness. The semicomatose and confused patient will combat restraint.

A considerate nurse often can eliminate the necessity of mechanical restraints. A chest restraint, permitting free movement of the arms and legs, will usually prevent the restless patient from falling out of bed. Encasing the hands in padded dressings will protect catheters and dressings and will encourage rest.

Only when attention to all these exigencies has failed is one justified in using drugs to control restlessness in a patient who has sustained head trauma.

Drugs. Use of narcotics, particularly morphine, in the treatment of head trauma has long been condemned on the premise that they mask changes in the state of consciousness and in the neurological signs, particularly of the pupils, which might permit the correct diagnosis of a progressive lesion of the brain. They also have been condemned on the premise that they tend to depress respiration. For the control of pain from associated injuries, the use of a reasonable amount of narcotics is justified. Eight milligrams of morphine sulfate intramuscularly will give relief. However, for the control of restlessness which arises directly from the cerebrum, chlorpromazine, 10 to 25 mg, at intervals of 4 to 6 hours, paraldehyde, or barbiturates appear more satisfactory.

SPECIAL STUDIES

ROENTGENOGRAMS

Open fractures of the skull require reduction, and in such cases roentgenographic examination should be made at the time of debridement and closure of the wound. It is rare for the course of treatment of a closed head injury to be influenced by the presence or absence of a fracture of the skull, but occasionally it is helpful to know whether or not a fracture line crosses a major vascular channel. In most instances, roentgenographic study of the skull should be deferred until more vital matters are under control and the patient is cooperative.

Most **depressed fractures** of the skull are associated with open injuries. A single, linear fracture depression usually does not exceed 1 to 3 mm and requires no surgical intervention. Closed comminuted fracture depressions are usually corrected as elective procedures for cosmetic reasons and because of the presumption that latent epilepsy may result.

Basilar fractures of the skull are difficult to visualize by roentgenography. **Displaced fractures** of the base of the skull may produce bleeding from the auditory canal, nose, or mouth.

CEREBRAL ARTERIOGRAPHY

Cerebral arteriography will be necessary to identify some expanding intracranial lesions. This requires special techniques, training, and experience. It should not be attempted by neophytes.

ECHOENCEPHALOGRAPHY

Determination of the position of the midline of the brain by a device that transmits ultrasonic waves through the skull to the intracranial structures is simple, safe, and requires no cooperation from the subject. It may be repeated at frequent intervals if progressive bleeding is suspected. But the technique requires an experienced operator. Artifacts are common and will mislead the uninitiated.

LUMBAR PUNCTURE

This is indicated in order to determine pressure when an intracranial clot is suspected and to ascertain the presence or amount of blood in the cerebrospinal fluid. It is hazardous and should not be performed if the patient is uncooperative. Furthermore, fluid pressure under such conditions is meaningless.

The patient is placed in the lateral recumbent position. A 3-inch No. 22 spinal puncture needle is used. Jugular compression tests may be harmful in brain lesions. They should be done only when one suspects injury to the spinal cord. Color, initial and final pressures, and amount of fluid withdrawn are recorded. Spinal fluid pressure above 150 mm of water is suspect; pressure above 200 mm of water indicates a pathologic lesion. In the elderly patient, the spinal fluid pressure may remain low despite the presence of a massive lesion.

SPECIFIC CONSIDERATIONS

HYPOTHERMIA, NORMOTHERMIA AND HYPOXIA

Brain trauma frequently produces a marked rise in temperature (an unfavorable prognostic sign) which increases metabolic demands on a brain already suffering from inadequate flow of blood. If the temperature of the body is lowered to normal or subnormal levels, the needs of the brain can be met even if the cerebral circulation is reduced by the injury. Treatment with mild hypothermia for days or weeks allows patients with very severe head injuries to survive; but hypothermia should be employed only by experienced personnel. It also requires constant qualified nursing attention.

SUBGALEAL HEMATOMA AND HYDROMA

Subgaleal hematoma in the majority of instances results from a linear fracture of the skull. Characteristically, it is discovered as a fluctuant mass of the scalp, hours or days after injury. At the same time swelling of the face may occur. Treatment is expectant—or aspiration with a 10 or 12 gauge needle. Incision and drainage may lead to infection. Aspiration will prevent the hyperpyrexia, intense pain, and tenderness that accompany spontaneous absorption. The signs and symptoms of spontaneous absorption simulate those of a subgaleal abscess.

Subgaleal hydroma is produced by leakage of cerebrospinal fluid and requires only a pressure bandage.

EXTRADURAL HEMORRHAGE

Extradural hemorrhage is most commonly produced by laceration of the middle meningeal artery associated with a linear fracture. It also occurs in association with lacerations of the sagittal and transverse dural sinuses produced by fractures traversing the site of these structures. The history is commonly as follows:

1. A blow to the head, usually in the temporal region, may or may not have produced unconsciousness.

2. If rendered unconscious the patient shortly regains his senses for a few minutes to several hours but again may lapse into coma.

3. The "lucid period" is marred by progressively severe headache and decreasing awareness.

4. Vomiting, brachycardia, and rising blood pressure may indicate increasing intracranial pressure.

5. Focal neurological manifestations such as convulsions, usually of the Jacksonian type, weakness of opposite face, arm, and leg, and dilatation of the ipsilateral pupil develop.

Patients with extradural hematomata are never entirely symptom free, for they do have headache during the lucid interval. Although they may be conversant, they tend to be confused and fall asleep if left alone.

Neurological abnormalities often can be demonstrated by careful examination during the early period of extradural hemorrhage. The most constant and reliable sign is a dilating and sluggish pupil on the side of the lesion. There may be increased reflexes on the opposite side with a positive Babinski sign and ankle clonus.

Echoencephalography is particularly useful in patients suspected of developing an extradural or subdural hematoma. Not only may a shifted midline be detected but occasionally the inner margin of the hematoma may be outlined; moreover, repeated examinations may be carried out every few minutes even if the patient is not cooperative.

Roentgenograms of the skull are very helpful in the diagnosis of extradural hemorrhage. One should look for fracture lines crossing grooves, for the middle meningeal artery and the sagittal and transverse dural sinuses, and for a displaced pineal calcification.

Surgical treatment of extradural hemorrhage prior to loss of consciousness will permit complete cure; thereafter, the mortality is very high. The following dicta may be useful:

1. Remember that the temporal area, the region of the middle men-

ingeal artery, is most frequently involved, and that the areas of the transverse and sagittal dural sinuses are less frequently involved.

2. Fracture lines seen in roentgenograms and in the area of scalp contusion help in localization. (Contrecoup fractures or middle meningeal artery tears do occur.)

3. Drill on both sides of the head (Fig. 8-2). Hematomata are bilateral in 25 per cent of all cases.

4. Nick the dura to look for subdural hematoma.

5. When clot is located, enlarge the bone opening and evacuate the clot by suction, scoops, and irrigation.

6. Control bleeding.
   a. Speed is not important.
   b. Tedious and time-consuming work is necessary to control all bleeding.
   c. Control bleeding from middle meningeal artery by electrosurgical coagulation or by plugging the foramen spinosum with cotton alone or impregnated with bone wax. Use of a tooth pick to plug the foramen also has been described.

7. Suture dura mater to the pericranium.

8. If signs of brainstem compression persist, explore to determine if the temporal lobe is herniated through the incisura. If herniated, the prolapsed structures should be elevated; rarely does the tentorium need to be sectioned.

Emergency room craniotomy for extradural hematoma may occasion-

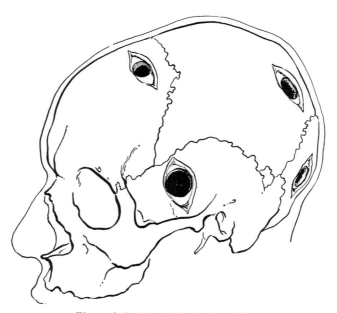

Figure 8-2 Burr holes in the skull.

ally be justified in a patient admitted in extremis with a history and findings indicative of an extradural clot. A drill hole is placed without the scalp being shaved and without sterile technique, if necessary. The establishment of an adequate airway is the only step that takes precedence over evacuation of the clot.

After the clot has been evacuated, the patient is transferred to the operating room, where hemostasis and closure are performed. Even a patient in extremis can usually be temporarily resuscitated by the intravenous administration of urea or mannitol (1 gm/kg of body wt dissolved in 100 cc of a 10 per cent solution of invert sugar). The resultant brain shrinkage provides about a 30-minute period of grace in which to prepare the operative site, put in a burr hole, and evacuate the clot.

SUBDURAL HEMATOMA

Acute subdural hematoma will cause changes similar to those of extradural bleeding of arterial origin and, indeed, may be more fulminating. Since the subdural space is so large, the lesion must be massive in order to produce symptoms. Symptomatic acute subdural hematomas are usually associated with cortical lacerations, with the bleeding coming from torn pial vessels. Less often, the sagittal bridging veins are torn. Because these patients have extensive brain damage their condition is precarious and the prognosis is poor. For this reason, surgical procedures should be as brief as is consistent with adequate definitive therapy.

1. Make 2 superior burr holes on each side.
2. Open the dura mater and evacuate the clot with irrigation and suction. Expose and coagulate the bleeding points.

SUBDURAL HYDROMA

Subdural hydroma is mentioned only because it may be found when the patient is explored for possible subdural hematoma. Adequate treatment usually consists in permitting the fluid to escape through the burr hole, after which it will continue to drain into the subgaleal space.

SUBARACHNOID HEMORRHAGE

Subarachnoid hemorrhage, with blood in the spinal fluid, is common in head injuries. If it arises from one of the larger arteries, such as the carotid, a rapid termination is usual. Often, after 8 or 10 days, signs of meningismus appear. Then spinal fluid drainage by lumbar puncture will lessen symptoms and speed convalescence.

INTRACEREBRAL, ECTOPIC, OR ABERRANT HEMATOMATA AND CEREBRAL SWELLING

It is difficult to evaluate clinically the patient who is unconscious from the moment of impact and whose condition then deteriorates, or the patient who develops progressive stupor without focal signs. In such cases the mortality rate is high. On the other hand, careful management will save many of these patients. Hemorrhage may be present in any part of the brain. Hematomata may form in unusual locations within the subdural space or, indeed, in the extradural space over the posterior fossa. It is not unusual for a patient to sustain head trauma as the result of a fall that has been initiated by a spontaneous cerebral vascular accident. None of these presents a characteristic clinical picture. It is necessary, therefore, to develop an orderly plan in order to make a correct diagnosis and to institute appropriate therapy.

In a patient who is deteriorating and who seems to be in imminent danger of death but shows no significant focal signs, an echoencephalogram will indicate the laterality of a space-occupying lesion, if one is present. A carotid angiogram on the suspected side may be necessary for precise localization. If these fail to indicate a hematoma, and no clinical localizing signs are present, intravenous urea or mannitol to reduce cerebral edema and, in young people, hypothermia offer the best prognosis. "Woodpecker" surgery is no longer advisable in such cases except that a suboccipital burr hole is indicated to rule out a posterior fossa or subdural or extradural hematoma if the pulse is slow. Angiography is preferable to pneumoencephalography in such cases.

Occasionally a patient will show marked increase in intracranial pressure and will appear in imminent danger of death without presenting focal neurological signs. The angiogram, in such cases, suggests temporal lobe swelling and transtentorial herniation. In such cases, resection of the edematous and contused temporal lobe may be a lifesaving procedure. These patients are suffering from herniation of the uncus, a condition which should be corrected, if possible, or the tentorium should be incised.

ANESTHESIA AND HEAD INJURIES (SEE CHAPTER 5, ANESTHESIA)

Indications for anesthesia are the same, whether the lesion be open or closed. Local anesthesia is preferable except in the restless patient. In this case, intravenous Pentothal sodium supplemented with oxygen is adequate. There is, however, no contraindication to any general anesthetic agent. The injured brain tolerates anesthesia well if adequate oxygenation is maintained.

DEFINITIVE TREATMENT

ROENTGENOGRAMS

If the patient is to have a major surgical procedure or debridement for a head wound, roentgenograms of the skull are advisable while the patient is on the way to the operating room. If the patient is restless and good films cannot be obtained, a general anesthetic should be given and maintained for the completion of the procedure. Unless roentgenograms of the skull are available to the operating surgeon, intracranial foreign bodies—bone or metal—may be missed during the exploration and be the nidus for a subsequent infection.

CLOSURE OF SCALP LACERATIONS

For closure of simple lacerations in the emergency room or operating room, the essentials are adequate lighting and instruments, local anesthesia (1 per cent procaine or Xylocaine), and, frequently, an assistant to help control bleeding. All open fractures require the facilities and assistance available in a major operating room, for it may be necessary to remove debris or bone and to control hemorrhage from the dura mater and brain.

1. Be sure the patient's general condition warrants closure of the wound.

2. Shave scalp widely around the wound.

3. Cleanse the skin around the wound with soap and water, and irrigate the wound with sterile salt solution.

4. Infiltrate the margins of the skin around the wound with 1 per cent procaine or Xylocaine through the normal scalp.

5. Incise about the margins of the laceration and remove debris and devitalized tissue.

6. Explore the exposed surface of the skull for fractures.

7. If no fracture exists, close the wound snugly with one layer of interrupted tantalum or stainless steel sutures. If desired, a galeal row of silk can be used and a cutaneous row of scalp sutures, especially if the wound appears clean and has been seen early.

8. Consider the indications for antibiotic agents and tetanus toxoid and tetanus immune globulin.

OPEN FRACTURES OF THE SKULL

In the operating room and after scalp cleansing and draping, the following procedures should be carried out in addition to the therapy outlined for simple lacerations:

1. Remove foreign bodies (distant metallic foreign bodies are occasionally not removed).

2. Remove all macerated brain tissue with a suction tip.

3. Elevate depressed fragments of the cranium.

4. Remove loose fragments of bone.

5. Make hemostatis complete to prevent hematoma formation.

6. Close wound in layers. It is especially important to close the dura mater.

7. Administer antibiotics for prophylaxis. Penicillin and streptomycin or one of the tetracyclines are used.

8. Treat excessive restlessness when present.

9. Get the patient out of bed and ambulating as soon as he is able and is willing to cooperate. If this is delayed more than a few days, physical therapy in the form of active and passive exercises should be initiated. Prolonged bed rest is conducive to traumatic neuroses.

10. Prevent posttraumatic neuroses; if they have already developed, treat the symptoms. Occipital headache and dizziness may be due to injury, delay in ambulation, or possibly to cervical root trauma. Cervical traction may relieve symptoms produced by the latter.

LEAKAGE OF CEREBROSPINAL FLUID

Fortunately, most cranial cerebrospinal fluid fistulas close spontaneously. The prognosis of cranial injury with cerebrospinal fluid leakage is more guarded than that of injury without leakage. Leakage of fluid from either the nose or the ear constitutes a special problem. When displacement of bone persists, spontaneous closure of the dura mater may be delayed or may not occur. Unless roentgenograms reveal a definite protrusion of bone into the subdural space or a marked depression in the frontal sinus area, one is justified in waiting 10 to 12 days to see if the fistula will close. If the leak persists, surgical closure should be considered. Antibiotic agents help to prevent meningitis.

Chapter 9

Spine and Spinal Cord

INTRODUCTION

Aside from rare, penetrating, small-missile or knife-blade wounds, spinal cord injuries are usually associated with disc ruptures, fractures, or fracture-dislocations of the vertebral column.

It should be emphasized that associated fractures or fracture-dislocations and spinal cord lesions cannot be managed separately. Surgeons must be continually aware of the danger of causing additional spinal cord damage by injudicious manipulation of the patient with a skeletal injury. For this reason, in any injury produced by high speed vehicles, the suspicion of a spinal fracture, particularly cervical, should be entertained and eliminated before measures are used that might complicate such an injury.

Patients with wounds of the face or head and shoulder, and all patients unconscious from head trauma should be suspected of having associated cervical spine injuries. The head and neck should be immobilized in supine position with sand bags *on a rigid surface* (e.g., spine board, wooden door, or something similar) until anteroposterior and lateral x-rays of the cervical spine can be obtained.

Patients suspected of having injury to the thoracic or lumbar spine should be placed either in prone position with padding under the head or in supine position with padding under the spine at the site of injury.

EXAMINATION

The principal symptom of fracture of the spine is acute local pain which may radiate into the arms, about the chest or abdomen, or into the lower extremities.

Detailed examination should be carried out without moving the patient's spine. Prominence of spinous processes, local tenderness, pain on attempted motion, edema, ecchymosis, visible deformity, and muscle spasm are of special diagnostic significance and help to localize the site of injury.

Extremities must be examined carefully for sensory disturbances, reflex changes, and muscle weakness.

TYPICAL NEUROLOGICAL FINDINGS

Motor involvement is determined by voluntary muscle contractions or involuntary response to painful stimuli. Autonomic disturbances are indicated by lack of sweating, altered vasomotor responses, lack of bladder and rectal control, and priapism. Typical findings are as follows:

1. Injury of C2 or C3:
   a. Complete respiratory paralysis.
   b. Complete flaccidity and areflexia.
   c. Death in a few minutes unless artificial respiration is maintained.
2. Injury of C5 or C6:
   a. Paralysis of intercostal respiration; diaphragmatic respiration continuing without abdominal muscle action.
   b. Quadriplegia; complete loss of motor power in trunk and lower extremities; preservation of shoulder girdle function and perhaps some deltoid, pectoral, and biceps action.
   c. Initially absent deep tendon reflexes with possible exception of biceps reflex; absent abdominal, cremasteric, and plantar reflexes.
   d. Anesthesia below the clavicles; anesthesia of at least the ulnar half of the upper extremities.
   e. Bladder and bowel retention; priapism.
3. Injury of T1 to T12:
   a. Paraplegia.
   b. Initially absent deep tendon reflexes in the lower extremities; absent cremasteric and plantar reflexes; upper abdominal reflexes may be preserved in low thoracic lesions.
   c. Anesthesia below the dermatome level on the trunk corresponding with level of cord damage.
   d. Bladder and bowel retention; priapism.
4. Injury of L1 to L5:
   a. Partial flaccid paraplegia, the extent depending on which roots of the cauda equina are involved.
   b. Above L2, knee and ankle jerks and plantar reflexes are absent; cremasteric reflexes present. Below L2, knee jerks are present.

c. Anesthesia of perineum, sacral area, and lower extremities may be spotty and asymmetrical.

d. Bladder and bowel retention at least temporarily but perhaps with some retention of sensation.

SPECIAL DIAGNOSTIC MEASURES

Immediately after the patient reaches the hospital a thorough but gentle examination of the neck is imperative. Although the physician or attendant should note any contusions, ecchymosis, or lacerations in the region of the cervical spine, all manipulation of the spine should be avoided until x-rays have been obtained.

A quick neurological examination will demonstrate weakness or impaired sensation of the extremities if the spinal cord has been damaged. Cervical traction with a **head halter** using 10 or 12 pounds should be applied with the neck in neutral position to prevent its movement during the remainder of the examination (Fig. 9-1).

If the patient is not in shock, he may be carefully moved in halter traction and in the supine position on a rigid surface (e.g., spine board) so that anterior-posterior and lateral roentgenograms of the entire cervical spine may be taken. Frequently, adequate demonstration of the odontoid process of the second cervical vertebra, the ring of the first cervical

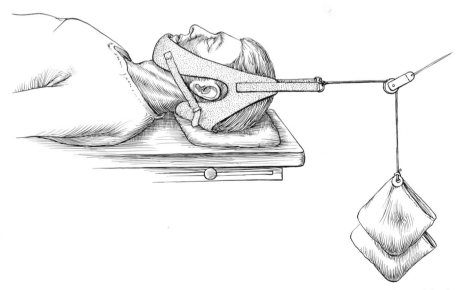

Figure 9-1 Halter traction in place. Note that direction of pull is in line with the vertebral column.

vertebra and the seventh cervical vertebra is difficult, yet these structures must be visualized by special techniques if necessary. If anterior-posterior and lateral films have revealed no evidence of fracture, oblique films of the cervical spine and a lateral view of the cervical spine in flexion and extension should be obtained with a physician in attendance. Roentgenograms are examined for:

1. Contour and alignment of the vertebral bodies.
2. Displacement of bone fragments into the spinal canal.
3. Linear or comminuted fractures of the laminae, pedicles, or neural arches. Bone damage is almost always more severe than even the best stereoscopic roentgenograms suggest.

Lumbar puncture should be used judiciously in the immediate period after spinal injury, for it may aggravate existing cord damage if the patient is carelessly manipulated during its performance.

Normal manometric tests are more significant than abnormal ones for many conditions such as dural tears due to depressed bone fragments, cord edema, and so forth may prevent a rise in pressure on jugular compression.

PATHOGENESIS OF INJURIES

Open injuries of the spinal cord in patients who do not die immediately are usually caused by knife blades, ice picks, or bullets and other missiles.

The types of trauma producing closed injuries of the dorsal and lumbar spine are usually different from those causing injury to the cervical spine.

CERVICAL SPINE

Injuries in this region may result from:
1. A blow on the top of the head with the cervical spine in the neutral position resulting in an explosion or blowout type of fracture of the vertebral body.
2. A flexion force applied to the cervical spine with fracture of the posterior elements or tearing of the posterior stabilizing ligaments with or without compression fracture of the anterior structures of the spine.
3. An extension force applied to the cervical spine with fractures through the vertebral bodies and tears of the anterior and posterior longitudinal ligaments with associated compression of the posterior elements.

Dislocations may be associated with either of the last two mechanisms. Regardless of the mode of injury, significant damage to the cord may occur.

Symptoms of cervical spine injury include pain, limited motion of the neck, and spasm of the neck muscles producing abnormal postures of the head. It should be emphasized, however, that **neck motion should not be determined before an x-ray study of the cervical spine has been made.**

The cervical spine frequently is injured in the absence of fracture or dislocation. An increasingly common type of trauma is that sustained by a passenger in an automobile that is struck from behind. The body of the passenger is thrown forward, leaving the head unsupported and resulting in hyperextension followed by hyperflexion of the neck. Thus, tears of the ligamentous structures of the cervical spine may occur with or without associated injury to the intervertebral discs.

DORSAL AND LUMBAR SPINE

The most common site of fracture or dislocation of the dorsal or lumbar spine is in the region of the dorsolumbar junction. By far the most frequently injured vertebrae are D12 and L1. A common mechanism of this injury is hyperflexion, that is, a sudden forward bending produced by a fall in which the spine is sharply flexed, or by a fall with the victim in a sitting position so that force is transmitted from the pelvis upward through the spine. The type of fracture produced by this mechanism is a symmetrical or asymmetrical compression of the vertebral body.

Fractures and fracture-dislocations of the pedicles, laminae, and facets are usually the result of major anteroposterior forces with or without a rotational component. These fractures are much less common and are difficult to diagnose even in roentgenograms.

The spinous process and transverse process may be fractured by direct blow, by hyperflexion injury which has produced a fracture of the vertebral body, or by violent contractions of the back muscles.

COMPRESSION AND CONCUSSION OF THE CORD

Disc rupture, fracture, or fracture-dislocation may produce compression without division of the spinal cord or cauda equina.

Concussion of the spinal cord results from severe trauma to the spine without actual mechanical compression or disruption of either the bony spine or the cord. There is possibly temporary or momentary dislocation of the intervertebral disc. The injury is accompanied by temporary interruption of function which does not ordinarily require specific therapy.

Spinal cord compression is commonly produced by the following skeletal injuries:

Compression Fracture of the Vertebral Body: This type of injury occurs with forced flexion of the spine and may lead to severe angulation of the spine or to posterior displacement of an intervertebral disc into the spinal canal. Compression fractures occur most commonly in the middle or low cervical region as a result of falls or blows on the head, and in the thoracolumbar region (T12 and L1) as a result of falls in the sitting position.

Fracture-Dislocation: Displacement of one vertebra forward upon another is usually accompanied by fracture and is likely to produce temporary or persistent compression of the spinal cord. Such a fracture-dislocation may be reduced spontaneously but may leave residual neurological signs. Dislocations are common at:

a. C1 and C2, in which case there is often a fracture of the odontoid process.

b. C2 and C3, in which there is often locking of the displaced fragments, which are very difficult to reduce without operation.

c. C5 and C6, and C6 and C7; these injuries are commonly produced by diving accidents.

d. T12 and L1; these are produced by severe blows against the back and by falls in a twisted position.

Depressed Fractures: These injuries are usually due to local blows directly over the spine. Cord injuries result when comminuted fragments of the lamina, spinous process, or pedicle are driven into the spinal canal. Depressed fractures may occur in any part of the spine and are most commonly associated with cord injury when they occur in the thoracic region.

Ruptures of the Intervertebral Disc: Any sudden force applied to the spine may cause a tearing and protrusion of the fibrocartilaginous substance between the vertebral bodies. If the protrusion is posterior, the spinal cord may be compressed; if lateral, the nerve roots may be compromised. Such injuries are not seen in roentgenograms of the spine, but may be visualized by myelography or discography.

DEFINITIVE THERAPY

OPEN INJURIES OF THE SPINAL CORD

Open injuries of the spinal cord are rare except in war wounds. In addition to the risk of neurological damage, the patient is subject to hemorrhage, infection of the wound, and meningitis. Puncture wounds rather than gaping lesions are the rule. The point of entry through the skin may be at some distance from the point of injury to the cord. If the invading missile has penetrated thoracic or abdominal viscera, treatment of the visceral lesion usually takes priority.

Definitive therapy is as follows:

1. Wounds of entry away from the midline are explored and debrided as in any other soft tissue wound.

2. Laminectomy is indicated for the following:

a. Wounds over or near the spine.

b. Persistent spinal fluid leakage, indicating a gaping laceration of dura mater, or a bone or a foreign body keeping a small dural tear open.

c. Roentgenographic evidence of bone or foreign body within the spinal canal which could cause compression.

d. Severe, persistent radicular pain following injury to the cauda equina.

CONCUSSION OF THE SPINAL CORD

Management of concussion of the spinal cord includes only careful attention to skin, bladder, bowel, nutrition, and physical rehabilitation (see instructions later in this chapter).

Recovery often begins within a few hours and is maximal, if not complete, within a few weeks.

FRACTURES

Definitive care of spinal injuries depends upon the location, the nature, and the extent of the injury particularly as the latter relates to injury of the spinal cord.

FRACTURES OF THE CERVICAL SPINE

Although skeletal traction is the most comfortable and the most effective form of immobilization of the cervical spine, a head halter (Fig. 9-1) is satisfactory in the emergency room until such time as a fracture or dislocation has been demonstrated.

Skeletal traction should be applied in all cases of cervical spine fracture except when there are (1) avulsions of the spinous processes, (2) chip fractures or "dew drop" fractures of the anterior margin of the bodies of the vertebra, or (3) fractures across the base of the odontoid without displacement of the vertebra and without associated neurological abnormalities. Dislocations accompanying fracture should be reduced by traction alone.

Crutchfield tongs are applied to the parietal bosses in line with the tips of the mastoid processes. The direction of the traction or line of pull should be in the axis of the cervical spine. Crutchfield tongs are readily inserted under local anesthesia while the patient is on a stretcher or a bed. After the scalp has been shaved, two small drill holes are made through the outer table of the skull on either side of the vertex. The tongs are inserted, and the locknut is made secure. A rope is led from the tongs over a pulley projecting from the head of the bed. Countertraction is achieved by elevating the head of the bed on 12-inch blocks. The security of the Crutchfield tongs should be checked daily, preferably by the same physician. If the displaced fragments are not brought into alignment after traction has been applied, the line of pull may be readjusted to bring them into proper position.

The weight applied for traction should depend to some extent upon the size of the patient. The result of traction should be evaluated frequently by roentgenograms and the dynamic effect of the traction regulated by adjusting the amount of weight applied as well as the direction of pull. In children, 5 to 20 pounds is usually sufficient to reduce a fracture-dislocation within a few hours, while in adults, 12 to 60 pounds may be necessary. However, the increase in traction should be regulated depending upon the position of the fracture or dislocated fragments. When acceptable alignment has been obtained, the amount of traction should be reduced to that sufficient to maintain the position of the fragments.

Fracture dislocation of the cervical spine with complete motor and sensory loss is associated with a poor prognosis for return of function. This injury requires **immediate** treatment by skeletal traction as previously described.

After reduction by traction, the alignment may be difficult to maintain. In such cases an anterior interbody fusion is advisable and may shorten the period of convalescence.

Surgical intervention may be required if there is any evidence of cord damage. In patients with clinical evidence of complete interruption of spinal cord function a lumbar puncture should be made. If the dynamics indicate a complete or partial block, a myelogram should be carried out immediately to demonstrate the extent and location of the block. Depending upon the presumed mechanism of injury and the location of the block anterior or posterior to the spinal cord, the spinal canal should be decompressed either by anterior decompression and fusion or posterior laminectomy and decompression followed by immediate spinal fusion.

If the patient does not have complete functional interruption of the spinal cord but has evidence of a progressive neurological deficit, lumbar puncture and myelogram are imperative, and, depending upon the findings, either an anterior or posterior decompression with fusion should be done.

If the patient has evidence of partial interruption of spinal cord function which is improving, further diagnostic and neurological procedures are not indicated but the traction should be maintained and the patient should be carefully observed. As long as the improvement continues, nonoperative treatment should continued.

If improvement ceases at a time when there is considerable neurological deficit, spinal puncture and myelogram may be carried out to determine the presence of spinal cord block or compression and appropriate treatment instigated. It should be recognized that a posterior disc protrusion may occur without radiographic evidence of its presence. For this reason, the *judicious use of spinal puncture and myelography is particularly important in these cases and requires expertise.*

FRACTURES OF THE DORSAL AND LUMBAR SPINE

Patients with **undisplaced uncomplicated fracture** of the lower dorsal or lumbar spine should be placed on a firm bed until the immediate reaction to injury subsides.

Correction of **compression fractures** of the dorsal or lumbar spine usually should not be attempted. The patient may be supported in a well-fitted plaster of Paris body cast or a well-fitted back support to prevent flexion of the spine and may be allowed to ambulate as soon as symptoms of back pain and abdominal distention have subsided. Early ambulation in a well-fitted back support is particularly desirable for elderly patients.

Intelligent, cooperative, adult patients may ambulate without the support of a body cast or back brace as long as they are given careful instructions regarding the nature of their fracture and the mechanism that produced it. They need to be told how to get out of bed by turning on their side and coming up to a sitting position while carefully maintaining the spine in hyperextension during this movement as well as when standing, sitting, and walking. Back strengthening exercises should be started early.

Fracture dislocations of the dorsal and lumbar spine with neurological involvement *should be investigated immediately by spinal puncture and myelography.* If a block is present, a decompressive operation followed by spinal fusion with rigid internal fixation should be performed. It is dangerous to attempt to manipulate such injuries because of possible additional damage to the spinal cord.

Depressed fractures of the neural arch, pedicles, or laminae, if associated with evidence of cord involvement (particularly in the thoracic region), should be treated by early laminectomy. Roentgenograms may be helpful in showing bone fragments in the spinal cord. A myelogram may be valuable.

Protrusions of intervertebral discs may be demonstrated only by myelography or discography. Depending on the site and extent of the protrusion, therapy may be (1) immobilization by a cervical collar, (2) decompressive foraminotomy, (3) laminectomy with removal of fragments in the canal, or (4) anterior interbody fusion.

Laminectomy: This operation may be performed under local or general anesthesia, usually with the patient in prone position, but it requires a full complement of neurosurgical equipment and experienced personnel.

Open injuries must have adequate excision, extensive laminectomy to assure removal of all foreign bodies and bone fragments (especially those in the spinal canal), and watertight closure of dura to prevent leakage of spinal fluid. Hematomata must be evacuated.

Fractures demand cautious exposure to avoid further cord damage by displacement of comminuted bone fragments. All loose fragments that might impinge on the cord or cauda equina should be removed.

The dura mater is not opened unless it already has been lacerated. Tears in the dura produced by penetrating bone fragments should be closed tightly.

SPECIAL CARE OF PATIENTS WITH SPINAL CORD LESIONS

SKIN

Special measures for skin care should be initiated as soon as the diagnosis of spinal cord injury has been established. In transections, **pressure areas** leading to ischemic necrosis develop with surprising rapidity. It is imperative, therefore, to change the position of the paralyzed parts at least every two hours. As soon as possible, the patient should be placed on an alternating pressure air mattress or, if such is not available, a foam rubber or air mattress, with great care being taken to protect the sacrum, trochanters, malleoli, and heels. If a Stryker frame or Foster bed is available and the patient's skeletal status permits its use, frequent changes of position are greatly facilitated.

The entire area of anesthetic skin should be lightly massaged with alcohol, dried carefully, and powdered at least once daily. Bed coverings should be kept dry at all times and as free from wrinkles as possible. After bowel movements or enemas, the perineum and sacral area should be thoroughly cleaned and dried. Frequent application of tincture of benzoin helps to protect the skin in areas of pressure.

BLADDER

Retention of urine develops at once after every severe cord injury, and, because of sensory paralysis, there may be no discomfort. It is important, therefore, to insert a urethral catheter under aseptic conditions (see Chapter 14 for technique) within a few hours after injury to prevent overdistention of the paralyzed bladder. Repeated catheterization should be avoided.

Suprapubic cystostomy is indicated only by associated injuries (see Chapter 14). The "needle" and "trocar" types are expeditious emergency measures for experienced personnel only.

BOWEL

Paralytic ileus is a frequent, early, and distressing complication of all types of spinal injury. The insertion of a nasogastric tube with constant suction and the administration of intravenous fluids for 1 to 2 days usually will relieve this distressing sequel. After cord transection, fecal retention ensues. Enemas should be started early and administered at regular intervals to encourage automaticity. Manual relief of fecal impaction may be necessary.

PHYSICAL AND PSYCHOLOGICAL REHABILITATION

Adjustment of patients with severe spinal cord damage should begin as soon as possible. It can be started in the emergency facility with proper positioning of extremities, personal reassurance and encouragement by the physician, and development of insight into the possibilities of adequate living even with severe disability.

Chapter 10

Face

GENERAL CONSIDERATIONS

Although facial injuries are properly located far down the list of thera-peutic priorities in multiple system injuries, two considerations require serious reflection:

1. Although the facial injury itself may not threaten life, it is fairly common for such injuries to threaten the patient's life by compromising the airway. (Also, a striking facial injury may occupy the attention of the examining physician, while more occult and life-threatening injuries may not be noticed.)

2. It must be recognized that compromise or delay in treatment may lead to permanent deformity. It is axiomatic, therefore, in the absence of other life-threatening injuries, that prompt treatment be instituted to eliminate or minimize permanent deformity, cosmetic defects, or func-tional disability. Careful examination for evidence of other injuries with special attention to possible brain damage and cervical spine and spinal cord injuries is required and should be repeated frequently.

INITIAL TREATMENT

Severe injuries of the face require immediate investigation of the upper airway. Foreign material in the oropharynx is relatively common. Vomitus and broken dentures and teeth in the posterior pharynx must be removed promptly. Retrodisplacement of the tongue as a result of injury to the central nervous system or collapse of the mandibular arch as a result of fractures must be relieved. Interstitial swelling of the tongue with obstruc-tion may occur after blunt or sharp trauma. Direct trauma to the larynx or tracheal cartilages, although a less common cause of respiratory obstruction, must be considered. Respiratory support is necessary in the case of brain stem injury or severe cerebral injuries.

Supportive emergency measures include:

1. Anterior traction of the fractured mandible and tongue.
2. Continual pharyngeal suction.
3. Endotracheal intubation.
4. Emergency tracheostomy — *good* lighting, proper instruments and at least one assistant are minimum requisites.
5. Mechanical ventilatory support (Ambu bag, respirator)

Hemorrhage in the facial areas should be treated with direct pressure since clamping of the larger vessels under ordinary emergency department conditions involves the risk of clamping one of the contiguous facial nerves or their branches, resulting in paralysis. Evidence of shock in patients with facial injuries should prompt a thorough search of other body areas for injuries which are more commonly related to shock. Pain associated with facial injuries is often mild, even when the injury is extensive. It is rarely necessary to use narcotics. In fact, they are often contraindicated because they interfere with continuous monitoring of the status of the central nervous system which is desirable in head injuries.

EXAMINATION

SOFT TISSUE INJURIES

Lacerations, avulsions, and abrasions about the head and neck are usually evident. Intraoral lacerations, produced by fractured dentures or pipe stems or by tongue bites, must be looked for immediately. Bleeding from these injuries is often brisk and, if the patient's mental status is depressed, they may be the cause of bleeding into the trachea. Bleeding about the head and neck can be controlled with pressure. Devitalized or badly contused tissue should be removed since this is the greatest source of facial wound infection. All possible viable tissue should be saved. The ordinary laceration will heal without infection if the surrounding tissue is well nourished.

The following soft tissue injuries will require operating room repair under optimum conditions: (1) parotid gland or duct, (2) facial nerve, (3) nasolacrimal injury with interruption of the canaliculus, sacculus, or nasolacrimal duct, (4) moderate soft tissue loss, and (5) extensive lacerations requiring debridement and accurate closure.

Deep laceration from the midportion of the cheek back to the ear should arouse strong suspicion that injury has occurred to the facial nerve, parotid gland, or parotid duct. Careful search and examination for injuries to these areas is indicated. Transoral probing of the parotid duct will facilitate diagnosis of parotid duct injury. Nasolacrimal injury should be suspected when blunt or sharp trauma has occurred near the medial canthus and epiphora. Fluorescin or radiopaque dye may be used to evaluate the integrity of the ducts. In case of doubt, such injury should be assumed to exist, and repair planned accordingly.

FRACTURES

The facial skeleton is constructed so that, through sequential small bone failures, it can absorb a tremendous amount of impact energy while affording maximum protection against concussion of the cranial vault. Recognition of these small bone fractures is essential if healing is to occur with proper contour of the face and its associated structures. Diagnosis of these fractures involves a combination of clinical inspection, palpation, and radiographic examination. Interpretation of facial radiographs, even in the hands of experts, frequently is difficult. Careful clinical examination of the face will usually detect fractures with significant displacement of fragments.

FRACTURES OF THE MANDIBLE

The keynotes in diagnosing fractures of the mandible are: (1) malocclusion or displacement of the mandible to one side and (2) pain in front of the ear when biting down, indicating condylar fracture. Frequently, the patient will mention the fact that his teeth do not fit together properly. This usually indicates a fracture of the mandible or maxilla. Digital palpation of all but the condyle and coronoid of the mandible is easily carried out intraorally and externally and will usually localize the fracture, especially if displacement is present. A fracture of the horizontal ramus on one side of the mandible often is associated with a corresponding fracture of the condyle or neck on the opposite side. Anesthesia of the lower lip suggests a fracture through the mental foramen or interruption of the inferior dental nerve in its canal.

FRACTURES OF THE ORBIT

Ordinarily irregularities of the orbital rim are present in orbital fractures. Isolated blowout fractures, although unusual, may occur in the presence of an intact orbital rim when the floor of the orbit is disrupted by pressure transmitted by the globe itself. This results in retrodisplacement and inferior displacement of the eye often associated with limitation of motion of the globe in the plane of upward gaze. Diplopia frequently is present.

Differentiation of zygomatic fractures and LeForte II fractures (Fig. 10–1) requires intraoral investigation. The former will show considerable discomfort when pressure is applied behind the zygomatic arch from the intraoral position; the latter maxillary fracture will usually display some "drawer type motion" when the anterior alveolar process is grasped and pressure is exerted in a to-and-fro motion. Disarticulation of the fronto-zygomatic suture is seen with trimalar fractures and with craniofacial separation. Diplopia frequently attends the limitation of extraocular motion found when the inferior rectus and inferior oblique muscles are entrapped in an orbital floor fracture. There may be disruption of the medial canthal ligament with apparent widening of the intercanthal distance. The nasal bridge is also flattened and widened in this type of injury.

In all such instances careful investigation for possible ocular or intra-ocular injury is indicated. Depression of the zygomatic arch often produces pain on motion of the jaw or limitation of motion due to impingement of the coronoid process on the fractured zygomatic arch in addition to an external depression in the area.

FRACTURES OF THE MAXILLA

Disruption of the medial portion of the orbital floor can produce entrapment of the inferior rectus muscle, resulting in diplopia and a step deformity at the infraorbital rim. Hypermobility of the maxillary segment elicited by efforts to move the anterior alveolar process indicates a maxillary fracture (Fig. 10–1). If this motion is observed concomitantly with motion of both infraorbital rims, a craniofacial separation has occurred (LeForte III). If only the medial section of the infraorbital rims move during this examination, it is probable that a LeForte II type of fracture has occurred. If the entire orbital complex remains stationary while the alveolar process is being moved, a LeForte I type of fracture has occurred through the pyriform aperture. Anesthesia over the distribution of the infraorbital nerve commonly accompanies these fractures since the fracture line is usually through this foramen. It is an important diagnostic sign.

FRACTURES OF THE NOSE

Nasal fractures are usually more evident clinically than radiographically. Nevertheless, x-rays should be taken if injury is suspected. The injury may depress the dorsum of the nose, displace it to one side, or simply result in epistaxis and marked swelling over the nose without apparent skeletal deformity. Crepitus and hypermobility of the nasal pyramid are usually evident in these fractures. Inspection for hematoma or dislocation of the septum should be made. In any injury of the naso-orbital complex, inspection for possible cerebrospinal rhinorrhea is indicated. If there is a question as to whether the clear material obtained is serum, cerebrospinal fluid, or mucus, glucose determinations should be obtained Cerebrospinal fluid glucose is approximately half that of the serum glucose level. Mucin content can also be determined to clarify the type of drainage.

In children, minor displacement of nasal bones will result in growth changes and ultimate deformity unless corrected at the time of the initial injury.

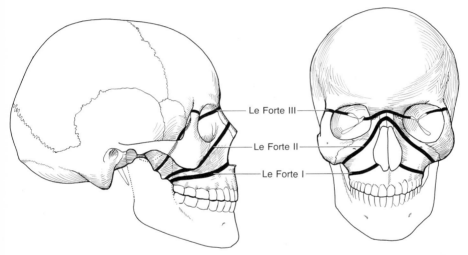

Figure 10–1 Fractures of the maxilla. Mobility of the maxilla when pushing or pulling on the anterior alveolar process indicates a fracture of the maxilla. In a LeForte III fracture, the whole of each infraorbital rim moves with the maxilla. In a LaForte II fracture, only the medial section of each infraorbital rim moves with the maxilla. In a LaForte I fracture, the whole orbital complex remains stable.

ROENTGENOGRAPHIC EXAMINATION FOR
FACIAL INJURIES

It is unwise to rush the patient to the x-ray department until a possible concomitant major injury (skull or cervical spine), which would make movement of the patient hazardous, has been evaluated. Complete roentgenograms should be obtained, however, when the patient's condition permits. Special views must be obtained for accurate diagnosis of facial bone injuries. In spite of proper roentgenograms, fractures of thin bones, such as the maxilla, ethmoid, and nasal bones, can be missed because of superimposition of shadows. **Usually, the bony injury is more severe than indicated by roentgenographic examination.**

The following roentgenographic views are recommended:

1. Lower jaw: lateral, oblique, and posteroanterior. Include additional views of the condyles.

2. Nasal bones: Lateral views taken with soft tissue technique.

3. Facial bones of the central third of the face: stereo-Waters view with horizontal shift; submento-occipital view to show zygomatic arches in relief; stereoscopic views to clarify superimposed bony shadows; tomography when necessary to clarify orbital floor and condylar fractures.

In viewing the roentgenogram, the principal things to look for are: (a) comparative size of the antra, (b) discontinuity of the antral wall, (c) clouding of one or both antra, indicating fracture with hemorrhage, (d) irregularity of the floor of the orbit, (e) irregularity of the orbital rim, (f) difference in distance between the coronoid and malar bones, (g) fracture of the zygomatic arch, and (h) separation of the frontomalar suture line.

OPTIMUM TIME FOR PRIMARY REPAIR

Primary repair of facial bone fractures should be carried out as soon as the patient's general condition permits, preferably within the first 12 hours following injury. Replacement of bone fragments should never be delayed longer than 7 days except in rare circumstances. Beyond this time limit, fibrous fixation of the bony fragments makes accurate reduction difficult or impossible.

ANESTHESIA

In cooperative patients, anesthesia may be administered by regional block for simple fractures. Infra-orbital, supra-orbital, or mental nerve blocks, as well as field blocks or local infiltration are useful. Topical anesthetics may be used on the nasal mucosa or in the conjunctival sac, provided proper precautions for sensitivity reactions are observed.

General anesthesia is frequently necessary in adults and is essential in children. (See also Chapter 5, Anesthesia.)

GENERAL PLAN FOR CARE OF THE WOUND

If local anesthesia is to be administered, the skin is cleaned, grease is removed with benzene, and the skin is prepared with an antiseptic after nerve blocks have been completed. The wound is irrigated with saline. After careful exploration, all dirt, hair, clothing, and other foreign bodies are removed. Dirt and carbon particles produce permanent "tattooing" of the skin if they are not completely removed at the initial debridement.

Facial fractures are repositioned and stabilized as necessary with interosseous wires, pins, interdental wiring, or arch bars to provide a stable skeleton for additional repairs.

Fractures of the teeth and alveolar process or dental lamina as well as loose teeth are indications for splinting the area in order to save teeth that might otherwise be lost. Although often necessarily delayed until more urgent repairs are carried out, early realignment of the alveolar process provides the highest probability of dental salvage.

Injuries of specialized structures are repaired, including the facial nerve, lacrimal system, parotid gland and duct, and cartilages of the nose and ear.

The remaining soft tissues such as muscle, skin, and subcuticular layers are closed, with emphasis on nontraumatic handling of tissues and accurate approximation. Fine suture material should be used. All foreign material should be removed and dead space obliterated.

Elastic bands should be applied between the maxillary and mandibular arch bars, if indicated, in order to immobilize bony parts in proper relationship with each other.

TREATMENT OF SPECIFIC INJURIES

FRACTURES OF THE MANDIBLE

The most important consideration in fractures of the mandible is the re-establishment of proper dental relationships and adequate bony contact of the bony fragments to ensure healing and immobilization. The majority of fractures of the jaw can be treated by closed methods by applying arch bars or interdental wiring between the teeth of the mandible and maxilla secured with rubber bands. The maxilla can be used as a physiologic splint for mandibular fractures.

In some fractures of the mandible the pull of the masticator muscles may produce distraction of the fragments which cannot be managed by closed methods. These "unfavorable" fractures will require open reduction and stabilization of the fragments with interosseous wires or K-wires in addition to intermaxillary stabilization of the teeth.

Fractures of the mandibular condyles should almost invariably be treated by interdental wiring alone without open reduction even with poor position. The condylar fractures and displaced segments will unite and remodel, resulting in less limitation of motion than those that are openly reduced and fixed under direct vision.

In edentulous patients the mandibular fragments should be splinted to dentures by circumandibular wires if the dentures are available and unbroken. Every effort should be made to obtain the dentures either from the accident site or from the home in order to use them as splints to re-establish the proper arch of the mandible. Fractured dentures often can be repaired for use.

Fixation of a fractured mandible with a Barton bandage should be discouraged because if the mandibular arch is unstable this type of dressing tends to produce a retruded position of the mandible. Occasionally, a Barton bandage may be all that is suitable because of the magnitude of the patient's other injuries. When mandibular substance has been lost as a result of blast injuries, it is essential that the remaining fragments be stabilized in their normal position by dental splints or K-wires to maintain the mandibular arch. If this is not accomplished, collapse, shortening, and permanent deformity of the mandibular arch will result.

Occasionally it is necessary to drain injuries of the mandibular area using external drains. This is particularly true in injuries with obviously nonviable tissue or when oozing from extensive contusion is anticipated.

FRACTURES OF THE MAXILLA

Fractures of the middle third of the face are the result of either direct or transmitted force. Blows which have their initial impact on a portion of the mandible can be transmitted to produce fractures of the maxilla and impaction of bones at the level of the pyriform aperture, orbits, or ethmoid sinuses. Overlying facial lacerations are often absent and the amount of edema at the time of initial observation in the emergency department may be slight. Careful examination, intraorally and externally, is essential if proper diagnosis is to be made. X-rays, particularly the Waters-stereoscopic view, will identify the larger bone fragments. Open reduction with direct interosseous wiring of the fragments will usually be necessary. Interdental wiring is also necessary for fixation to the mandible to restore the normal dental relationship.

If the patient is edentulous it will be necessary to wire the denture or an acrylic spacer directly to the alveolar process and through the pyriform aperture in order to hold it securely and maintain adequate jaw space. In craniofacial dysjunctions (LeForte III, Fig. 10–1), the maxillary complex will require suspension from the zygomatic processes of the frontal bone to prevent facial elongation. Wires are passed behind the zygomatic arch to the arch bars and placed on the maxillary teeth. The fixation point should not be located too far anteriorly because tilting can occur. The proper fixation is located between the second bicuspid and the first molar. Although fractures of the mandible heal in 4 to 6 weeks, fractures of the maxilla require 3 to 6 months for stable consolidation.

Crushing injuries of the interorbital area often produce comminution of the bony fragments. Fitting together the individual fragments is impossible and manipulation of these bony fragments may deprive them of their tenuous blood supply with subsequent resorption of bone, producing permanent deformities. Securing one medial canthal ligament to the contralateral one should be accomplished by a wire suture passed transnasally. Subcutaneous hematomas and scarring in the medial canthal area are often extensive. Prompt and accurate reduction of fractures and canthal ligament security are the primary objectives of initial treatment.

FRACTURES OF THE ZYGOMA

Fractures of the malar bone or zygoma are common injuries and are nearly always the result of a direct blow that produces fractures in three areas: the lateral orbital rim, the zygomatic arch, and the infraorbital rim. The fracture usually occurs through the infraorbital foramen, resulting in anesthesia over the lateral side of the nose. Usually blood in the antrum produces opacity of the sinus on x-ray films. Entrapment of the inferior rectus muscle in the fracture site is a common finding. One fragment has a tendency to be displaced backward and rotated outward. Loss of the sharp definition of the infraorbital rim with a step deformity is common in this injury.

Although simple reduction by using an elevator in the antrum placed through a Caldwell-Luc incision often can be accomplished without external incisions, more accurate reconstitution of the orbital floor and rim can be obtained through an infraorbital incision with direct wiring. If the orbital floor is badly comminuted or absent, support must be provided with a thin piece of Silastic or a thin iliac bone graft. After reduction, gentle traction on the conjunctiva of the globe should be used to ensure that there is no limitation of eye motion as a result of entrapment of the extraocular muscles. Reduction of the fracture and release of the entrapped muscle should be done as soon as possible to minimize subsequent fibrosis of this tiny muscle resulting in permanent limitation of motion.

FRACTURES OF THE NOSE

Nasal fractures are usually the result of direct trauma and usually involve more than one fracture within the nasal pyramid. The dorsum of the nose may be impacted in a posterior direction or displaced to either side. The inability to correct all of the nasal deformity at the time of initial injury is sometimes frustrating. The following corrections can and should be made in the emergency treatment of nasal fractures:

1. Elevation of a depressed nasal dorsum with a guarded instrument.

2. Repositioning of a laterally displaced nose in its proper anatomical position. This may require overcorrection, in order to loosen impacted fragments followed by repositioning in the midline.

3. Repair of badly torn nasal lining.

4. Repositioning of a dislocated septum. Dislocated septa are common injuries and are easily reduced if recognized at the time of the original injury. The repair of these injuries at a later date is considerably more difficult and the results are often less than optimal.

5. Aspiration and drainage of septal hematomas. Evacuation of these hematomas can rarely be accomplished with a needle, and an incision in the mucosa usually will be required in order to eliminate them completely. Nasal dressings should include vaseline gauze packing for 1 to 2 days. An external splint made of light aluminum, plaster, or plastic, held securely to the face with tape, completes the dressing.

SPECIAL STRUCTURES

EAR AND NASAL CARTILAGE

Repair of multiple lacerations both of the nose and of the ear are time-consuming. They generally require a three-layer closure. In the case of the ear, comparison with the uninjured side is valuable during anatomical repair. It is helpful to fix the cartilaginous pieces into their proper positions and then proceed with soft tissue repair. The prominence and importance of these features in facial appearance and expression justify all efforts to obtain precise repair. Postoperative splinting by wet cotton dressings is helpful in preventing otohematomas.

PAROTID AND SUBMAXILLARY GLANDS AND DUCTS

Proper repair and management are necessary to prevent the two most common wound complications following these injuries, namely, cyst formation and salivary fistula. The parotid is made up of tough glandular material, and extensive debridement of the gland itself usually is not required. The capsule of the gland accepts sutures well. If the parotid is severely contused, drainage of the gland is indicated even when the larger ducts are intact. The parotid duct is repaired most easily over a plastic stent that is brought out through the orifice of the duct. Sutures should be of chromic catgut since nonabsorbable material could provide a nidus for calculus formation. Sialoadenograms can be carried out by injection of 3 cc of radiopaque material through a polyethylene tube into the parotid duct. This provides useful information regarding the integrity of the duct and the gland.

Lacerations of the ducts of the submaxillary glands are relatively uncommon. They usually do not require formal repair, but produce fistulas into the mouth, causing no further trouble.

EYELIDS

Both vertical and horizontal lacerations of the eyelids can produce serious sequelae. In vertical lacerations, notching and contracture can cause severe deformity if the repair is not carried out carefully. Horizontal lacerations in the upper lid can result in division of the levator muscle or section of its tendinous insertion or lacerations of the globe at or above the conjunctival fornix.

Repair of the eyelids requires careful approximation of the conjunctiva and tarsus in one layer using absorbable material. Knots should be placed external to the tarsus away from the conjunctival surface to prevent irritation of the globe. The orbicularis oculi muscle is then reapproximated after which the skin is closed. Stepping procedures to interrupt a vertical healing interface can be carried out; however, when moderate tissue loss is present, these procedures have a tendency to use up additional lid tissue. This may be impractical if a lid deficit exists.

In general, careful layer repair with 6–0 or 7–0 sutures, taking small bites, will suffice for the initial repair. Tarsal repairs after partial lid loss may require closure under some tension, but this is not necessarily incompatible with an acceptable result.

Loss of conjunctiva often can be repaired using flaps from the conjunctival fornices. In the case of large upper lid avulsions, lower lid flaps often can be used to correct upper lid defects. The reverse of this, swinging upper lid tissue to fill in full-thickness lower lid defects, should not be attempted. The lower lid should be reconstructed, using nasal cartilage-mucosa grafts with local skin flaps.

In large defects of the lid, it is necessary to provide a moist clean environment for the globe to prevent desiccation. This can be accomplished in a steam croup tent or by a cover glass which is taped in an airtight manner to the skin of the face about the orbit after ointment has been inserted into the eye.

LACRIMAL APPARATUS

Lacerations of the medial portions of the eyelids may involve the lacrimal canaliculi leading from the upper and lower lids to the sacculus; or the sacculus itself may be injured. When the sacculus is injured or punctured, usually the superficial leaf of the medial canthal ligament also has been divided; this structure should be repaired. Small sutures in the sacculus usually will lead to adequate healing and repair. Injuries to the anterior wall of the sacculus may require no repair. Injuries to the canaliculus can be repaired by threading a suture of 5–0 nylon or other monofilament material through each open end of the canaliculus and bringing it out through the skin medially and laterally to the laceration. The overlying soft tissues are then repaired.

Eye

EXAMINATION

A detailed history should be taken with regard to the circumstances of any ocular injury. Vision should always be recorded when the patient is first seen. If vision-testing charts are not available, the examiner can compare vision by holding up a hand or fingers, alternatively covering one eye and then the other.

The eye should always be examined carefully for possible damage when a physician treats any injury to the eyelids or adnexa. Once involvement is ascertained, further manipulation of the eye or eyelids is contraindicated. Improper handling of the injured eye may convert a relatively trivial injury into one that is extremely serious and may result in blindness. In addition, a physician should be aware of the possibility of associated intracranial injury. A penetrating wound in the region of the eye not infrequently involves the cranial cavity because the roof of the orbit is fragile.

Except to determine the presence of ocular injury, examination of an eye should be deferred until adequate anesthesia, good lighting, and satisfactory facilities are available. A facial nerve block with local anesthesia should be employed so that the patient cannot squeeze his eyelids together and thus cause herniation of ocular contents. The orbital rim should be palpated. Ocular rotations should be tested in various positions. Diplopia suggests injury to cranial nerves or the orbit.

LACERATION

Immediate treatment is to immobilize the injured eye as soon as possible. This is accomplished best by patching both eyes and moving the patient by litter. No attempt should be made to remove what appears to be a foreign body or a blood clot because of the danger of injuring intraocular structures. The iris may be indistinguishable from the blood clot, and the contents of the eyeball may be extracted. Any manipulation of an injured eye causes pain, with resultant squeezing of the lids and a tendency toward further damage. All lacerations must be regarded as contaminated. Therefore, broad-spectrum antibiotics should be given parenterally as soon as possible after injuries of the globe. Prophylaxis is important because infection usually causes permanent damage to the visual apparatus. The possibility of an intraocular foreign body should always be considered, and its presence excluded by careful examination including roentgenographic study.

Small corneal or scleral lacerations, without incarceration of ocular contents, may be left unsutured. More extensive lacerations require careful apposition with fine 6–0 or 7–0 silk or 6–0 chromic catgut sutures. If iris or uveal tissue is incarcerated, replacement or excision is indicated prior to suturing.

Injury to the lens requires special consideration. A rapidly developing cataract may be followed by serious complications, such as irritative iridocyclitis, secondary glaucoma, and even loss of the eye if not properly managed. Sympathetic ophthalmia is a constant threat following wounds involving the uveal tract. It probably results from an allergic response to uveal pigment in the contralateral eye as a result of the disorganization of pigment-containing cells of the injured eye. The only satisfactory treatment is prevention, which is achieved by prompt enucleation when indicated.

An injured eye can be safely observed for two weeks. After that time, if wound healing is delayed because of incarceration of uveal tissue, or if an intraocular foreign body is present and irritation continues, enucleation usually should be done. Many considerations are involved, such as residual visual function and the overall condition of the eye. Even eyes with severe lacerations to the ciliary body may survive. If this likelihood exists, they should be sutured and given a trial period of two weeks. A wound through the ciliary body perpendicular to the limbus carries a better prognosis than one parallel to the limbus because fewer blood vessels are cut and there is less danger of massive hemorrhage. Intracranial injury and the presence of a foreign body should always be excluded.

CONTUSION

Contusion of the eyeball is a common cause of loss of vision. Blunt injury, directly to the eye or transmitted from the impact of a high velocity fragment, can be devastating. Sudden blunt force to the anterior portion of the eyeball results in tears of the iris, ciliary body, or other ocular structures. Occasionally, rupture of the eyeball itself is seen.

Hemorrhage into the anterior chamber, or hyphemia, resulting from blunt trauma, is serious and quite common. Even a small amount of blood in the anterior chamber immediately after an injury is a grave prognostic sign. Severe bleeding may occur 3 to 5 days later, with persistent elevation of intraocular pressure or profound staining of the cornea with blood pigment. Intraocular pressure may be reduced by diuretics and intravenous urea. If the elevated pressure persists, irrigation with fibrinolysin may be helpful in removing the clot from the anterior chamber.

Other results of blunt trauma to the eyes include traumatic iridocyclitis, dislocation of the lens or rupture of the lens capsule, tearing of choroid with choroidal hemorrhage, and retinal detachment.

CHEMICAL BURNS

Acid burns are less dangerous to the eye than alkali burns which cause the most serious chemical burns. Alkali appears to combine with the tissues, apparently in an active form, causing progressive damage over a long period of time.

Chemicals damage the eye by injuring the eyelids, conjunctiva, and cornea. The extent of the damage depends on the nature of the chemical and the length of time the substance is in contact with the ocular tissues.

Immediate and copious lavage with nonirritating fluid is of paramount importance. Isotonic saline usually is used in hospital emergency departments. Plain tap water or any nonirritating material should be used immediately after the injury. A rubber-bulb irrigating syringe is ideal for flushing conjunctival cul-de-sacs. Lavage should be continuous for 20 to 30 minutes when the patient is first seen and repeated every half-hour. Local and systemic antibiotics should be instituted immediately in an effort to avoid secondary infection. Steroid ophthalmic ointments and solutions may help prevent inflammation and secondary scarring. Atropine may be indicated. The prognosis is always guarded.

The serious sequelae of chemical burns are corneal ulceration accompanied by corneal opacities, necrosis, or perforation. The conjunctiva may develop scar with the development of symblepharon (adhesion of the lids to the eyeball).

Chapter 11

Neck

Injuries to the neck frequently affect the many important structures which traverse the neck longitudinally. These include the spinal column, esophagus, trachea, carotid and jugular vessels, and the vagus nerves. These structures are protected by the heavy neck muscles which are invested with thick fascial envelopes that blend to form a rigid cylinder around the vital structures. However, bleeding underneath the fascia can cause pressure with collapse or obstruction of the trachea or esophagus.

An injury to the neck can directly affect three major systems necessary for life: the respiratory system, the cardiovascular system, and the central nervous system. (Injuries to the central nervous system are discussed in Chapters 8 and 9.) These three systems must be thoroughly examined when the injured patient is being evaluated. First priority should be given to the respiratory system because respiratory obstruction can often be cleared quickly with a minimum of effort. Next in priority is the cardiovascular system, and then the central nervous system.

INJURIES TO THE AIR PASSAGE

Respiratory obstruction may result from aspiration of blood or a foreign body, from direct trauma to the larynx or trachea, from edema resulting from injuries to adjacent structures in the neck or floor of the mouth, from increased pressure in the neck caused by hemorrhage from an artery of any size, or from injury to the recurrent laryngeal nerves.

Injuries to the trachea or larynx, inflicted by blunt objects, may produce life-threatening edema even as late as 48 hours after the injury. Tracheostomy then, may become necessary at any time. Patients with this type of neck injury, if not closely watched by competent attendants, may strangle as a result of edema. The gradual development of hypoxia may be too subtle to be recognized before fatal anoxia sets in. The early signs may be restlessness, occasionally mistakenly attributed to pain, followed by increased activity of the accessory muscles of respiration with inspiratory indrawings of the suprasternal notch, supraclavicular fossa, and epigastrium, followed by cyanosis and respiratory and circulatory arrest. Ideally the patient s condition should be diagnosed in the early stages of restlessness.

The first step is to quickly check the upper airway to the level of the larynx and to manually correct any obstruction. If this fails to relieve the obstruction and if a laryngoscope or bronchoscope and endotracheal tube are available, access to the trachea can be accomplished swiftly in less than a minute or two. If a tracheostomy is needed, an elective tracheostomy is best, but this requires a minimum of 15 to 30 minutes and should be done under good operating conditions. If an immediate access to the trachea is needed and no endotracheal tubes, bronchoscopes, or laryngoscopes are available, then an emergency tracheostomy should be performed.

EMERGENCY TRACHEOSTOMY

If a true emergency tracheostomy is necessary, suction, light, and a few simple instruments along with a knife should be at hand. The patient's head should be slightly extended and held in the midline and the thyroid and cricoid cartilages identified; this brings the cricothyroid membrane into prominence and a quick incision can be made through the skin, subcutaneous tissue, and membrane directly into the lower larynx (Fig. 11-1). This temporary operation can be done in less than a minute with a minimal loss of blood. As soon as the airway is established the patient should be prepared for an elective tracheostomy which should be done as soon as is practical in order to minimize damage to the larynx, particularly to the vocal chords.

ELECTIVE TRACHEOSTOMY

This procedure is done best in an operating room with a complete complement of lights, suction, instruments, and operating table. However, it can be done at the bedside with the patient's head raised, extended, and fixed. Skin preparation should be done and the position of the thyroid cartilage identified. A transverse skin incision should be made at the level of the second or third tracheal ring. After the skin incision, the fascia and muscles should be divided in a longitudinal direction and the thyroid isthmus retracted or divided.

A tracheal hook is extremely useful in grasping the trachea and delivering it into the wound. Many surgeons, particularly those who work a good deal with children, prefer to place stay sutures in the trachea at this time and leave them in for 48 hours or longer to give ready control or

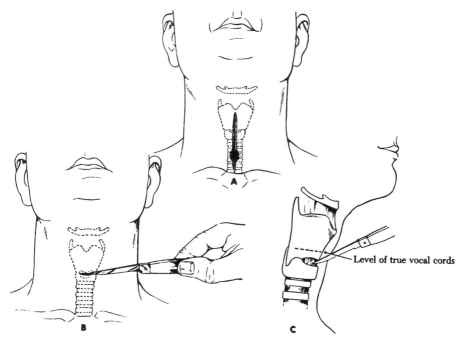

Level of true vocal cords

Figure 11–1 Emergency tracheostomy. *A*, Site of incision and tracheal opening in the usual emergency procedure. *B*, Cricothyroid laryngotomy, anterior view. *C*, Cricothyroid laryngotomy, lateral view.

access to the tracheostomy opening. Small right angle retractors, one for each side of the trachea, are also very useful. Care should be taken to carry the dissection directly over the trachea and not to one side, and to identify and preserve or ligate any vascular structures crossing the trachea. After the cervical fascia is divided most of the dissection, to the level of the trachea itself, can be accomplished bluntly. When the trachea is reached it should be firmly grasped with a tracheal hook or by stay sutures, before it is opened. Arguments exist as to whether a portion of a tracheal ring should be excised or not. If a portion of ring is excised there is less possibility of complete obstruction if a tracheostomy tube slips from the trachea before a fibrous tract is formed, but loss of a portion of ring may increase the incidence of tracheal scarring and posttracheostomy narrowing.

The tracheal rings should be identified and care taken not to place the tracheostomy too high or too low. The most common error, especially in children, is to place the opening too low. If the opening is made between the second and third trachea rings and the third ring is divided, difficulties with low or high placement are avoided.

The tracheostomy tube should be selected carefully. It should fit the trachea snugly, without compressing the side walls and should be of sufficient length to extend into the trachea to the level of the fifth or sixth ring. Most tracheostomy tubes are metal but some excellent tubes of flexible plastic materials have recently been developed. To secure the tube in place it is best to affix a strap to the tube externally and pass it completely around the neck, fastening it with a square knot. Some surgeons also prefer to suture the tube to the skin opening. After the tube is in place, light packing should be placed around it. This can be removed in 24 hours. The tracheostomy tube should not be changed for 48 hours until a fibrous tract has begun to form so that the tube can be easily replaced.

VASCULAR INJURIES

Most of the injuries to blood vessels are the result of trauma caused by sharp instruments or missiles. Occasionally, however, injuries result from blunt trauma. Since the blood flow through the neck is only exceeded by that of the aorta and vena cava injuries to the blood vessels in the neck can be rapidly exsanguinating. The patient may show evidence of massive external hemorrhage or severe respiratory distress or cardiovascular collapse.

First attention must be given to the control of hemorrhage. The best method is to apply direct pressure, compressing the bleeding vessel against the spine. Bleeding from a major vein, such as the jugular, innominate, or subclavian, also exposes the patient to possible air emboli. If this is suspected, the patient should be turned so that he is lying on his left side, to trap the air in the right auricle, while pressure is simultaneously applied. Complete severance of a major artery in the neck—carotid, subclavian, or innominate—will usually exsanguinate the patient within two or three minutes; therefore, most of the patients who arrive at the hospital will be bleeding from a branch of one of these large vessels.

The innominate, subclavian, and internal jugular veins can be safely ligated on one side, and usually the subclavian artery can be safely ligated. The ligation of the innominate or carotid arteries, however, is dangerous and may lead to cerebral ischemia.

Bleeding in the neck should be approached by a wide surgical exposure. Preferably, incisions in the neck should be transverse, but as far as healing is concerned, an incision can be made safely in any direction. It may be necessary to split the sternum or divide the clavicle to expose the vessels at the root of the neck, and occasionally thoracotomy is necessary. If the bleeding is not massive it is preferable to expose the vessel proximally and distally to the suspected point of injury and then attack the bleeding point directly. Laceration of a major vessel should be closed with the technique outlined in Chapter 19.

EMBEDDED FOREIGN BODIES

Patients with perforating wounds, lacerations, and superficially embedded foreign bodies do not warrant immediate roentgenographic studies. However, a penetrating wound with a possible foreign body lodged in the neck warrants roentgenographic study to determine the probable course of the missile, its site of lodgment, and the likely damage resulting therefrom. Two views, anteroposterior and lateral, are taken. They should include the base of the skull and the clavicles. Studies of the skull or chest are made if the direction of the wound indicates that they are needed to enable a complete evaluation of the extent of the injury. It is extremely important to mark the left and right sides correctly on the films. Missiles which enter one side of the neck may lodge on the opposite side and may do more damage at the site of lodgment than on the side of entrance. Thus, surgical care may be more urgent on the side opposite the external wound. Misinterpreting a roentgenogram with regard to the site where a missile is lodged may result in a futile and possibly disastrous effort to improve the condition of the patient.

INJURIES TO THE PHARYNX AND ESOPHAGUS

These injuries may be noted on inspection, or their presence may be suspected because of the course taken by a missile, or they may become obvious when complications develop. Since the pharynx and the esophagus heal readily, the only treatment necessary for a small wound is exposure of the site of the wound, with decompression of the fascial spaces or mediastinum and drainage. In lacerations and perforations of more than a few millimeters the edges of the mucous membrane may be everted, which may lead to the formation of a mucous fistula. Therefore, large rents require suture of the mucous membrane and reinforcement with a supporting tissue in order to prevent persistent leakage of secretions. After necessary care at the site of injury, the skin is closed loosely and a drain is put into the fascial space. Feeding through a nasal catheter is desirable for a period of a few days to a week. In extensive wounds, it may be necessary to do a cervical esophagostomy or a gastrostomy to maintain adequate nutrition. Occasionally, these wounds, particularly floor-of-mouth wounds, become infected with pus developing within the muscle sheath with dissection to the hyoid bone, causing upper airway obstruction. These should be drained externally through a transverse midline incision.

Chapter 12

Chest

GENERAL CONSIDERATIONS

Because of obvious anatomical and physiological conditions, a large number of persons with thoracic injuries die before there is an opportunity to render medical aid. Another group of patients with thoracic injuries survives even if untreated. Others survive for a limited period but succumb unless early and proper treatment is available. In the initial management of thoracic injuries, one is concerned with the correction of conditions which produce disturbances of cardiorespiratory physiology, as well as with the control of hemorrhage and with the prevention of infection. Insufficient aeration of the blood, reduced cardiac output, and death may result from any one or any combination of the following factors:

1. Obstruction of the respiratory passages.

2. Impairment or failure of the neuromuscular-skeletal system of chest wall and diaphragm.

3. Loss of normal negative intrapleural pressure and occupation of the pleural spaces by blood or air.

4. Injuries of the heart or mediastinum and accumulations of blood or air in pericardial sac or mediastinum.

Maintenance of uninterrupted and unimpaired respiratory function is essential and is the ultimate objective of all treatment of thoracic trauma.

SITUATIONS DEMANDING EMERGENCY MEASURES

RESPIRATORY OBSTRUCTION

Assure a pharyngeal airway by clearing the pharynx of blood and mucus and, if necessary, pull out the tongue. In a comatose patient it may be necessary to hold it out with a safety pin and fasten it to the jacket. When possible, a tongue suture taped to the cheek is better.

Relieve laryngeal obstruction by emergency tracheostomy if the situation demands it (Chapter 11, Neck).

OPEN CHEST WOUNDS

Open or so-called sucking wounds of the chest produce profound alterations in intrathoracic physiology (Fig. 12–1). Because of the opening in the chest wall, negative intrapleural pressure is replaced by atmospheric pressure. With inspiration, air is sucked into the pleural space and air is pulled also from the lung of the affected side to the lung of the uninjured side. When the opening is large, the lung completely collapses and the mediastinum shifts to the uninvolved side. It also swings even more to the uninvolved side with inspiration. This collapse of one lung and compression of the other leads to very poor aeration of the blood and to hypoxia. It also leads to reduced return flow of blood to the heart and to reduced cardiac output. Smaller wounds permit less air to enter the pleural cavity with each inspiration and, if occluded promptly, will not lead to such profound changes.

All penetrating injuries of the chest wall should be treated as open, or sucking, wounds until careful inspection or actual debridement proves them to be otherwise. Open wounds must be closed effectively as soon as possible. Simple closure with the palm of the hand may prove lifesaving in a large sucking wound until a more adequate dressing can be applied. As an emergency measure, a simple dressing of gauze securely bound on with adhesive tape is usually adequate. Occasionally, in very large wounds, it may be necessary to suture the dressing to the edges of the wound to maintain it in position. Blood and serum from the wound will quickly soak the dressing and will tend to render it impervious to air. These wounds should not be closed by suture until the patient has been removed to a hospital where facilities for indicated surgery are adequate and until the wound has been debrided.

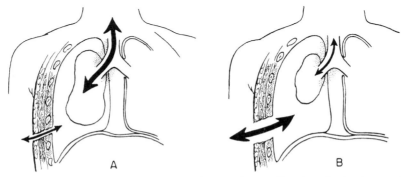

A   B

Figure 12-1 Open pneumothorax. *A,* An opening smaller than the trachea produces relatively little respiratory interference. *B,* An opening larger than the trachea produces gross disturbance of respiratory function. (From Noer, R. J.: The management of acute chest injuries. Postgrad. Med., *23*:A45, April, 1958.)

TENSION PNEUMOTHORAX

Tension pneumothorax occurs when air enters the pleural space with inspiration and cannot escape with expiration through the wound in the trachea, bronchus, lung, or chest wall. This condition is relatively rare as a direct sequel of trauma but it is an emergency when it occurs. The pressure in the pleura increases as the air accumulates, until it completely collapses the lung and pushes the mediastinum to the other side. Death results if the condition is not promptly relieved.

Diagnosis: The diagnosis of tension pneumothorax is based on the physical findings of massive pneumothorax plus positive pressure in the intrapleural space. If a needle attached to a syringe is inserted into the second interspace anteriorly, the plunger will rise in the barrel of the syringe. This pressure can be demonstrated better and can be measured if the needle is attached to a manometer or to the pneumothorax apparatus.

Treatment: The treatment of tension pneumothorax consists in providing an outlet valve for this air under pressure. After emergency aspiration, a catheter should be inserted through the second interspace in the midclavicular line anteriorly (Fig. 12–2). Air should be allowed to pass out through the catheter with expiration but prevented from passing in with inspiration. A flutter valve made of a condom or a large Penrose drain may be used temporarily (Fig. 12–3). The catheter should be attached to a water seal bottle as soon as possible (Fig. 12–4).

Massive hemothorax or pneumothorax occasionally demands emergency aspiration to save life or to render the patient transportable. Management of both conditions will be discussed elsewhere. Aspiration should be accomplished rapidly and the patient should be promptly trans-

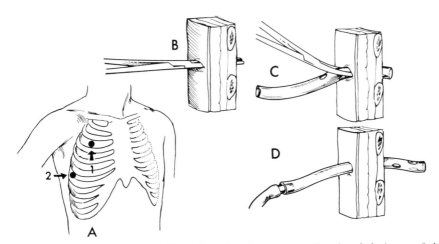

Figure 12–2 Hemostat technique for tube thoracostomy for closed drainage of the chest. *A,* Sites for insertion: upper-anterior for air, lower-lateral for fluid. *B, C, D,* Steps in introduction of the tube. (Modified after Netter, CIBA Clinical Symposia, 1971.)

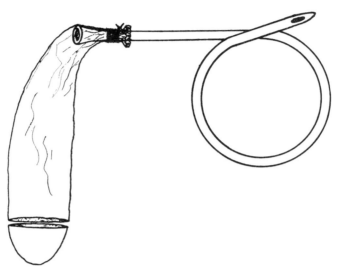

Figure 12-3 Flutter valve made by tying condom to catheter (closed end of condom is cut away). It may be tied to a needle if catheter is not available. In either instance, the condom is placed beneath a dressing on the chest.

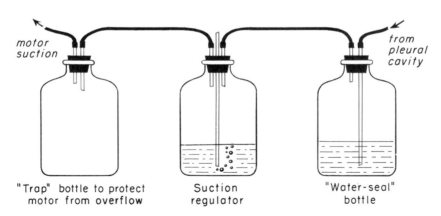

motor
suction

from
pleural
cavity

"Trap" bottle to protect   Suction   "Water-seal"
motor from overflow   regulator   bottle

THREE-BOTTLE SUCTION SET

Figure 12-4 Closed drainage of the chest. From right to left, a water seal bottle may be used alone with catheter drainage of the pleural space by patients' own ventilatory activity; a second bottle may be added for regulated motor suction on the catheter; a third bottle may be added to protect the motor from overflow.

ported to a hospital where facilities for thoracotomy and definitive care are available. Such patients, particularly those with pneumothorax, may suffer from transportation by plane. Unless the flight is at low level or the cabin is pressurized, air in the pleural cavity will tend to expand with increasing altitude.

FLAIL CHEST

With multiple rib fractures, large segments of the chest wall may move paradoxically with respiration, and inadequate pulmonary ventilation may lead to fatal anoxia. Large, mobile segments should be partially stabilized by a pressure dressing consisting of a pad and adhesive strapping and by placing the patient on the injured side. Complicating hemopneumothoraces may require attention. Tracheostomy (see Chapter 11) may be necessary. (For further discussion of the flail chest see p. 140 of this chapter.)

ROUTINE INITIAL MANAGEMENT OF WOUNDS AND INJURIES OF THE CHEST

EXAMINATION OF THE PATIENT WITH A CHEST WOUND OR INJURY

A complete but rapid examination of the patient is always indicated. All clothing should be removed. One must determine not only the extent of the thoracic injuries but also the extent of any concomitant or associated injuries of other parts of the body. The color of the lips and skin, the presence or absence of dyspnea and, if it is present, its degree may be noted as the pulse is palpated and counted and the blood pressure taken. Collapse or distention of the veins of the neck and the upper extremities should be noted. The position of the trachea in the suprasternal notch may be determined by palpation. The symmetry or lack of symmetry in expansion of the chest should be noted. Inspection is likely to be the most neglected part of the examination; much can be learned by a few seconds' observation of the patient's thoracic walls during breathing.

The location of the wounds of entrance and exit should be observed, if possible. The position of the patient at the time the wound or injury was incurred should be ascertained. Inspection, palpation, percussion, and ascultation of the chest should yield information as to the presence or absence of fluid or air in either pleural cavity, fluid in the pericardial sac, widening of the mediastinum, bulging and crepitus in the suprasternal notch indicative of mediastinal emphysema, and any evidence of hemorrhage from wounds of the chest wall or elsewhere. The position of wounds of entrance and exit and the position of the patient at the time he was wounded will frequently determine whether or not there is a possibility of a mediastinal or diaphragmatic injury requiring thoracotomy.

Examination of the abdomen may also be helpful in determining the presence or absence of a thoraco-abdominal wound. Tenderness and rigidity in the abdomen may be secondary to a chest wound. Intercostal nerve block usually relieves the pain and rigidity in such situations; with an intra-abdominal injury, such relief is less pronounced and is likely to be absent.

Rapid examination of the patient and the appraisal of his wounds should enable one to estimate the probable extent of blood loss. Roentgenographic examination of the chest should be made as soon as shock is controlled.

EARLY RESUSCITATIVE MEASURES

As the examination is made, indicated resuscitative measures should be promptly instituted.

1. The wound dressing is inspected and made adequate.

2. The litter is left level except for the dyspneic or cyanotic patient. Unless the blood pressure is below 80, such a patient is more comfortable if the head and chest are elevated.

3. Replacement of blood loss should be started immediately, as discussed in Chapter 3. Autotransfusion of filtered blood obtained by aspiration of hemothoraces is most satisfactory if the blood is not older than 12 hours and if it is not contaminated by contents of the gastrointestinal tract.

4. Intercostal nerve block should be done as soon as possible to relieve pain and promote coughing and clearing of the tracheobronchial tree.

5. If the patient cannot clear his tracheobronchial tree by coughing, endotracheal aspiration by nasotracheal catheter should be carried out. The technique of this procedure will be described in a later section.

6. Hemothoraces and pneumothoraces may be aspirated immediately after intercostal nerve block.

CHEST WALL PAIN AND INTERCOSTAL
NERVE BLOCK

If an opiate has not been administered, a small dose of morphine, 8 to 15 mg in an adult, is given intravenously. When the pain is severe, each of the intercostal nerves of the involved area is injected with 5 ml of 1 per cent procaine or 0.5 per cent Xylocaine, just below the inferior costal margin, posterior to the angle of the rib, with care not to enter the pleura (see Chapter 5). Injection is made two interspaces above and two below the obvious area of injury. With relief of chest wall pain the patient is frequently able to clear the trachea and bronchi of blood and mucus by coughing. This should be encouraged. Adhesive strapping is inadvisable, except when needed for the stabilization of certain flail chest walls.

RESPIRATORY OBSTRUCTION FROM
BLOOD AND MUCUS

Respiratory obstruction due to retention of mucus and blood in the tracheobronchial tree may be caused by:

1. Severe chest wall pain.
2. Abnormal mobility of segments of the chest wall or a ruptured diaphragm.
3. Intrathoracic wounds with accumulations of blood and air in the pleura.
4. Depression of the cough reflex through unconsciousness, or the administration of excessive amounts of opiates.
5. Associated wounds of the neck, jaws, face, or brain.

(It should be remembered that one of the normal responses to chest injury is increased tracheobronchial secretion, and that removal of these added secretions, in addition to blood and material that may have been aspirated, is of paramount importance.)

NASOTRACHEAL CATHETER SUCTION

If intercostal nerve block and coughing do not suffice to clear the tracheobronchial tree, the trachea and main bronchi are aspirated immediately with a nasotracheal catheter (Fig. 12–5). A fairly stiff catheter, 16 to 18 French, is used. The insertion of a glass "Y" between the suction source and the aspirating catheter will give the operator better control of the suction; by raising and lowering his finger from the open end of the "Y," adherence of the catheter to the walls of the tracheobronchial tree can be prevented (Fig. 12–6).

The patient is placed in a sitting or semisitting position with the back supported and the head and neck dorsally extended and the tongue out. The lubricated catheter is passed through the nose into the pharynx without suction. The patient is instructed to take a deep breath, and during inspiration the catheter is passed into the trachea. Success is signified by violent coughing and hoarseness. If the patient gags, this indicates that the catheter is in the esophagus, not in the trachea. Suction is applied intermittently as the catheter is passed into the tracheobronchial tree. It may be passed into the right main bronchus by inclining the head laterally onto the left shoulder. It may be passed into the left bronchus by reversing the maneuver.

ENDOSCOPIC ASPIRATION

The use of a simple direct laryngoscope, of the type used by anesthetists, makes aspiration of the tracheobronchial tree under direct vision easy. These instruments are inexpensive, and can be folded into a small space and made a part of the armamentarium in every physician's bag or office. Their use will frequently permit effective cleaning of the tracheo-

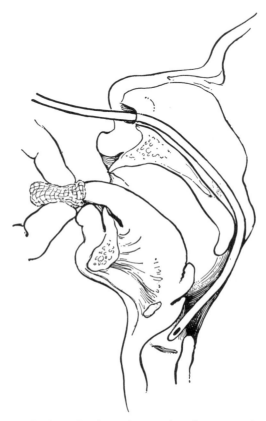

Figure 12–5 Introduction of catheter into trachea for nasotracheal suction. Tongue pulled forward to raise epiglottis, opening passageway for catheter. (From Haight and Ransom: Ann. Surg. 1941, *114*:255. Courtesy of Annals of Surgery.)

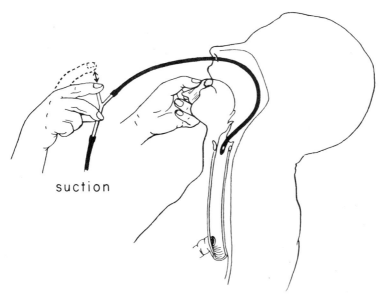

suction

Figure 12-6   Catheter aspiration of the tracheobronchial tree. (From Noer, R. J.: The management of acute chest injuries. Postgrad. Med. *23*:A45, April, 1958.)

bronchial tree in circumstances where "blind" aspiration is ineffective and bronchoscopy not practical.

In some patients, effective aspiration can be accomplished only by means of the bronchoscope.

TRACHEOSTOMY

If relief of chest wall pain, endotracheal catheter aspiration, and bronchoscopic aspiration do not succeed in keeping the tracheobronchial tree free of mucus and blood, a tracheostomy should be performed (see Chapter 11). It is most often necessary for patients in coma, for those with associated maxillofacial wounds, and for those with flail chests. It not only will permit adequate aspiration of blood and mucus, but also will serve to reduce residual or dead air space in the respiratory system.

HEMOTHORAX

Hemothoraces should be aspirated promptly. Aspiration is best accomplished with a 16 gauge needle and a vacuum bottle. If a vacuum bottle is not available, a syringe and a 3 way stopcock may be used instead. The needle is usually inserted in the sixth or seventh interspace in the posterior axillary line.

All blood should be withdrawn from the pleural cavity, the aspiration being interrupted only when the patient complains severely of a tight feeling or pain in the chest. As much as 2000 ml of blood may be aspirated at one time without distressing the patient. There was no evidence during World War II that early aspiration prolongs or brings about recurrence of hemorrhage. The old teaching that aspirated blood should be replaced by air has been abandoned, since it not only does no good, but is actually harmful through delaying re-expansion of the lung. Aspiration of hemothoraces may have to be repeated in a few hours and must be repeated at 24-hour intervals until less than 50 ml of blood are obtained by aspiration.

If blood continues to accumulate after repeated aspiration, institute closed drainage of the chest immediately (see preceding discussion under Tension Pneumothorax and Figs. 12–2 and 12–4).

If blood reaccumulates rapidly, bleeding may be continuing from a partially divided intercostal or internal mammary artery. Continued bleeding from the lung itself is rare because of the low pressure in the pulmonary artery. Continued bleeding rarely comes from a completely divided intercostal vessel, but it is frequent when the intercostal vessel is only partially divided. In such rare cases, **thoracotomy may be indicated to control the hemorrhage.** It should be done if blood in the pleura accumulates very rapidly and if the administration of 500 to 2000 ml of blood leads to only transient improvement or no improvement in the blood pressure.

Occasionally, massive, **clotted hemothorax** is encountered. It usually results from rapid, profuse hemorrhage from the pulmonary vessels, the blood filling the pleura so rapidly that it clots before becoming defibrinated by the respiratory movements. The bleeding soon subsides, and will have stopped by the time the patient is seen, if he survives. The blood cannot be aspirated through a needle; **thoracotomy should be done to evacuate the clot,** if it is large, and to repair the blood vessel if bleeding recurs.

PNEUMOTHORAX

Aspiration of pneumothoraces usually is accomplished best through the second interspace anteriorly in the midclavicular line. The air may be aspirated by vacuum bottle, by syringe and 3-way stopcock, or with the pneumothorax apparatus. All air should be withdrawn. If air tends to reaccumulate after the chest wall wound has been closed, a catheter should be inserted through the second interspace anteriorly and connected with a water seal bottle (Figs. 12–2 and 12–4). If air continues to escape in large quantities, it is probable that there is a wound of the trachea or of a bronchus which will require thoracotomy for closure. Bronchoscopy may establish the diagnosis preoperatively.

WOUNDS OF THE CHEST WALL

Debridement of chest wall wounds is best done under positive pressure anesthesia. An incision is made parallel to the ribs and of sufficient length to expose the entire wound tract down to the pleura. All devitalized tissue is excised. Dirt, foreign bodies, and loose rib fragments are removed. Indriven rib fragments are elevated or removed. In the usual small, penetrating, and perforating wounds, care is exercised not to enlarge the opening in the pleura. Some air nearly always enters this pleural opening, but positive pressure anesthesia reduces the amount. A small catheter attached to a suction machine and inserted through the pleural opening will be of value in evacuating air and blood from the pleura during debridement and during wound closure. The musculofascial tissues should be sutured to provide an airtight closure. The catheter is withdrawn as the last stitch is tied. It is not necessary, and may be impossible, to suture the pleura itself. If the wound has been badly contaminated, the skin should be left open.

Open, or sucking, chest wall wounds should have very thorough debridement. If the wound of the pleura is not small, foreign bodies should be removed from the pleura, and lacerations of the lung which continue to leak air or to bleed should be repaired by suture. A modest enlargement of the chest wall wound may be made to facilitate these procedures and in some instances to repair a wound of the diaphragm, or to survey accurately the intrathoracic damage. Frequently, however, when exploration or intrathoracic surgery is indicated, the chest wall wound should be debrided and closed and a thoracotomy incision should be made. Before the wound is closed, the pleura should be thoroughly irrigated with copious quantities of warm physiological salt solution. A catheter inserted in the sixth or seventh interspace in the posterior axillary line should be connected with a water seal bottle (Fig. 12–4) to care for oozing or exudation which is likely to continue, and to promote early re-expansion of the lung following closure of the thorax. This is particularly important if a laparotomy for abdominal wounds is to follow the thoracotomy. If there is continuing air leak from the lung, insert a catheter in the second interspace anteriorly (Fig. 12–2) and connect it with a water seal. Catheter drainage through the fourth or fifth interspace in the midaxillary line has proved effective for either air or blood.

FRACTURED RIBS AND FLAIL CHEST

Rib fractures are of greater or lesser significance depending upon the degree to which they interfere with respiration. Closed fractures of 1 to 3 ribs usually cause limitation in breathing and coughing due to pain on motion of the thorax. Reference has already been made to the use of intercostal nerve block which helps in the removal of tracheobronchial secretions and permits free thoracic motion unhampered by pain at the site of fractures. Severe crushing injuries of the chest with multiple rib fractures in several places introduces yet another factor which may be of immediate life-threatening proportion. A "floating" segment of the thoracic wall may be produced so that the paradoxical respiration already referred to in the case of pneumothorax can here be produced by another mechanism. The fractured segment moves in and out with respiration, and if the area is of sufficient size, it may critically interfere with aeration of the underlying lung. Stabilization is essential.

The introduction of positive pressure respirators has completely changed the treatment of the "flail chest." A variety of machines are available, any of which, when properly used, will supply an appropriate amount of air under proper pressure synchronous with respiration. Or the machine can be well used to provide the entire ventilatory function. Since full respiratory function can be maintained by one of these machines attached to a tracheostomy tube, the abnormal mobility of the chest wall is no longer of consequence and the patient can be maintained in adequate oxygenation until such time as his thoracic wall stabilizes. Widespread experience with the treatment of flail chest by positive pressure respiration has clearly demonstrated that this method of treatment is superior to any other previously proposed.

There are, however, certain inherent dangers in the use of these machines:

1. A leak at or around the tracheostomy may produce increasing amounts of subcutaneous emphysema.

2. Without adequate pleural decompression when indicated, a tension pneumothorax can be produced. It is essential to use proper closed drainage by tube thoracostomy when indicated (Figs. 12–2 and 12–4).

3. In certain centers there has been a marked increase in staphylococcal and pseudomonas pneumonia subsequent to the use of these machines. Meticulous cleansing of all elements of the machine is most essential, and bacteriologic cleanliness can only be achieved by placing the entire machine in a gas sterilizer. This is a somewhat expensive but practical technique. The cost of prolonged hospitalization of only a few patients for pneumonia that need not have occurred will quickly offset the cost of a gas sterilizer.

Should the positive pressure respirator be unavailable, the floating segment of chest wall can be stabilized by passing a towel clip around the central portion of the flailing segment and applying continuous light traction to the clip. A cord attached to a weight (usually not more than about 5 pounds) can be passed through a pulley on an overhead frame and attached to the towel clip. This allows motion of the chest wall while stabilizing the segment. This was standard therapy before the advent of the positive pressure respirators. Although it is less effective, it is still useful. Minimal amounts of flailing often can be handled simply with a sand bag placed against the segment.

Fractures of the sternum with displacement may require open reduction with steel wire holding the fragments in position.

Oxygen therapy and other supportive measures are necessary for patients with severe thoracic injuries.

CARDIAC INJURIES AND TAMPONADE

Cardiac tamponade most often results from penetrating and perforating wounds of the heart, when blood fills the pericardial sac and either cannot escape or cannot escape as fast as it enters. When it can escape freely into the pleura, the signs and symptoms are those of hemorrhage and hemothorax and not those of tamponade. Cardiac tamponade rarely occurs when a blunt object strikes the chest, as in the steering wheel injury.

DIAGNOSIS

The diagnosis is made upon characteristic physical findings: the veins of the head, neck, and upper extremities are distended, the blood pressure and pulse pressure are low, the pulse rate is comparatively slow, and the heart sounds are faint or absent.

TREATMENT

Aspiration: In patients who survive long enough to reach a hospital, 90 per cent of all cardiac wounds can be managed with pericardiocentesis. **The pericardial sac should be aspirated at once.** This may be done by inserting a 16 gauge needle with a short bevel close to the left sternal border in the fifth interspace, with careful avoidance of the internal mammary vessels.

Many writers feel that it is safer to use the left costoxiphoid route (Fig. 12–7). This procedure requires a needle 10 cm long. The skin should be punctured with a sharp pointed knife 2 cm below the costal border adjacent to the xiphoid. The needle is inserted at an angle of 45 degrees

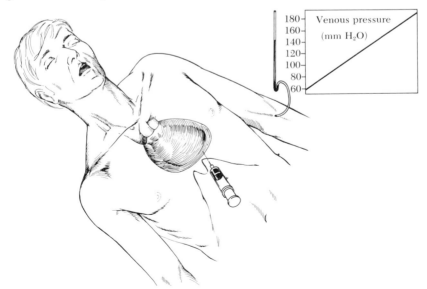

Venous pressure (mm H_2O)

180
160
140
120
100
80
60

Figure 12–7 Cardiac tamponade. Treatment by pericardiocentesis. (Modified after Netter, CIBA Clinical Symposia, 1971.)

to the abdominal wall and is passed upward and backward for 4 or 5 cm or until the point seems to enter a cavity. The plunger is gently withdrawn and, if no blood is obtained, a stylet is inserted to be certain the needle is not plugged. The needle is then carefully passed further until blood is obtained or until cardiac pulsations are felt. The removal of even a few ounces of blood is followed by dramatic improvement. Aspiration will rarely be prevented by the clotting of blood in the pericardial sac. When this does occur, thoracotomy is usually necessary.

If aspiration is successful and there is no recurrence of the signs of tamponade, pericardiotomy will not be necessary. If, after a considerable lapse of time, tamponade recurs, aspiration should be repeated. When tamponade recurs rapidly, immediate pericardiotomy and cardiorrhaphy are indicated.

Surgical Treatment: Wounds of the heart not infrequently require operative attention. The advent of better resuscitative techniques and the availability of blood and blood substitutes have greatly enhanced the likelihood that severe cardiac injuries will reach the operating room alive or amenable to resuscitation upon arrival. Extracorporeal circulation with one of the several pump oxygenators now available is desirable in the repair of critical injuries to the myocardium. Wherever possible it would be desirable for any medical center receiving considerable numbers of critically injured patients to have available a pump oxygenator with a team competent to operate it in an emergency. The latter is essential however. Repair of a critically injured heart is not a suitable place in which to acquire experience with the pump oxygenator. The pressures and demands of the urgent situation may make its operation even more difficult than in the well-planned elective cardiotomy.

Wounds of the heart should be operated upon promptly under the following circumstances:

1. When tamponade cannot be relieved by pericardiocentesis because of clotting of blood within the pericardial sac.

2. When tamponade, owing to failure of the wound to seal off, continues or recurs rapidly.

3. When bleeding continues into the chest cavity or to the outside.

CARDIORRHAPHY: If differential pressure anesthesia is available, a transpleural approach through a long incision in the third or fourth intercostal space anteriorly is preferable. If additional exposure is necessary, the adjacent cartilages may be divided at the sternum. The internal mammary vessels are ligated and the prepericardial areolar tissue and pericardium are incised. The pericardium is opened widely, blood is removed by suction, and the wound in the heart is located. Bleeding is controlled by pressure over the wound with the index finger of the left hand, and a deep traction suture is passed beneath the compressing finger. Slight traction on this suture will largely control bleeding while the approximating sutures are placed and tied. The traction suture is then removed. Cardiorrhaphy is done best with interrupted sutures of medium, No. 3–0 or No. 4–0, silk on a slender, curved needle. Apical traction sutures should be employed only when the wound is difficult to expose. The pericardium is closed with a few widely spaced, interrupted sutures.

In rare instances, the patient with wounds perforating the peri-cardium and heart will survive for a considerable period. In such cases there may be confusion and delay because of the combination of signs of cardiac tamponade and massive hemothorax. This combination indicates a grave prognosis, but, if conditions permit, thoracotomy and cardior-rhaphy should be undertaken immediately. The transpleural approach through a long, posterolateral, intercostal incision can be executed rapidly, and it gives more adequate exposure for repair of the posterior heart wound than does the anterior incision.

Contusion of the heart probably occurs more frequently than is realized; and rupture of one of the cardiac chambers may occasionally occur as the result of heavy blows or crushing force over the precordium. The latter possibility should be kept in mind with steering wheel injuries and other crushing injuries of the chest. Myocardial contusion may be so extensive as to require the same treatment as a fresh coronary occlusion. As in coronary occlusion, changes do not appear on the electrocardiogram until 12 to 24 hours after injury. Extensive surgery or too much activity during this period may be fatal. Such occurrences are rare, but their pos-sibility always should be kept in mind.

Rarely does one see a patient in whom a **foreign body** (missile) is retained in the myocardium or in one of the cardiac chambers. Unless emergency pericardiotomy and cardiorrhaphy must be performed to control cardiac tamponade, the foreign body should not be removed until the patient has been properly prepared and proper facilities for such surgery have been provided.

THORACO-ABDOMINAL WOUNDS

DIAGNOSIS

In every chest wound it is important to rule out the possibility of an abdominal wound. The diagnosis has frequently been overlooked. Study of the location of wounds of entrance and exit is helpful. When either wound is below the level of the fourth anterior rib, diaphragmatic injury should be suspected. The possibility of herniation through a diaphragmatic tear must always be borne in mind. The scout film of the abdomen will usually suffice to make this diagnosis, and should always be obtained if there is any reasonable possibility of severe diaphragmatic injury.

In penetrating wounds, the relation of the wound of entrance to the lodging place of the missile, as demonstrated by roentgenogram, may yield important information. Shock is apt to be more severe in thoracoabdominal injuries than in thoracic injury alone. Abdominal pain, tenderness, and rigidity not relieved by intercostal nerve block are significant. The associated wound is especially dangerous because of the likelihood of bacterial contamination, both of the peritoneum and of the pleura. **Early operation is therefore necessary.**

PREOPERATIVE CARE

Preoperative preparation should include all measures outlined in the section on early resuscitative measures, page 134.

OPERATION

The operation should be performed under endotracheal anesthesia, with a competent anesthesiologist and good facilities for intrathoracic surgery. Most thoraco-abdominal wounds can be approached by thoracotomy or thoracolaparotomy. When the abdominal component of the wound is confined to the upper portion of the abdomen, all of the necessary surgery on the left side can be accomplished through the thoracotomy incision. With a reasonable extension of this incision into the abdominal wall, all of the abdominal contents with the exception of the pelvic colon, a fixed cecum, and perhaps lower descending colon can be dealt with. When laparotomy, in addition to thoracotomy, is necessary the chest should receive care first. Otherwise, a wound in the diaphragm may produce pneumothorax when the abdomen is opened, or the pre-existing thoracic pathology may prejudice life. In right thoraco-abdominal wounds, the diaphragm must be repaired through the thoracotomy incision. Drainage of liver wounds should always be established beneath the diaphragm. When the abdominal part of the wound is confined to the right upper quadrant, necessary surgery may be accomplished by extending the incision into the abdominal wall for a few inches beyond the costal margin.

In the Korean War, Army surgeons preferred to debride and repair the chest wall wounds, to establish intercostal drainage with a large tube or catheter connected to a water seal bottle, and then to repair the abdominal wounds and the diaphragm through the laparotomy incision. Some surgeons report excellent results with this plan of management in civilian thoraco-abdominal wounds. When facilities for positive pressure endotracheal anesthesia are not available, this procedure is certainly the one of choice.

MEDIASTINAL EMPHYSEMA

PATHOGENESIS

Mediastinal emphysema may occur with tension pneumothorax. Such a combination usually indicates a serious underlying injury. Air gains access to the mediastinum through perforation of the esophagus, the trachea, or mediastinal portions of the main stem bronchi. Also, air may dissect along bronchovascular sheaths and gain access to the mediastinum from the lung.

DIAGNOSIS

The diagnosis of mediastinal emphysema is made by hearing the so-called "mediastinal crunch" with the stethoscope and by visualizing the air by roentgenogram. In cases where air dissects up into the base of the neck, distinctive crepitation is easily elicited. When tracheal or bronchial tear is suspected, initial bronchoscopy may establish the diagnosis before thoracotomy does.

TREATMENT

Treatment should be directed toward correction of the underlying lesion. If tension pneumothorax is present, a catheter is inserted into the pleural space through the second interspace anteriorly and is connected to a water seal bottle (Figs. 12–2 and 12–4). If air is present in sufficient quantity to cause labored respirations and circulatory impairment, a collar type of incision should be made at the base of the neck and a finger should be introduced into the superior mediastinum. This permits the ready escape of air. If the air in the mediastinum is the result of laceration of the esophagus, trachea, or main stem bronchus, open thoracotomy and indicated repair are necessary.

ESOPHAGEAL WOUNDS

PATHOGENESIS

Injury of the esophagus may result from missiles or instruments which traverse the mediastinum, from trauma by the esophagoscope, and spontaneously from vomiting.

DIAGNOSIS

Esophageal injury should be suspected in any transmediastinal wound, and suspicion of such an injury is an indication for open thoracotomy. Substernal pain, leukocytosis, and fever following endoscopic examination of the esophagus, or vomiting, particularly after an alcoholic binge, may be the first indication of a perforation of the esophagus. When there has been no injury of the trachea, bronchi, or lung, the demonstration of air in the mediastinum by roentgenogram, particularly when it shows the typical onion peel distribution, is most suggestive of esophageal perforation.

Esophageal perforation may be demonstrated by roentgenography or fluoroscopy after the patient has swallowed Iodochloral or Lipiodol. **Barium must not be used.** Further evidence of perforation may be obtained after the patient has swallowed 5 ml of tincture of methylene blue in 30 ml of sterile water; the blue fluid is then recovered by thoracentesis. This also may help the surgeon locate the injury at operation.

TREATMENT

Treatment is open thoracotomy, opening of the mediastinal pleura, closure of the perforation with two layers of fine, interrupted sutures, and drainage of the pleural space with two intercostal catheters, one in the second interspace anteriorly and one in the sixth or seventh interspace posterolaterally, connected to water seal bottles. Antibiotics should be used intrapleurally and in large doses parenterally.

Chapter 13

Abdomen

GENERAL CONSIDERATIONS

The abdomen is subject to almost every type of injury. Wounds of the abdominal viscera may occur with or without the wounding agent penetrating the abdominal wall. Penetrating wounds may be caused by any missile. Nonpenetrating injuries may occur from blunt force ranging from a bump into a piece of furniture or a blow of the fist to severe crushing injuries, falls, or blast injuries. Even innocent medical procedures can cause abdominal injury; the stomach, rectum and urinary tract may be damaged by diagnostic instrumentation, and any organ may be injured during surgical operation. Fractures of the bony pelvis may be accompanied by injuries to the soft tissues of the pelvis, particularly the bladder and the urethra (see Chapter 14).

When death occurs from wounds of the trunk below the diaphragm the causes are predominantly due to hemorrhage or peritoneal inflammation. Injuries to both solid and hollow viscera occur in both penetrating and nonpenetrating wounds. Injuries from missiles follow the general rules of wound ballistics; that is, very high velocity missiles may have small wounds of entrance, larger wounds of exit, and a disproportionately greater internal disruptive effect than do low velocity missiles.

The first consideration in treating abdominal wounds is to ease pain, combat shock, and dress the wound with a sterile dry dressing to prevent further contamination. Narcotics are to be used only in patients with severe pain, and they should not be used in patients who might require follow-up abdominal examination. Probing or other manipulation of the wound is avoided at this early stage. No efforts should be made to replace prolapsed viscera; it is sufficient to apply a moist dressing.

147

PLAN OF MANAGEMENT

When the patient arrives in the emergency department, his respiratory and circulatory status should be immediately assessed and appropriate corrective measures taken (see Chapters 3 and 5). A nasogastric tube is inserted into the stomach and the contents are aspirated. An indwelling Foley catheter is utilized to follow urinary output as a guide to fluid replacement. If intraperitoneal injury is obvious large doses of intravenous antibiotics should be used.

After the aforementioned supportive measures have been instituted and after a careful physical examination has been completed, if intraperitoneal injury is obvious, or if the patient's condition cannot be stabilized because of continued blood loss, then immediate celiotomy must be performed. If, on the other hand, the patient's condition appears stable and if the diagnosis is not clear, then a course of observation with careful monitoring of the patient and further diagnostic studies is appropriate.

DIAGNOSIS

Penetrating Abdominal Wounds

Penetrating wounds of the abdomen should be divided into groups according to the offending agent (missile vs. stab wound) and whether or not the patient is in shock.

All bullet or missile wounds of the abdomen need exploration despite the absence of shock or any indications of peritonitis. If the wound of entrance is posterior or located in the flank, the retroperitoneal organs (particularly the duodenum and colon) should be examined carefully. Immediate exploration is also mandatory for patients with stab wounds of the abdomen and obvious signs of blood loss or peritonitis. Diagnostic studies, other than physical examination (including digital palpation of the rectum and insertion of a nasogastric tube and a Foley catheter) should be limited.

Roentgenograms of the abdomen and the chest will help locate the path of a missile and demonstrate associated thoracic injury. Roentgenograms, however, should be obtained only if the patient appears stable after initial resuscitative care.

Stab wounds of the chest which are located at or below the level of the fifth intercostal space and which penetrate the ribs should arouse suspicion of possible intra-abdominal injury. If a diaphragmatic injury is suspected, tubes for closed thoracic drainage should be inserted before the abdomen is opened in order to avoid tension pneumothorax and death under anesthesia.

Most stab wounds of the abdomen should be explored. Those without signs of blood loss and obvious intraperitoneal injury present difficult problems. If the peritoneal cavity has been entered, operation is indicated. The wound should be carefully inspected to determine the extent and direction of the injury. Probing the wound is frowned upon. An acceptable diagnostic method is thorough exploration of the wound under local anesthesia with all preparations made for laparotomy if perforation of the peritoneal cavity is found.

NONPENETRATING WOUNDS

In contrast to penetrating wounds, diagnosing nonpenetrating wounds of the abdominal viscera may be difficult. A period of observation frequently is necessary to permit diagnostic signs to develop.

A good history of the injury is important, but this frequently is not available in cases of alcoholism, shock, and unconsciousness. Numerous pertinent physical signs may be present and should be looked for:

Peritoneal irritation and internal hemorrhage and contusions and abrasions of the abdominal wall are significant.

Fractures of the lower third of the chest frequently are accompanied by subdiaphragmatic injury. Pain in the shoulder indicates lesions below the diaphragm.

Peristalsis may be absent. Nausea and vomiting may occur. Abdominal distention and localized tenderness may be present.

Paradoxic respiratory motion in the abdomen may be present with rupture of the diaphragm or flail chest. Peristaltic sounds in the chest may indicate a rupture of the diaphragm with abdominal viscera in the chest.

Blood may be present in the vomitus, stool, or urine.

Four-quadrant paracentesis can be an important diagnostic measure (Fig. 13-1). This may be of particular value in the unconscious patient who is unable to show signs of peritoneal irritation. In the female a culdocentesis may be performed. The aspiration should be performed in all four quadrants of the abdomen with a short bevel 18-gauge spinal needle. The rectus muscles should be avoided because of the possibility of lacerating the inferior epigastric artery. A peritoneal tap is diagnostic even when it yields only 1 ml of blood or fluid. *Negative aspirations do not, however, rule out visceral damage.* Repeated examinations at 2- to 4-hour intervals may yield significant findings.

Peritoneal lavage is another technique that some consider helpful in the diagnosis of blunt abdominal trauma. After the bladder has been emptied, a dialysis tube is inserted through the lower midline of the abdomen under local anesthesia. Care should be taken to avoid bleeders in the subcutaneous tissues.

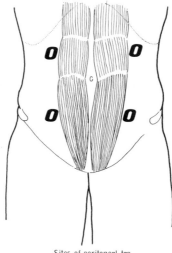

Sites of peritoneal tap

Figure 13–1 Potential sites of peritoneal tap. If one chooses to do a peritoneal tap it is wise to do it in four quadrants of the abdomen. The marked sites point out that the best places to insert the needle are just lateral to the rectus muscles.

If aspiration reveals no gross blood or fluid, 1000 ml of lactated Ringer's solution (300 to 500 ml in children) is infused into the abdomen. The bottle is lowered to create a siphon effect and the fluid is collected. The color of the returning fluid is significant. As little as 75 ml of blood will color the perfusate salmon pink.

One should examine the fluid for white blood cells, bacteria, and fecal content. An elevated amylase suggests pancreatic injury or perforation of the duodenum or the small bowel. In the latter situation the fluid may contain intestinal contents.

Roentgenographic examination may disclose the presence of free air or fluid, immobility of the diaphragm on the affected side, displacement of hollow viscera, or obliteration of the renal and psoas shadows. Retroperitoneal emphysema may be present in injuries of the duodenum or of the extraperitoneal rectum. A negative roentgenogram does not rule out an intra-abdominal lesion.

In some instances evidence of intraperitoneal injury may not be apparent for many hours or even days after the injury. In rupture of the small bowel, with minimal hemorrhage and soiling, the onset of bacterial peritonitis may be the first sign. A similar situation occurs with injury to the mesenteric blood vessels; signs of necrosis of the bowel may not appear for several days and paralytic ileus may be the first evidence.

Delayed rupture of the spleen may occur 2 weeks or even longer after the accident. It usually is due either to early plugging of the splenic wound by blood clot or omentum, with late autolysis, or to subcapsular hemorrhage which may not be evident until the capsule suddenly ruptures from internal pressure.

Repeated examinations are essential in all cases of suspected nonpenetrating injury.

OPERATIVE TREATMENT

INCISION

Since abdominal wounds require thorough exploration, the initial incision should be one that can be extended to any portion of the abdomen. A midline vertical incision is the most useful; it may be extended upward, downward, or laterally. It can be made more rapidly than most other incisions and closure usually is fast and solid.

As soon as the peritoneal cavity has been opened blood should be removed by the most expeditious means. Any major bleeding points should be searched for quickly. If there is serious abdominal hemorrhage one should look for injury to the larger blood vessels. The small intestines should be eviscerated rapidly and adequate exposure obtained to identify easily the bleeding points. Most operative deaths occur because of delay in controlling hemorrhage. The ideal approach is to quickly open the abdomen, find the bleeding area, and arrest the hemorrhage. Then time can be taken to obtain good exposure and to transfuse the patient so that he can withstand further blood loss that may be encountered as the bleeding point is being repaired. Major injuries to the superior portion of the liver require thoracoabdominal incision.

After the hemorrhage is controlled, the liver, spleen, biliary tree, and retroperitoneum are systematically examined along with the intestinal tract. Particular attention is paid to the posterior surface of the stomach and the duodenum as well as the retroperitoneal colon.

SPLEEN

The spleen is the intra-abdominal organ most frequently injured by blunt trauma. Splenic injury often is associated with rib fractures on the left. Penetrating injuries of the left thorax should also arouse suspicion. The clinical features of splenic injury include signs of blood loss, abdominal pain in the left upper quadrant, and pain in the left shoulder. The white blood cell count is often markedly elevated (20,000 to 30,000 per cu mm) after splenic injury. Roentgenographic findings include an increased density in the left upper quadrant, obliteration of the left renal and psoas shadows, and an elevated left hemidiaphragm. Displacement of the stomach bubble and downward displacement of the colon are often seen.

It is difficult to diagnose slow or delayed hemorrhage with subcapsular hematoma. Eventually the condition manifests itself, in some cases, days to weeks after the injury. A falling hematocrit associated with left upper quadrant pain and possible shoulder pain should make one suspicious. An IVP and upper GI series may show displacement of the stomach and kidneys. The treatment for splenic injury is splenectomy. Drains usually are not necessary unless there is evidence of oozing or associated pancreatic injury.

LIVER

Injuries to the liver, like those of the spleen, are most often associated with blunt trauma to the abdomen and lower thorax but usually on the right side. Injuries of sufficient force to lacerate the liver often are associated with injuries to other organs. Pain usually is localized to the right upper quadrant.

Hemostasis is a major problem in hepatic injuries. Most wounds should be treated conservatively. Small wounds and perforations, that are not bleeding at the time, should be treated by drainage alone. Hemorrhage, associated with large lacerations, requires suture control with large chromic catgut on atraumatic needles. Horizontal mattress sutures often will suffice. Packing the wounds with Gelfoam and other such hemostatic agents should be avoided if possible. These materials, along with other foreign bodies, present a nidus for infection. Partial and temporary hemostatic control may be obtained by manual compression of the portal vein and hepatic artery at the foramen of Winslow. Hepatic blood flow cannot, however, be interrupted for more than 15 minutes at a time. Temporary gauze packing may aid in stopping hemorrhage. Some surgeons use gauze packs when all other hemostatic methods fail, but the incidence of infection and rebleeding when these packs are removed is great. Therefore, many surgeons are turning to partial and often complete resection of the lobe of the liver when faced with persistent hemorrhage.

All severe liver trauma requires T-tube decompression of the common bile duct. Hemobilia is detected very early with T-tube drainage. This complication can occur from days to weeks after liver injury and is almost always associated with intrahepatic abscess. In all severe hepatic trauma, the possibility of associated injuries to the diaphragm and thorax must be kept in mind.

External drainage with Penrose and sump drains is necessary to prevent bile from collecting.

BILE DUCTS

Blood or bile in the subhepatic space at celiotomy suggests injury to the structures in the hepatoduodenal ligament and requires thorough

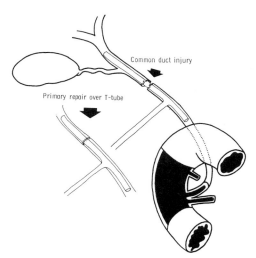

Figure 13-2 Technique for repair of common duct injury. A T-tube is inserted into the common duct at a site away from the injured area. The injured area is then sutured over the arm of the T-tube.

exploration of the hepatic artery, portal vein, and extrahepatic biliary tree. Unrecognized biliary injury can lead to bile peritonitis and its attendant problems. Bile staining without an obvious source of injury requires operative cholangiograms. Vascular injuries in the hepatoduodenal ligament should be repaired primarily. One should attempt to salvage the hepatic artery at all costs, even if a saphenous vein graft has to be employed. If hepatic artery reconstruction fails, the vessel must be ligated. In this situation large doses of antibiotics and a stable postoperative blood pressure are prerequisites for survival.

Injuries to the cystic duct and gallbladder are treated by cholecystectomy. Wounds of the hepatic or common duct are sutured carefully over one arm of a T-tube inserted in the common duct through an incision above or below the wound. Complete transection of the common bile duct may be repaired by end-to-end anastomosis over a T-tube with interrupted sutures (Fig. 13-2). Often repair or anastomosis is impossible due to extensive loss of tissue. Cholecystoenterostomy or choledochoenterostomy must then be employed. The anastomoses should always be drained thoroughly since the incidence of leakage is high.

PANCREAS

Primarily because of an increased number of automobile accidents, upper abdominal trauma and associated pancreatic injury are being seen with increasing frequency. An elevated serum amylase suggests pancreatic

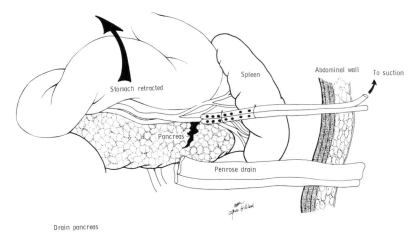

Drain pancreas

Figure 13–3 All injuries of the pancreas should be drained. Two drains are desirable: (1) a Penrose and (2) a sump. These should be inserted through two stab wound sites in the lateral abdominal wall.

injury and in itself is an indication for celiotomy. Later, a persistently elevated amylase suggests pseudocyst formation. Isolated pancreatic injury is uncommon because of its anatomic location. It often is associated with trauma to other organs, namely the stomach, duodenum, and liver and to major blood vessels in the area of the portal vein, vena cava, and the superior and inferior mesenteric arteries and veins.

The two principles of treatment are hemostasis and drainage. The pancreas can be explored thoroughly by inspecting the body and the tail through the lesser sac; the head of the pancreas can be evaluated by reflecting the right colon and mobilizing the retroperitoneal duodenum. Hemostasis in the pancreatic substance should be obtained with figure-of-8 nonabsorbable sutures. Simple wounds are treated with sump drainage for at least two weeks (Fig. 13–3). Extensive injuries to the body and tail of the pancreas can be handled satisfactorily by distal pancreatectomy and splenectomy. If the pancreas has been transected at its neck, this injury has been treated successfully by suturing both ends of the pancreas into the side of a Roux-en-Y loop of jejunum. This obviates attempts at pancreatic duct reconstruction which have been notoriously unsuccessful. Severe injuries to the head of the pancreas accompanied by injuries to the duodenum and biliary tree should be treated with a pancreaticoduodenectomy. A hallmark of surgical treatment of the pancreas is adequate long-term drainage.

STOMACH

In most injuries of the stomach, blood is present in the nasogastric aspirate. All defects are managed by two-layer closure. It is important to look for and repair wounds of the posterior gastric wall. Wounds of the cardiac end of the stomach may require a thoracoabdominal incision, although they often can be exposed and treated by dividing the triangular ligament of the left lobe of the liver.

SMALL INTESTINE

Injuries to the duodenum are often the result of stab wounds or crushing injuries associated with blunt abdominal trauma. These wounds frequently are associated with injury to the pancreas, bile ducts, and vena cava. In blunt abdominal trauma the injury may not be apparent for 12 to 18 hours. Abdominal roentgenograms may show retroperitoneal air, and a Gastrografin swallow may demonstrate perforation of the duodenum. Retroperitoneal hematoma and bile staining in the area of the duodenum make it mandatory to mobilize the duodenum extensively for adequate exposure of its posterior surface and adjacent structures.

Small clean wounds may be treated with simple closure accompanied by nasogastric suction. Severe wounds in the first portion of the duodenum may be treated by Billroth II distal gastrectomy with the injured portion of the duodenum being resected along with the distal stomach. Wounds in the fourth part of the duodenum may be resected in conjunction with direct end-to-end or end-to-side anastomosis with a loop of jejunum.

Severe wounds in the second and third portions of the duodenum and concomitant pancreatic injury present the surgeon with an extremely difficult problem in management. Primary closure frequently is followed by fistula formation. If associated pancreatic injury is not severe, the laceration should be closed and gastroenterostomy with a decompressive duodenostomy should be done. If the wound is massive and associated with pancreatic and biliary tract injury, a pancreaticoduodenectomy is the treatment of choice.

In all duodenal injuries the area must be drained adequately and the gastrointestinal tract decompressed by a nasogastric tube or gastrostomy. Feeding jejunostomy should be considered if a fistula develops or if the patient has to be maintained without oral alimentation for several weeks.

Intramural hematoma of the duodenum should be suspected in patients who develop obstruction after an episode of blunt abdominal trauma. Roentgenograms may demonstrate a "coiled spring" appearance of the second and third portions of the duodenum. Treatment consists of incising the seromuscular coat, evacuating the hematoma, and decompressing by tube duodenostomy.

The small intestine is injured most frequently as a result of penetrating wounds of the abdomen. Surgical treatment involves closure of the holes or resection with anastomosis when the damage is extensive. In the case of missile wounds an even number of holes must be counted unless a tangential wound can be demonstrated. It is often difficult to visualize a perforation on the mesenteric side of the small intestine. With small bowel injuries copious peritoneal irrigation and the administration of antibiotics parenterally are adjunctive measures.

LARGE INTESTINE

Wounds of the colon are less frequent but more serious than wounds of the small bowel. In simple lacerations and small wounds produced by low velocity missiles, the treatment consists of careful debridement and an inverting double-layer closure (Fig. 13-4). Major damage to the bowel is best treated by exteriorization or primary closure with proximal colostomy (Fig. 13-5).

Exteriorization of a defect in the right colon should be avoided; these wounds, along with extensive injuries to the cecum, should be treated by right colectomy and ileocolostomy. Ileostomy should be avoided if at all possible.

Exteriorization is reserved for wounds of the transverse and left colon in which primary repair or resection seems unwise. When the terminal

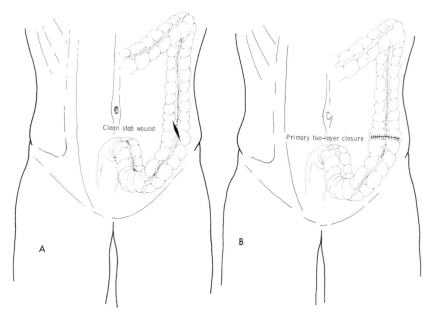

Figure 13-4 Although extensive wounds of the colon should be treated by exteriorization, certain clean stab wounds (*A*) in civilian practice are best handled with a primary two-layer closure (*B*).

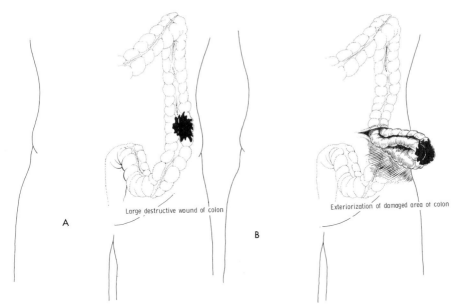

Figure 13–5 In large, dirty or destructive wounds of the transverse, descending and sigmoid colon (*A*) the best method of treatment is exteriorization of the damaged portion of colon as a loop colostomy (*B*). This should be performed through a stab wound separate from the abdominal incision.

colon is too short to be exteriorized onto the abdominal wall following resection of the distal left colon, it may be closed and left in the peritoneal cavity. The proximal colon then is used for colostomy. When a colostomy is made it should be brought out through a separate incision, never through the site of injury or operative incision. As in small bowel injuries, extensive irrigation with saline is indicated. Systemic antibiotics are essential. In the contaminated abdomen one should drain the areas of extensive retroperitoneal damage often seen with injuries to the colon.

RECTUM

Wounds of the extraperitoneal rectum should be repaired and a proximal diverting colostomy should be performed. Drainage of this area by a presacral route is mandatory. This can be accomplished through an incision anterior to the tip of the coccyx through the fascia propria (Fig. 13-6). In wounds of the anorectum, the sphincter muscles should be repaired and wide drainage established. Extensive perineal wounds require a diverting colostomy.

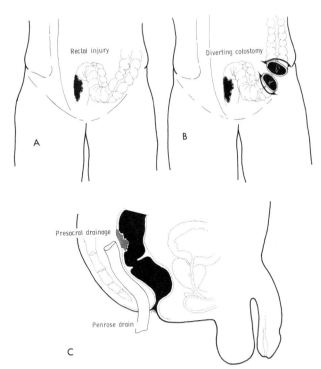

Figure 13-6 Wounds of the rectum (*A*) are particularly dangerous unless they are managed appropriately. The fecal stream must be kept away from the wound by a diverting separate stoma colostomy done preferably in the sigmoidal region (*B*). It is mandatory that the presacral area be drained. This is best accomplished by use of a Penrose drain inserted just anterior to the tip of the coccyx (*C*) through the fascia propria.

CLOSURE OF THE ABDOMEN

Before closure of the incision there should be careful inspection to make sure that no continuing hemorrhage is present. All foreign bodies, tissue fragments, and blood clots should be removed. The abdomen should be irrigated thoroughly with large quantities of saline. Some surgeons prefer the use of an antibiotic solution for irrigation.

Celiotomy wounds should be closed in layers and also with through-and-through stay sutures, since these wounds have a high incidence of dehiscence. In some instances, through-and-through closure alone with heavy suture material may be more prudent. Through-and-through sutures should be left in situ for about three weeks. In cases of extensive loss of substance from the musculofascial structures of the abdominal wall, closure may be accomplished by mobilization of the skin and by suturing only the skin, leaving the hernia to be repaired at a later date. If there is appreciable tissue damage around the wounds of entrance and exit, these areas should be debrided.

POSTOPERATIVE CARE

Detailed postoperative care is essential to the successful management of abdominal wounds. The temperature, pulse, respiration, and blood pressure should be checked at regular intervals.

Deep breathing exercises are encouraged to prevent atelectasis. Leg exercises are employed to prevent deep venous thrombosis. The patient is turned frequently from side to side to prevent pulmonary complications. As peristalsis returns, the nasogastric tube should be clamped periodically to determine when nasogastric suction can be discontinued safely.

Usually there is an appreciable loss of fluid into the peritoneal cavity, the lumen, and the wall of the bowel. This hidden sequestration of a large volume of fluid into the interstitial space requires replacement. Adequate quantities of lactated Ringer's solution should be administered in addition to the other daily fluid requirements. Blood should be given when indicated.

An indwelling urethral catheter serves as an adjunct to accurate measurement of hourly urinary output This assists in replacement of fluid. In most instances, parenteral antibiotic therapy is continued for at least five days after operation. A combination of penicillin and streptomycin has been the regimen of choice. If this proves ineffective, a broad spectrum antibiotic is indicated. Early ambulation is encouraged.

Chapter 14

Genitourinary Tract

Successful repair of injuries to the genitourinary tract is dependent upon early diagnosis, since the success rate of primary repair is markedly decreased with the passage of time and the extent of urinary extravasation and abscess formation.

WHAT PATIENTS SHOULD BE SUSPECTED OF HAVING GENITOURINARY INJURY?

Any patient who receives blunt trauma to the perineum, genitalia, abdomen, back, or flank, and who evidences hematuria of any degree, decreasing urinary output, unexplained abdominal tenderness, mass, or paralytic ileus, should be suspected of having injury to the genitourinary tract.

Any patient with a penetrating wound of the abdomen, flank, genitalia, or pelvis must be considered as having a genitourinary tract injury until otherwise indicated, whether or not there is hematuria.

Any pedestrian who has been struck by a motor vehicle may have genitourinary injury regardless of physical or laboratory findings, because of the extremely high incidence of urinary and renovascular injury in this type of accident.

Any patient who has unexplained edema of the lower abdomen or genitalia should be suspected of having genitourinary injury.

INJURIES TO THE KIDNEY

The kidney is most often injured by blunt trauma to the upper abdomen or posterior chest. Injuries to the renal artery with resultant subintimal dissection and thrombosis most often result from contrecoup damage in auto-pedestrian accidents.

DIAGNOSIS

EXCRETORY UROGRAM

Indications: The following may be considered as indications of kidney injury:

(1) blunt abdominal trauma with any degree of hematuria or history of hematuria; (2) auto-pedestrian injury; (3) unexplained ileus or abdominal pain; (4) all penetrating abdominal wounds; (5) fracture of the lower ribs or the transverse processes of the lumbar vertebrae; and (6) flank mass or costovertebral angle tenderness.

Technique: High-dose infusion technique (1 ml of contrast medium per pound of body weight) should be used because of decreased excretion during or after shock. When available, tomography should be used routinely with the infusion intravenous pyelogram to demonstrate parenchymal lacerations of the kidney that might not be apparent on the conventional radiograph.

Findings (Fig. 14–1): The following findings are important in the diagnosis of kidney injury:

(1) negative shadow within parenchyma or tomography indicating parenchymal laceration, (2) extravasation of the contrast medium; (3) obliteration of the psoas shadow; (4) lumbar scoliosis away from the injured kidney.

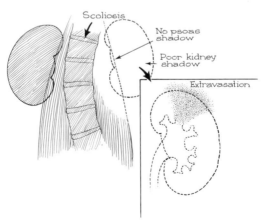

Figure 14–1 Positive findings on excretory urogram indicative of renal injury: absence of the psoas shadow, absence or diminishment of the renal shadow, lumbar scoliosis away from the site of injury, and extravasation of contrast medium.

RETROGRADE PYELOGRAMS

Retrograde pyelograms are very useful in delineating injury to the collecting system but they are less accurate than excretory tomography or renal angiography in demonstrating parenchymal injury. While retrograde pyelograms have been unpopular in the past, they are useful adjuncts and should be made without hesitation when clearly indicated.

RENAL ANGIOGRAPHY

Indications: Renal angiography should be considered when there is (1) inadequate parenchymal delineation with nephrotomography, or (2) a suspicion of renal arterial injury (failure of excretion on excretory study). Unilateral traumatic thrombosis of the renal artery will be discovered only if angiography is used routinely when the kidney does not excrete contrast medium on an excretory study. Early diagnosis is of paramount importance.

Technique: The transfemoral route is preferred because better pictures can be obtained and the injured patient does not have to be moved and manipulated. A "flush shot" of the aorta to delineate the celiac axis outflow should be obtained, as this may demonstrate injury to the liver or spleen. In addition, all accessory renal vessels can be identified, making any subsequent operation easier. A selective renal arteriogram can then be done if needed.

Findings: Positive findings of intimal thrombosis, vascular disruption, and parenchymal laceration are demonstrated in Figure 14-2.

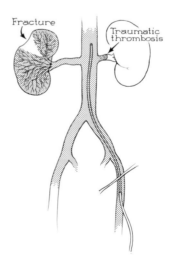

Figure 14-2 Diagrammatic representation of positive angiographic findings in renal trauma. *Right:* triangular filling defect indicative of renal parenchymal laceration. *Left:* traumatic thrombosis secondary to intimal laceration of the left renal artery.

TREATMENT

Preliminary resuscitation and supportive therapy are detailed in the chapter dealing with shock.

SURGICAL TREATMENT

Indications: (1) **Penetrating renal injuries** generally call for surgical treatment since about 85 per cent are associated with significant injury to the intraperitoneal viscera.

(2) **Nonpenetrating injuries** may also require surgical treatment. In past years there was a justified hesitancy to explore patients with nonpenetrating injuries of the kidney because techniques in hemorrhage control had not been perfected. At the present time hemorrhage can be controlled, and the need to remove a kidney solely for the control of hemorrhage rarely occurs. A number of kidneys will, of course, have to be removed because the extent of the renal injury precludes healing and a functioning organ.

Exploration of the injured kidney is a safe procedure and should be carried out without hesitation when indicated. This is especially true when there is involvement of major intrarenal vessels or when the collecting system is involved. Such injuries usually will be manifested by one or a combination of the following signs: (a) a period of hypotension; (b) flank mass or tenderness; (c) evidence of significant hemorrhage or disruption of parenchyma on the angiogram or nephrotomogram; (d) occlusion of the renal artery on the arteriogram; (e) significant extravasation on the

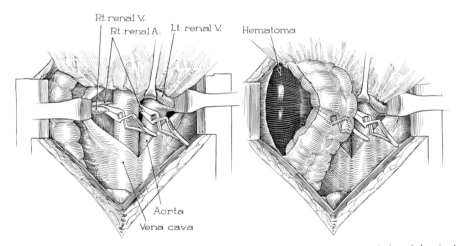

Figure 14–3 Surgical approach to the injured kidney. Exposure of the abdominal aorta and left renal vein through an incision in the posterior parietal peritoneum. Application of noncrushing vascular clamps to the appropriate renal artery and vein. Mobilization of the injured kidney and release of the perirenal tamponade only after vascular control.

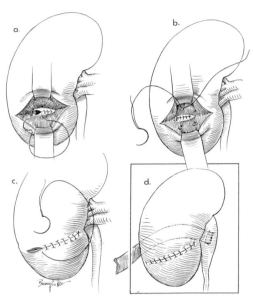

Figure 14–4 Technique of repair of simple renal laceration. *a*, Water-tight closure of the collecting system following adequate debridement of injured tissue. *b*, Suture ligation of all visible bleeding vessels. *c*, Reapproximation of the renal cortex and capsule. *d*, Penrose drain pyelostomy, or evacuation of blood clots where there has been extensive hematuria.

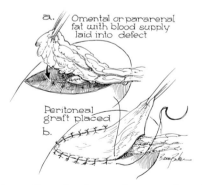

Figure 14–5 Technique of repair of extensive parenchymal defects where primary closure is not feasible. *a*, Placement of live fat to obliterate dead space. *b*, Re-establishment of capsular integrity with a free graft of peritoneum.

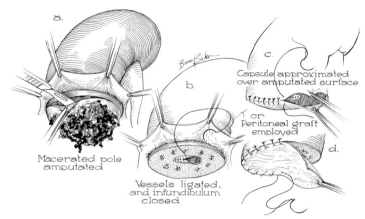

Figure 14–6 Surgical technique for treatment of extensive renal polar injury. *a*, Guillotine amputation of injured tissue. *b*, Suture hemostasis and primary closure of collecting system. *c*, and *d*, Alternate methods of re-establishing capsular integrity.

IVP; (f) evidence of extrarenal collection of blood or urine on the IVP or KUB.

Technique: See Figures 14-3 to 14-6.

NONOPERATIVE TREATMENT

Indications: Minor cortical lacerations and renal contusions not associated with significant bleeding can be treated nonsurgically.

Regimen: (1) Strict **bed rest** for a minimum of 10 days to decrease the possibility of secondary hemorrhage.

(2) **Antibiotics** to prevent infection of the perirenal hematoma with formation of a perinephric abscess.

(3) **Observations** for some of the following signs predicting failure of conservative treatment: (a) temperature elevation—signs of perirenal infection; (b) secondary hemorrhage (expanding flank mass, anemia, tachycardia); (c) IVP prior to discharge; (d) hypertension of renal origin secondary to perirenal fibrosis or vascular injury, resulting in renal ischemia (patient must be watched for several weeks).

INJURY TO THE URETERS

Ureteral injuries of surgical etiology are decreasing as surgical proficiency increases. Ureteral injuries secondary to external violence, however, are increasing parallel to the overall increase in incidence of body trauma and are manifested usually as intraperitoneal irritation. The ureters may be injured by penetration of a foreign body or occasionally avulsed by the contrecoup effect.

DIAGNOSIS

Extravasation when seen on an excretory urogram is suggestive. However, ureteral injury can be present even though the IVP is normal. If the IVP is normal and ureteral injury is suspected, retrograde or bulb pyelogram should be made.

TREATMENT

See Figures 14-7 and 14-8.

INJURIES TO THE BLADDER AND PROSTATIC URETHRA

The **bladder** in its empty or near-empty state is located deep in the bony pelvis and is resistant to injury. The distended bladder, however, is easily ruptured, most commonly from striking a steering wheel during deceleration in an auto accident (Fig. 14-9). Injury to the **prostatic urethra,** almost invariably, is caused by the shearing effect at the rigid attachment of the apex of the prostate to the membranous urethra, in association with fracture of the bony pelvis. Rarely, this injury may result from severe straddle trauma (Fig. 14–10).

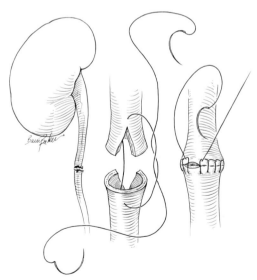

Figure 14-7　Technique of repair of injured ureter. Spatulation of opposing surfaces of the ureter after debridement of injured tissue. Meticulous water-tight closure of the ureter employing 5–0 chromic catgut.

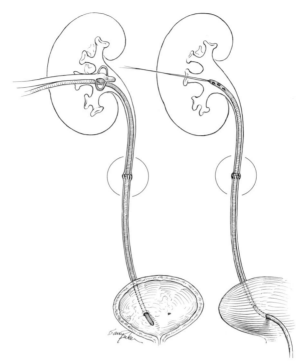

Figure 14-8   Alternate techniques of placement of splinting ureteral catheters where ureteral tension, infection, or other factors might result in failure of primary healing.

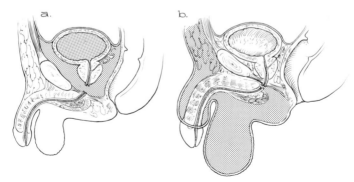

Figure 14-9   *a*, Typical location of hematoma and urinary extravasation in injuries to the extraperitoneal portion of the bladder or prostatic urethra. *b*, Typical route of urinary extravasation and blood collection with injury to the urethra distal to the urogenital diaphragm.

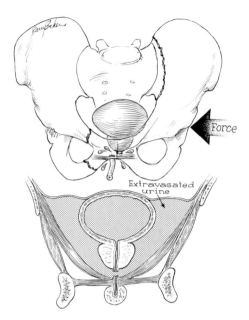

Figure 14–10   Typical mechanism of injury to the urethra at the junction of the prostatic apex and the membranous urethra. Note the shearing force applied to the urethra as the pelvic girdle is fractured.

DIAGNOSIS

PHYSICAL EXAMINATION

Ruptured Bladder: A board-like rigidity of the abdomen with hypotension and an inability to urinate are frequently seen in this condition.

Prostatic Urethra: There are signs of a ruptured bladder plus fluctuance in the area of the prostate on rectal examination, due to a collec-

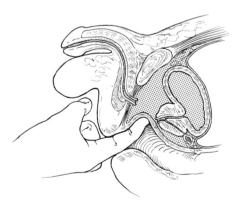

Figure 14–11   Rectal-digital findings with complete laceration of the prostatic urethra: striking absence of the prostate to palpation and balloon-like consistency of the pelvic hematoma.

tion of blood or urine in this area. With complete severance of the prostatic urethra, there is striking absence or displacement of the prostate on rectal palpation (Fig. 14–11).

RADIOGRAPHIC STUDY

The two most important radiographic studies are the retrograde urethrogram and the retrograde cystogram. Too often, adequate delineation of the urethra is missed because of the hasty insertion of a urethral catheter which may bypass a significant urethral laceration. In trained hands, the retrograde urethrogram is an innocuous and easily performed study and should be carried out whenever vesical or urethral injury is even slightly suspected. This study is obtained by placing the patient in the oblique position on the x-ray table and gently and slowly inserting into the urethral meatus 30 ml of viscous contrast medium (Fig. 14-12). Regular intravenous medium serves this purpose well.

If retrograde urethrography reveals no intrinsic injury, vesical injury can be evaluated by means of retrograde cystography. The patient's meatus is prepared with a suitable antiseptic solution and the penis is isolated by sterile drapes. A No. 14 or 16 Foley catheter is introduced with sterile forceps or with sterile gloves (Fig. 14-13). It is important that the catheter not be forced, and it must be remembered that if there is prostatic,

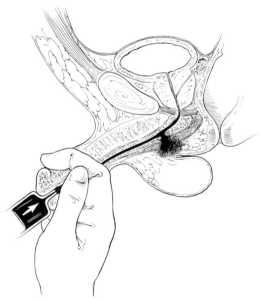

Figure 14–12   The technique of retrograde urethrography. The tip of a large syringe is impacted into the urethral meatus and viscous contrast medium injected in a retrograde manner.

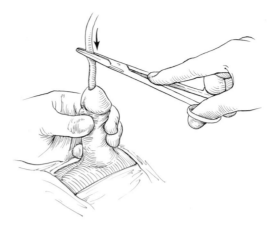

Figure 14-13 Technique of sterile catheterization. After thorough preparation and draping of the genitalia, a catheter is introduced with a sterile forceps.

urethral, or vesical laceration the catheter may pass from the urinary tract into extravesical tissue planes or the peritoneal cavity.

The bladder is filled with a contrast medium (a 10% solution of IVP medium is excellent) under gravity by inserting the barrel of an Asepto syringe into the end of the Foley catheter and pouring contrast medium into the syringe held as high above the patient as the Foley catheter will permit until flow stops or the patient complains of a full bladder (Fig. 14-14). An anteroposterior x-ray is obtained, the contrast medium is drained from the bladder, and a second anteroposterior x-ray is obtained immediately to demonstrate any medium that might have extravasated anteriorly or posteriorly.

TREATMENT

BLADDER

Prompt diagnosis and surgical treatment is of unusual importance in a patient with a ruptured bladder, since the mortality rate rises rapidly with delay in operation (see Fig. 14-15).

PROSTATIC URETHRA

1. **Primary anastomosis** of the severed urethral margins from above is preferred and should be done when possible (Fig. 14-16).

2. **Vest sutures** should be carried from the apex of the prostatic urethra through to the perineum where primary suturing is not possible.

3. A **Foley catheter** should be inserted and kept under slight traction for 24 hours and left indwelling for 14 to 45 days, depending on how soon the surgeon feels healing may have occurred.

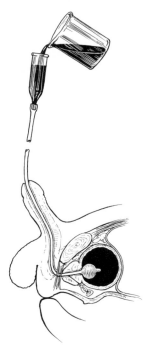

Figure 14-14 Technique of retrograde cystography.

4. **Diversion of urine** should always be accomplished by suprapubic cystostomy in the male because the urethral catheter may become dislodged accidentally, or its removal may be dictated by the onset of urethritis. In the female a urethral catheter is the only form of diversion usually required.

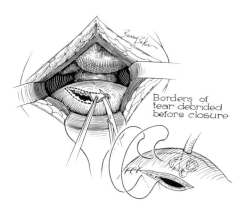

Borders of tear debrided before closure

Figure 14-15 Technique of debridement and repair of ruptured bladder with absorbable suture in contact with urine.

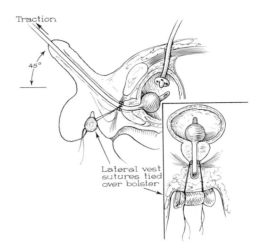

Figure 14–16 Diagrammatic representation of technique of repair of membranous urethra with illustration of primary approximation and placement of Vest perineal traction sutures.

5. **Adequate evacuation** of hematoma and bone fragments and pro-longed **extraperitoneal drainage** of the perivesical space should be carried out.

6. A simple **suprapubic cystostomy** may be done by a nonurologist, and repair of the laceration later by a urologist. However, primary repair is preferred if there is a urologic surgeon available.

INJURIES TO THE ANTERIOR URETHRA

Usually a straddle injury is responsible for this type of injury.

DIAGNOSIS

Diagnosis is based on physical examination, urethrography, and pan-endoscopy.

TREATMENT

OPERATIVE TREATMENT

All but the most minor puncture wounds of the urethra should be treated by exploration with primary excision and repair to obviate dense fibrosis and stricture resulting from nonsurgical treatment of urethral laceration (Fig. 14-17). The principles of treatment include:

1. Precise **delineation** of the location and extent of injury by urethrog-raphy and urethroscopy.

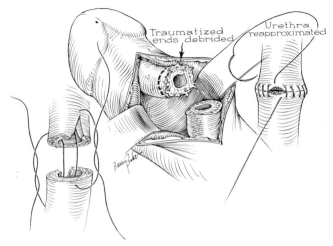

Figure 14–17 The injured anterior urethra is mobilized from the corpora cavernosa. The injured ends are debrided, spatulated, and closed in a water-tight fashion.

2. Wide **mobilization** of the urethra from the cavernous bodies, allowing debridement and reanastomosis under no tension.

3. Spatulated water-tight **reanastomosis.**

4. Adequate periurethral space **drainage.**

5. Proximal **urinary diversion** (by suprapubic cystostomy) only if primary healing is not expected or water-tight anastomosis is not obtained. If water-tight anastomosis is obtained and primary healing anticipated, a Foley catheter is employed for 24 to 48 hours.

NONOPERATIVE TREATMENT

Indications: Contusion or very minor puncture type wounds or nicks of the urethra do not require surgery.

Regimen: Such injuries can be treated with antibiotics alone, or with incision and drainage of periurethral hematoma with antibiotic therapy and use of an indwelling Foley catheter for 7 to 10 days or until external tract is healed.

INJURIES TO THE PENIS AND SCROTUM

TREATMENT

AMPUTATION

This procedure is explained in Figure 14-18.

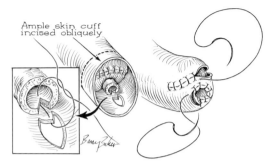

Figure 14–18 Repair of the amputated penis. Corporal bodies are oversewn with horizontal mattress sutures. A new spatulated urethral meatus is created as demonstrated.

FRACTURE OR LACERATION OF CORPUS CAVERNOSUM

The operative procedure for this type of injury can be seen in Figure 14–19.

AVULSION OF PENILE AND SCROTAL SKIN

Initial Care: There should be minimal debridement of skin in order to leave all possible tissue and reduce secondary grafting. Scrotal skin will regenerate if any remnant is left intact.

Definitive Care: If any remnant of scrotal skin remains intact, scrotal regeneration usually will occur. During this period of time simple topical care of the granulating surface should be carried out. Grafting of penile skin with split-thickness graft should be accomplished at an appropriate time. Skin grafts over the testes usually are unsatisfactory. If spontaneous regrowth of scrotal skin does not occur, the most satisfactory management of the testes is implantation into the subcutaneous tissue of the medial aspect of the thigh (Fig. 14–20).

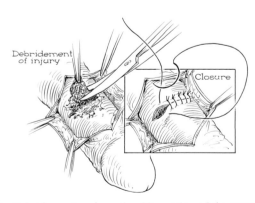

Figure 14–19 Debridement and repair of laceration of the corpus cavernosum.

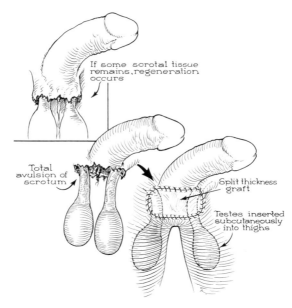

Figure 14–20 Expectant treatment where remnant of scrotum remains. With total avulsion of the scrotum, the testes are implanted into the medial aspect of the thigh.

INJURIES TO THE TESTES

SURGICAL TREATMENT

Any laceration of the tunica albuginea of the testes should be treated by debridement and primary repair to obviate secondary hemorrhage, infection, and necrosis. Any viable part of a testis should be preserved for possible hormone production. The tunica vaginalis should be excised to prevent hydrocele.

Technique (Fig. 14-21): Devitalized seminiferous tubules or seminiferous tubules which cannot be covered by tunica albuginea should be

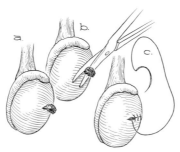

Figure 14–21 Excision of devitalized seminiferous tubules and primary reapproximation of tunica albuginea.

excised and hemostasis must be obtained. The tunical albuginea can be closed with a continuous suture of 4-0 chromic catgut.

NONOPERATIVE TREATMENT

Indications: Testicular contusion can be treated with a simple regimen.

Regimen: Bed rest, elevation, antibiotics, and icepacks should be used during the first 24 hours.

TORSION

Appendages: The diagnosis is to be considered in any patient with sudden onset of scrotal pain. The strangulated appendage may be demonstrated by thorough, gentle palpation of the scrotal contents and the demonstration of a small bluish, tender mass, usually at the upper pole of the testes or epididymis. The treatment is surgical excision.

Spermatic Cord: The absence of fixation of a testis to the inferior aspect of the scrotum provides the potential for *torsion of the testis* on its spermatic cord. The incidence of bilaterality of this defect is 30 per cent. **Diagnosis** is suggested by sudden onset of scrotal pain with or without coincidental trauma. It may occur at night during bed rest.

The testis lies horizontally and is retracted superiorly. In any patient in whom this diagnosis is entertained (even if epididymitis seems to be more likely) infiltration of the spermatic cord at the level of the external ring should be carried out with 1% lidocaine (Xylocaine) to allow careful palpation of the spermatic cord and scrotal contents (Fig. 14-22a). Most torsions of the spermatic cord of recent origin can, after infiltration of the

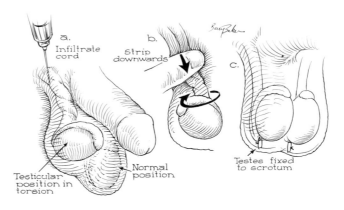

Figure 14-22   *a,* Cephalad displacement and lateral rotation of the testis with torsion of the spermatic cord. Technique of infiltration of the cord with local anesthetic is illustrated. *b,* Technique of nonoperative reduction of torsion of the spermatic cord. *c,* Definitive correction of the congenital deformity allowing torsion of the cord.

spermatic cord, be reduced by stripping the spermatic cord between the thumb and forefinger inferiorly from a point above the location of the torsion (Fig. 14-22*b*).

Definitive treatment is surgical exploration of the scrotum, excision of the tunica vaginalis, and suture fixation of the tunica albuginea of the testis to the inferior aspect of the scrotum (Fig. 14-22*c*). This must be done bilaterally because of the high incidence of bilateral torsion.

INJURIES TO THE VULVA AND VAGINA

Injuries to the vulva and vagina are uncommon due to the protected location of these structures. They occur most often in the prepubertal girl as a result of straddle falls, but they may be self-inflicted by insertion of various objects. Hematomas and lacerations are the most common sequelae.

HEMATOMAS

DIAGNOSIS

Hematomas are seldom serious, though ecchymosis may be extremely alarming. They are manifested by the presence of swelling and tenderness and, if large, by severe pain. In most instances, the hematomas are small and localized, although occasionally they may be extensive and extend from the vulva through the paravaginal tissues into the broad ligament. The skin over large hematomas is usually black, shiny, edematous, and susceptible to surface trauma. Rarely, the blood loss into tissue spaces may be severe enough to produce shock. Due to the dependent location of this lesion and the loose structure of the tissues, considerable edema may develop in the vulvar area following severe trauma.

TREATMENT

Small hematomas should be treated with analgesics and should be carefully observed for evidence of continued enlargment. The use of cold compresses immediately following the trauma is of some value.

Large hematomas may require more extensive treatment. When a large, fluctuant collection of blood is found, it should be evacuated either by aspiration or incision. The latter method is preferable in most cases. If an obvious bleeding vessel is seen, it should be ligated, but it is best not to explore the hematoma cavity extensively looking for obscure bleeding vessels. If there is a significant generalized ooze, the cavity of the hematoma should be carefully packed, or if it appears dry, a drain should be left in place for at least 24 hours.

LACERATIONS

DIAGNOSIS

Laceration of the vulva and vagina is most likely to occur from an injury received by falling violently on a slender object, such as a stake or picket fence. Occasionally the injury may extend through the vagina into the adjacent organs, such as the rectum, bladder, and urethra or may even extend through the cul-de-sac into the peritoneal cavity. Under these circumstances, hemorrhage may be quite severe. When multiple severe lacerations are noted in the vagina, a foreign body should be suspected as the cause and one should carefully search for remnants of glass, metal, or plastic. Anteroposterior and lateral x-rays, including the vaginal area, should be taken to locate radiopaque objects. Lacerations of this type may result in profuse hemorrhage and severe pain.

TREATMENT

Treatment should be directed toward restoration of normal anatomical relationships. Bleeding vessels should be ligated and tissue edges carefully reapproximated. Large traumatic areas should be thoroughly irrigated with sterile saline, and necrotic tissue debrided. Damage to adjacent organs, such as the bladder and rectum, must be looked for and repaired. If the peritoneal cavity has been penetrated, it should be explored for evidence of visceral lacerations and intra-abdominal bleeding.

No attempt should be made to forcibly examine a child. If there is considerable pain, bleeding, or evidence of laceration, she should be examined under anesthesia. Injuries should be repaired by careful approximation of the tissue edges utilizing small instruments and taking small bites of tissues.

SEXUAL INJURIES

Sexual injuries may be received during the process of defloration, in association with rape, or when foreign bodies are inserted into the vagina. In a large majority of cases, trauma to the lower genital tract is related to coitus. These injuries may involve the introitus, alone, or varying sites within the vagina. Vaginal lacerations resulting from coitus may be associated with initial coitus, with sexual contact during the postpartum period, following hysterectomy, or in the postmenopausal woman with a markedly atrophic vagina. The lateral vaginal walls are the structures most often lacerated. The next most common sites of vaginal injury are the posterior fornix, the posterior vaginal wall and the vaginal vault. Rarely, the laceration may extend into the broad ligament, the peritoneal cavity, or the rectum.

The majority of introital injuries associated with first coitus are minor in degree and are accompanied by minimal bleeding. Occasionally, the injury may involve extensive laceration of the hymenal ring and may extend into the vagina with associated profuse bleeding.

TREATMENT

These injuries are managed in the same fashion as "nonsexual" lacerations. Adequate hemostasis and reapproximation of tissues in an anatomical manner are of prime importance.

RAPE INJURIES

Rape injuries are usually much more extensive than defloration injuries, especially when they involve a virgin or young child. Frequently there is extensive trauma to the vulvar region, hymenal ring, and vagina, resulting in severe hemorrhage, hematoma formation, and laceration of the hymen. In children, these lacerations may be deep and extend into the rectum and even the bladder. Rarely, the cul-de-sac may be ripped through and the peritoneal cavity entered. If bleeding is extensive, it is usually best to anesthetize the individual and then carefully obtain hemostasis and repair the lacerated tissues.

It is vital that an accurate history and physical examination be performed on victims of alleged rape, since the examining physician may be called upon to give testimony in a court of law. Not only is it of extreme importance for the examining physician to note any evidence to substantiate the individual's claim of rape, but he must also look for such information as will indicate a false claim of rape. Rape is defined as unlawful sexual intercourse with a woman by force and against her will. Before a charge of rape can be substantiated, there must be medical evidence of lack of consent and proof of intercourse. The passage of the penis between the labia minora constitutes intercourse.

PROCEDURES FOR EXAMINING A RAPE VICTIM

The following procedures are suggested in evaluating a patient suspected of being raped.

1. Before the alleged victim is examined, **consent** must be obtained, preferably in the presence of a witness. If the patient is a child or is mentally deficient, the consent of parent or guardian is necessary.

2. The **time and place of the examination** should be recorded, as well as the length of time since the alleged assault took place. The emotional status of the patient should be noted.

3. Certain **pertinent data** such as the age, marital status, parity, and last menstrual period of the patient should be obtained. The date of last coitus should be noted if the patient is not a virgin. Inquiries should also be made as to whether the patient douched or bathed following the alleged rape. The person's clothing should be searched in search of

missing buttons, tears, and stains. All of the clothing should be carefully saved for the police to examine.

4. A **physical examination** should be conducted for signs of violence. This does not only include the genital area where lacerations and hematomas may be found, but includes the entire body. Bruises and scratches on the face and trunk should be carefully noted. Matted pubic hair should be noted, as well as the presence of any foreign hairs on the patient. The latter should be carefully saved and labeled. If the pubic hair appears matted, some of it should be obtained for laboratory examination to see if any semen is present. The presence or absence of the hymen should be noted as well as whether or not it is lacerated and bleeding. Vaginal lacerations should also be looked for.

5. **Laboratory studies** should be run on all material. It is preferable that all items be given directly to the clinical pathologist who will examine them. If this is not feasible, the technologist who will be doing the examination should sign a receipt for each specimen delivered to the laboratory.

> To check the **presence of sperm** a wet mount of secretions should be obtained from the vaginal fornices. If the vagina is dry, it may be irrigated with saline and a preparation made from this. Motile sperm should be looked for. These may be found in the vagina from 1/2 to 6 hours after intercourse, the average being 3 hours. Nonmotile sperm may be found for 7 to 12 hours and, exceptionally, for 18 to 24 hours. A dry smear, stained with methylene blue, Wright's stain, or Gram's stain also should be made in search of spermatozoa.

> The absence of sperm does not preclude intercourse, since the assailant may have been azoospermic or may have withdrawn before ejaculation. Dried stains on the clothing or the pubic hair may be examined for the **presence of seminal fluid**. Ultraviolet light produces a bluish fluorescence on seminal fluid stains, quite unlike that seen with material from the bladder or rectum. A vaginal aspirate and dried stains may be studied for acid phosphatase, which presumes the presence of seminal fluid. The finding of a positive fluorescence, plus a high acid phosphatase level (for an immediate answer, Phosphatabs-Acid, Warner-Chilcott, may be used) or a high creatinine phosphokinase level is good presumptive evidence of seminal fluid.

> If seminal fluid is present and if the assailant's blood was type A or B, the **A or B substances** will be in the seminal fluid, and the blood type of an alleged assailant can be compared to it.

> Dried stains of blood on the victim should be typed and compared with the **blood type** of the suspected assailant as well as the victim.

> **Foreign hairs** found on the clothing or body of the victim should be saved to be compared with the alleged assailant s hair.

> **Smears** and **cultures** and **serology** should be taken as indicated.

6. If possible, **photographs** should be taken of any bruise marks on the body of the patient as well as of lacerations and bruises in the genital area.

7. The use of **stilbestrol** (5 mg. four times daily for 5 days) may prevent a resultant pregnancy. The use of a concomitant drug to prevent the nausea often associated with the ingestion of stilbestrol is also advisable.

Special attention must be afforded the child who has been sexually assaulted. The immediate physical and emotional needs of the child must be met, as well as the needs of the parents. The response of the parents to this tragic event may well affect the psychosexual development of the child.

FOREIGN BODY INJURIES

In most cases, insertion of a foreign body into a nonvirginal or parous woman will not result in any significant injury. Occasionally, however, when this is attempted in a virginal female, there will be laceration of the hymenal tissues as well as the perineum. Molded "phalluses" used in homosexual activities or as a form of masturbation may produce severe laceration of the vagina. Glass objects such as soda bottles or drinking glasses may break within the vagina and produce severe damage to these tissues. Other sharp metal objects may also be introduced into the vagina and produce severe trauma.

TREATMENT

Careful inspection of the tissues must be made in search of residual foreign bodies. If it is known that a glass object has broken in the vagina, a careful search must be made for glass fragments before repair of the lacerated tissues is accomplished. All bleeding points should be ligated and necrotic tissues debrided. The tissues should be carefully reapproximated.

Chapter 15

General Principles of Fracture Treatment

THE FRACTURE LESION

The actual conditions at the site of the fracture are of great importance in establishing the general principles of treatment. These conditions may vary from a simple crack in the bone, with only the mildest disturbance of the surrounding tissue, to a lesion of the greatest severity, with marked displacement of the fragments and much damage to all of the neighboring tissues. The method of treatment will depend largely on the character of the bone lesion and the nature of the soft-tissue damage, as well as on the stage of pathological change. That is, the proper care may depend on whether the patient is seen immediately after injury, early in the course of swelling and infiltration, later at the height of the inflammatory reaction, or days or weeks after the injury.

Ordinarily, when a bone is broken, the endosteum and the periosteum are torn and the surrounding soft parts are damaged to some extent. Blood vessels and lymphatics are ruptured and the tissues become infiltrated and engorged with blood, lymph, and exudate. This causes swelling, pain, and circulatory disturbance, all of which are increased by handling of the extremity and movement of the bone fragments.

The infiltration and swelling of the soft parts increase rapidly during the first 8 to 24 hours, and by the end of this time the muscles and other soft parts have lost their elasticity and have become edematous. The circulatory disturbance caused by pressure from swelling and from thrombosed vessels produces edema, even to the extent of bullae and blebs beneath the skin surface. Reduction at this late stage necessitates the use of more violence, is more difficult to accomplish, and results in more damage than if done earlier.

Swelling that is unduly rapid or extensive indicates serious hemor-

182

rhage, and, if this occurs in a region with tight fascial covering, there may be serious vascular complications. Under these conditions circulation, sensation, and motor power must be checked carefully and frequently.

The extent and severity of these processes are greatly increased by motion of the bone fragments and muscle spasm due to pain before reduction. The type of emergency splinting is therefore important. The proper splinting procedures are explained in the section on Splints and Splinting.

When a fracture involves a joint, the hemorrhage into the joint cavity may be under great tension. This produces intense pain and restriction of motion. Aspiration of the joint may provide relief from the pain. Joint aspiration, if done, must be done under conditions of rigid asepsis.

When the patient is under an anesthetic, interposition of tissue can frequently be recognized by failure to get bony contact or crepitus. Its early recognition allows proper treatment and may eliminate the necessity for later operative procedures for resultant nonunion.

In addition to this picture of the fracture lesion, there may be associated injuries to contiguous muscles, nerves, joints, tendons, tendon sheaths, and viscera, which must be considered in both examination and treatment. The possibility of multiple fractures or of serious injury involving the head, chest, or abdomen should always be considered at the outset and should be kept in mind throughout the patient's course. (See Chapter 1.)

The effect of the fracture upon the patient as a whole is a vital part of the fracture lesion. Injury of any kind is upsetting to a patient and the degree of emotional response to injury is a variable to be assessed. Performance whether intellectual, physical, or economic can be seriously threatened by the disability of injury. Reassuring the patient and choosing the treatment best suited to the patient's individual needs so as to restore him as soon as possible to maximum possible performance are as important in the treatment of the injury as an understanding of its pathophysiology.

To be of clinical significance a fracture is defined as *a localized area of soft tissue and bone damage attended by secondary harmful effects upon adjacent regional structures and upon the patient as a whole.*

HEALING OF FRACTURES

The actual mechanism whereby calcium is deposited in the reparative tissues to form callus is not completely understood. However, the rest of the healing process is fairly well known. Most fractures will heal unless there is infection, mechanical obstruction, such as interposition of soft tissues, avascularity, or excessive motion. After the fracture lesion has appeared, the bone ends and the surrounding soft parts (endosteum, marrow, reticulum, bone chips, periosteum, and extraskeletal tissue which has undergone laceration) are bound together by the interlacing mesh of the fibrin formed from clotted blood always present at the site of fracture.

Within hours, perivascular connective tissue cells, round cells, and fibroblasts infiltrate the fibrin scaffolding in a centripital manner to begin the formation of a rich granulation tissue. Within the first two weeks, the mass of cells and tissue encompassing the ends of the fracture fragments becomes more organized and creates a sleeve of soft callus, thereby stabilizing the fragments.

At first the callus is rubbery, allowing a certain degree of movement of the fragments. If movement is sufficiently restricted, the elastic callus remains intact and becomes progressively stiffer as mineralization occurs, producing young, fiber bone. When movement is not restricted, the immature callus may be disrupted by shear or torsion, and, if disruption is repeated frequently, the stage may be set for the development of nonunion or pseudarthrosis. The bulk of the callus is related directly to the amount of instability, as is the differentiation of cartilage in the reparative tissue. Unstable fractures tend to produce larger amounts of callus. Where the coapted ends of a fracture are rigidly fixed, however, primary bony union takes place without external or internal callus and healing is characterized by intracortical bone formation.

With use and the action of normal stresses over a period of months, the provisional callus may be removed by remodeling and the normal anatomical features of the lamellar structure of cortical bone restored. This process may take a year or more. The time required for sufficient ossification to allow function depends upon the degree of solidarity demanded for the function of a given bone. Thus, the arm, which does not have to bear weight, can return to activity sooner than the leg which must be strong enough to bear weight; and the clerk can assume full function more quickly than the manual laborer with the same fracture. Furthermore a patient with a fracture of the metaphyseal region, which has a broad surface of trabeculae, many osteogenic cells, a good blood supply, and one fragment with a short lever arm, can be returned to activity earlier than one with a midshaft fracture which has few or none of these favorable factors.

The following clinical guides are derived from a study of the factors involved in fracture healing.

1. The healing of fractures is primarily a local phenomenon. A good blood supply to the fragments, adequate apposition of bone surfaces and adequate immobilization are the most important prerequisites for healing. Local circulatory impairment, inadequate apposition of fragments, inadequate immobilization of fragments, interposition of soft parts between the bone ends, extensive tissue necrosis, and infection have been shown to have a profoundly adverse effect on healing.

2. Advanced age, general disease, and general disturbance of metabolism should be considered factors affecting the patient's chances of survival, not factors interfering with the healing process.

3. Severe, prolonged negative nitrogen balance, excessive steroids, and avitaminosis C are known to affect bone healing adversely.

4. Fractures in children heal rapidly and nonunion is rare.

5. There is frequent difficulty with the healing process in certain locations, notably in the intracapsular portion of the femoral neck, the junction of the lower and middle thirds of the tibia, the proximal half of the carpal scaphoid, and the lower third of the ulna. Fractures at these points, therefore, require prolonged immobilization or special treatment — operative or otherwise — to increase the chances of union.

6. Distraction is detrimental to bone repair. The case for any influence of compression on *cortical* bone repair has not been documented. Optimal compression does, however, augment engagement and approximation of the bone ends which in turn favors the healing process. Rigid internal fixation promotes rapid, primary bone healing. There are but three common causes for a gap between the fragments of an internally fixed fractured bone — infection, motion at the fracture, and fixation in distraction.

7. When functional disabilities are not caused by failure of union, by bony deformity, or by direct nerve or vascular lesions, they result from fibrosis in soft parts injured at the time of fracture and intensified by prolonged or extensive immobilization of joints and muscles. These disabilities may be reduced by a judicious balance of minimal immobilization and maximum exercise of joints and muscles with due care not to interfere with the immobilization of the fragments throughout the healing of the fracture. In any given case, the methods of care which most nearly meet these requirements will produce the best convalescence and functional end result.

GOAL OF FRACTURE TREATMENT

The best method of treatment for any fracture is that which most nearly approaches the hypothetical ideal proposed by Dr. Clay Ray Murray. "Hypothetically, the ideal treatment for any fracture would be to 'wish' the fragments into place, hold them there by 'moral suasion,' and send the patient on about his business while the fracture heals."

"To 'wish' the fragments into place" implies that the primary tissue damage caused by the injury may be multiplied several times by secondary damage resulting from reduction maneuvers. Therefore, reduction, regardless of method, must be designed and carried out in such a manner as to minimize the inevitable secondary tissue insult.

To "hold them there by 'moral suasion'" implies that, of the multiple methods available for the treatment of most fractures, the best is that which, in addition to providing fixation, interferes least with the continuing function of the uninjured regional structures.

To "send the patient on about his business while the fracture heals" is to recognize that a fracture problem is actually the problem of an injured person. It is not necessary to make a fracture fit a favorite treatment. There are numerous methods available for the treatment of most fractures. These can and should be adapted to fit the needs of the patient as well as the fracture so that daily activities are interrupted as little as possible and full activities restored as soon as possible.

SPLINTS AND SPLINTING

The injured part may or may not have been splinted prior to the patient's arrival at the hospital. Additional tissue damage may occur during preparation for treatment as it may at the scene of the accident or during transport. Therefore, unsplinted injuries should be splinted, even for the short trip to and from the x-ray department, because adequate films will require positioning of the injured part by the x-ray technician.

UPPER EXTREMITY EMERGENCY SPLINTS

1. *Coaptation splints* (padded boards) may be used for injuries of the wrist and forearm. For injuries of the elbow, if extension of the elbow exceeds that of a right angle, a double coaptation splint should be applied rather than flexing the elbow to fit a sling before x-ray diagnosis of the injury (Figure 15–1*A*).

2. *Sling or swathe* may be used for injuries of the shoulder, arm, and elbow (Fig. 15–1*B*).

3. *Air splints* are preferred for injuries of the wrist and forearm and those around the elbow when the elbow cannot be flexed. The air splint is

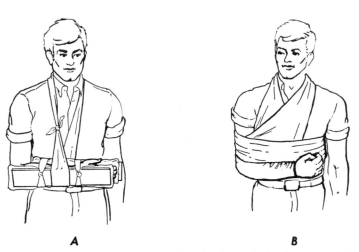

A   **B**

Figure 15–1   *A*, Coaptation splinting with padded boards for fractures of the forearm. *B*, Sling and circular bandage about the thorax for fractures above the forearm. (From Rhoads, J. E., Allen, J. G., Harkins, H. N., and Moyer, C. A.: Surgery, Principles and Practice, 4th Edition. Philadelphia, J. B. Lippincott Co., 1970. Reprinted with permission.)

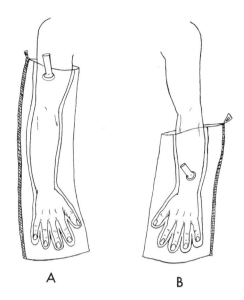

Figure 15-2   *A*, Air splint for fractures of the forearm and about the elbow when the elbow cannot be flexed. *B*, Air splint for fractures of the wrist.

closed over the extremity by a zipper and inflated by blowing air through the mouth tube. A twist of the tube closes the air valve. Air pressure from a mechanical pump can produce circulatory constriction and should not be used (Fig. 15–2).

LOWER EXTREMITY EMERGENCY SPLINTS

1. *Air splints* are preferred for injuries about the knee, leg, and ankle. Control of swelling and bleeding are ancillary benefits provided by the air splint (Fig. 15–3).

If the limb is angulated it is permissible and proper to restore alignment by gentle traction in the long axis of the limb before the splint is applied.

Rotary deformity of leg and ankle which can threaten circulation must be corrected at once by traction and gentle derotation.

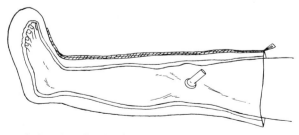

Figure 15-3   Air splint for fractures about the knee, leg, and ankle.

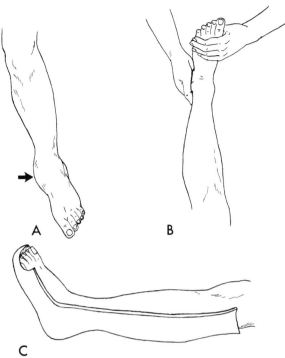

Figure 15-4 *A*, Ankle fracture with lateral dislocation of the foot and excessive stretching of the skin over the medial malleolus (indicated by arrow). *B*, Immediate reduction of the dislocation by gentle manual traction to relieve skin tension prior to definitive reduction of the fracture. *C*, Posterior moulded plaster splint to maintain the corrected position prior to x-ray and definitive treatment.

Gross lateral dislocation of the foot at the ankle requires immediate correction to avoid skin pressure from within on the skin of the medial ankle. At times a temporary posterior moulded plaster of paris is helpful in controlling ankle and foot displacements (Fig. 15-4).

2. *The Thomas splint* has been in use for many years to provide traction-countertraction on the lower extremity for injuries of the hip region and the shaft of the femur. The ring engages the ischial tuberosity for countertraction, and traction is applied to the distal end of the splint by means of an ankle hitch and "Spanish windlass" (Fig. 15-5).

The half-ring splint is more widely used. It can be adjusted to fit the right or left lower extremity. The half ring engages the ischial tuberosity and the ring is closed by a strap and buckle across the anterior thigh. Padding is placed beneath the strap to protect the groin vessels and nerves. Padding is also applied about the ankle to avoid circulatory constriction. The circulation of the foot is checked at frequent intervals.

Limb-support slings, padded-ankle hitch and traction strap for the Thomas and half-ring splints are commercially available. These accessories

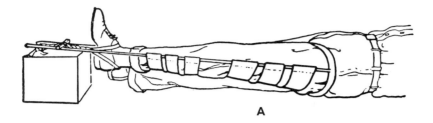

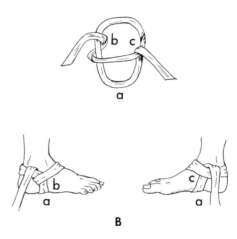

Figure 15–5 *A*, Thomas splint applied. Note ring pulled against ischial tuberosity. Padding should be applied about the ankle to avoid circulatory embarrassment. Circulation of the foot is checked at frequent intervals. *A*, Ankle hitch. Various knots can be used for this purpose; one of the simplest is a slip knot (b & c) with a retained loop (a). The slip knot (b & c) goes over the ankle and loop (a) acts as a stirrup. The hitch is tightened over padding and the two ends tied to the lower end of the Thomas splint and twisted with a tongue depressor to provide the so-called "Spanish windlass" traction.

are usually more efficiently applied and more uniformly effective than improvised accessories.

The method best suited for splinting of fractures of the *proximal end* of the femur in the emergency department is *Buck's skin traction* applied to the leg with the traction cord passed through a pulley attached to an extension bar at the foot of the stretcher. Countertraction is provided by the weight of the body. The advantages over the Thomas and half-ring splints are threefold:

1. The ankle hitch is eliminated.

2. There is no need to remove the Thomas and half-ring splints to obtain unobstructed x-ray views of the hip.

3. The stretcher can be wheeled over the x-ray table by adjusting the wheels, thereby making patient transfer unnecessary (Fig. 15–6).

The method best suited for splinting fractures of the *shaft* of the femur in the emergency department is the Thomas or half-ring splint utilizing *Buck's skin traction* as a substitute for the ankle hitch.

SPLINTING AN OPEN FRACTURE

The fragment of bone which protrudes through an open wound should be covered with a sterile dressing and left undisturbed until proper

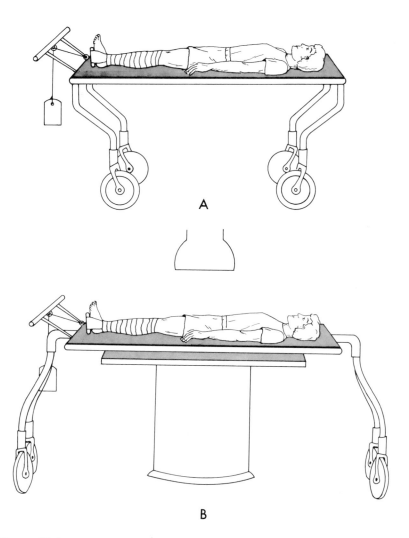

Figure 15–6 *A*, Buck's skin traction applied to the leg. This is the preferred method of applying traction to the lower extremity in the emergency department for splinting of fractures of the proximal end of the femur. *B*, The stretcher can be wheeled over the x-ray table by adjusting the wheels without disturbing the patient or the traction and provides unobstructed x-ray views of the hip.

definitive care is effected in the operating room. The best method of splinting is that which protects the fracture and the limb and does not disturb the wound.

Traction sufficient to draw extruded bone ends into the wound is contraindicated in the emergency department. However, severe angular and rotary deformities must be corrected if the distal circulation is compromised by the deformity.

VERTEBRAL INJURIES

1. *Neck injuries* can be stabilized by the use of head halter traction, manual traction, or the short spine board (Fig. 15–7*A*). The head and neck must be maintained in the neutral midline position in relation to the body. The patient should be turned "like a log." The neck should not be flexed, extended, or rotated. It should be stabilized in the long axis of the spine. (See Chapter 9.)

2. Injuries of the dorsal and lumbar spine are managed with the patient lying in a straight line on a firm surface such as a long spine board, thereby avoiding flexion or extension; again the patient should be moved "like a log." (See Chapter 9 and Fig. 15–7*B*).

The Committee on Trauma of the American College of Surgeons recommends the short and long spine boards as essential equipment for ambulances. They should be kept in the inventory of hospital emergency departments to be exchanged with arriving ambulances so that the patient need not be transferred from the spine board on which he arrives (Fig. 15–7).

PREPARATION FOR TREATMENT

In any emergency the saving of life comes first; treat impending asphyxia, hemorrhage, shock, and other life-endangering conditions before treating a fracture. (See Chapters 1, 2 and 3 and Fig. 15–8).

The patient who has had splints applied prior to arrival at the hospital should be examined immediately to make sure they are comfortable, efficient, and nonconstricting. Any constrictive dressing should be loosened immediately, but a tourniquet should not be removed until treatment for shock has been started and facilities to control hemorrhage are available. It is rarely necessary to remove adequate splints for a detailed assessment of the injury prior to roentgen examination, but inspection should be sufficient to rule out the presence of an open wound. A review of the roentgenograms makes unnecessary any extensive manipulations of the fracture until the stage has been set for definitive treatment.

The condition of the peripheral nerves and circulation distal to every extremity injury should be evaluated and *recorded* at the first examination. A detailed neurological examination is unnecessary. If the patient can flex

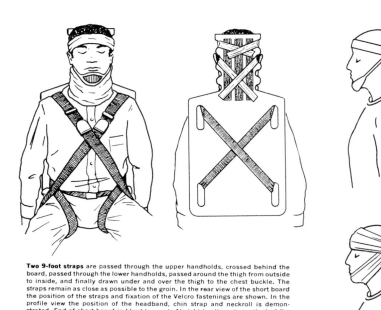

Two 9-foot straps are passed through the upper handholds, crossed behind the board, passed through the lower handholds, passed around the thigh from outside to inside, and finally drawn under and over the thigh to the chest buckle. The straps remain as close as possible to the groin. In the rear view of the short board the position of the straps and fixation of the Velcro fastenings are shown. In the profile view the position of the headband, chin strap and neckroll is demonstrated. End of short board is blunt-tapered. At right is alternate method of fixation.

Equipment for the short board consists of headband, chin strap and neck roll.

Headband (Fig. 1), which measures 42 inches, has:
a. Padded section;
b. Thin webbing 2 inches wide;
c. Strip of looped or pile Velcro.

Chin strap (Fig. 2), which measures 42 inches, has:
a. Regulation football chin strap;
b. Thin webbing 2 inches wide;
c. Strip of looped or pile Velcro.

Neck roll (Fig. 3), which measures 32 inches, has:
a. Foam rubber roll 8 inches wide and 6 inches in diameter, covered for protection first with plastic, then stockinette, both disposable and easily replaceable;
b. Thin webbing 1-inch wide;
c. Strip of looped or pile Velcro.

Ends (looped or pile Velcro) of straps grab strips of Velcro with hook surface affixed to back of head piece on the short board.

The neck roll is seldom used. It is necessary in rare fracture-dislocations of the neck in which the head is fixed in an awkward position. A heavy folded towel will serve well as a substitute.

Velcro is a fastener. It consists of two strips of nylon tape—one covered with minute hooks, the other with minute loops forming a pile surface—which lock securely when pressed together, open when peeled apart.

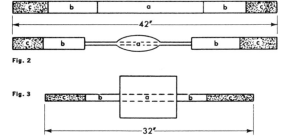

Fig. 1

42″

Fig. 2

Fig. 3

32″

A

Figure 15–7 *A,* Short spine board with head and neck support. *B,* Detail of short and long spine boards. (From American College of Surgeons: Bulletin May 1970.)

Illustration continued on opposite page.

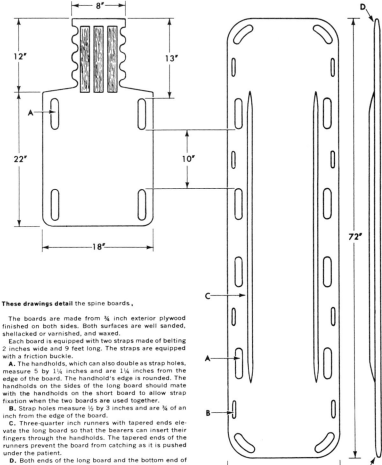

These drawings detail the spine boards.

The boards are made from ¾ inch exterior plywood finished on both sides. Both surfaces are well sanded, shellacked or varnished, and waxed.

Each board is equipped with two straps made of belting 2 inches wide and 9 feet long. The straps are equipped with a friction buckle.

A. The handholds, which can also double as strap holes, measure 5 by 1¼ inches and are 1¼ inches from the edge of the board. The handhold's edge is rounded. The handholds on the sides of the long board should mate with the handholds on the short board to allow strap fixation when the two boards are used together.

B. Strap holes measure ½ by 3 inches and are ¾ of an inch from the edge of the board.

C. Three-quarter inch runners with tapered ends elevate the long board so that the bearers can insert their fingers through the handholds. The tapered ends of the runners prevent the board from catching as it is pushed under the patient.

D. Both ends of the long board and the bottom end of the short board are blunt-tapered, so that the boards will slide as easily as possible when pushed under or behind the patient.

E. The edges of the head portion of the short board are serrated to allow an alternate method of fixation of the head. One or more 6-inch soft roller bandages are wrapped about the board, forehead and chin. The serrations prevent the bandage from slipping.

B

Figure 15–7   *Continued.*

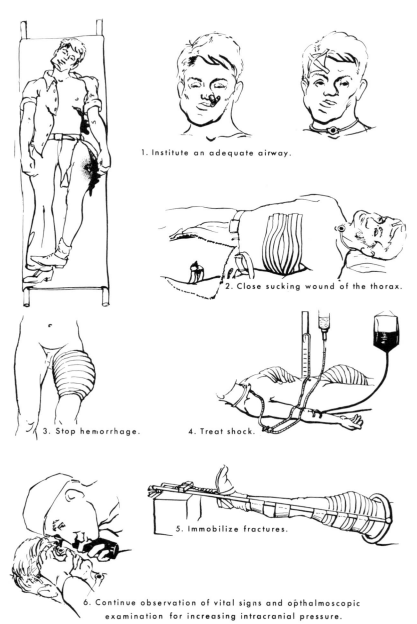

1. Institute an adequate airway.

2. Close sucking wound of the thorax.

3. Stop hemorrhage.   4. Treat shock.

5. Immobilize fractures.

6. Continue observation of vital signs and opthalmoscopic
examination for increasing intracranial pressure.

Figure 15-8   Treatment of multiple injuries. Priority of injury. (See Chapters 1, 2 and 3.
(From Rhoads, J. E., Allen, J. G., Harkins, H. N., and Moyer, C. A.: *Surgery, Principles and
Practice*. 4th Edition. Philadelphia, J. B. Lippincott Co., 1970. Reprinted with permission.)

and extend his toes, the major nerves of the lower extremity are grossly intact; if he can spread and flex his fingers and extend his thumb, functional integrity of the major nerves of the upper limb is indicated. Absence of the ability to carry out these motor functions warrants a more detailed examination, and if a nerve injury is recognized at the start, it will be unnecessary for the patient and surgeon to speculate later whether such an injury was produced by trauma or by the treatment.

An obvious injury is apt to captivate the attention of a casual examiner to the exclusion of less apparent concomitant lesions. A fracture of the femoral shaft can camouflage an associated dislocation of the hip; a fracture of the os calcis, a concomitant spine fracture; fractured ribs, a ruptured spleen; and the crushed pelvis, a serious genitourinary injury. Always order an x-ray of the pelvis in the presence of major lower limb trauma.

Examination of every injury should include a rapid survey of the entire patient. The patient should be entirely disrobed for this examination, and when necessary scissors should be used to remove clothing to avoid disturbing the patient or the splint.

An elaborate history is not always possible and rarely is necessary. The time, place, and details of the accident and description of intervening events should be recorded. Inquiries into the cardiovascular, renal, and respiratory status of the patient must be complemented by sufficient clinical and laboratory examination to determine the anesthetic risk and the agent of choice. The time of the last food intake must be ascertained. The important interval is that between intake and accident not between intake and anesthesia. Cessation of gastrointestinal function is one of the early responses to injury, and the stomach may not empty for many hours following even a minor painful injury. Unless the stomach is empty there is a risk that vomitus may be aspirated during inhalation anesthesia.

Emotional stress, as well as physical discomfort, must be alleviated as much as possible. A frank discussion with a conscious patient to apprise him of the facts of the injury and the implications of the projected plan of treatment to dispel uncertainties and to answer as many questions as possible promotes the patient's confidence in his doctor and quickly establishes patient and doctor as a team with a single goal and a mutually acceptable program.

REDUCTION OF FRACTURES

Force is unnecessary to the early reduction of a fracture and represents compensation for an error in technique or an attempt to overpower some anatomical obstruction which more often than not is unrecognized. Several factors will determine whether a fracture reduction will prove to be easy (atraumatic) or difficult (traumatic): (1) the time, (2) the anesthesia, (3) the displacing forces, (4) the choice of method.

THE TIMING OF REDUCTION

A fracture should be considered a surgical emergency. When reduction is done prior to or in the early stages of the inflammatory local response to injury with adequate anesthesia for muscle relaxation, the surrounding soft parts are in their most favorable condition to facilitate reduction. Delayed reduction with fixation and inelasticity of all the tissues provide the impediments common to delayed reduction. When "jelled" in malposition, these soft tissues must then be torn apart by force before reduction can be accomplished in contradiction to the principles of sound fracture treatment.

ANESTHESIA

Reduction in the early stages after injury requires adequate anesthesia for the obliteration of pain and muscle spasm; and, when treatment has been delayed, anesthesia makes possible disruption of the organized soft tissues. Modern methods of anesthesia can circumvent almost every contraindication formerly advanced to explain a delay in treatment except inconvenience to the surgeon. The multiplicity of agents and techniques now available make it possible to reduce fractures immediately, or within a few hours, without undue jeopardy to the brain, heart, lungs, kidneys, liver, or full stomach—wherever the risk may lie. (See Chapter 5).

THE DISPLACING FORCES

The deformity to be corrected in the reduction of a fracture is the resultant of many forces, including the direction of the injury, the manipulations of initial care, the splinting or the uncontrolled mobility of unsplinted bone fragments, the strength and direction of the muscles attached to each fragment, the presence or absence of loose bone fragments wedged across the main fracture gap, and the influence of soft tissues penetrated by or interposed between the bone fragments. The surgeon should assess and prorate the importance of all displacing forces prior to electing a method of reduction and proceeding with its implementation.

THE CHOICE OF METHOD

There are five general methods for the management of fractures (Fig. 15–9). Every means available for the treatment of any given fracture may be classified as one of these five methods. They are:

1. Closed reduction (or maintenance of reduction if the position is satisfactory) and immobilization, usually with a plaster cast.

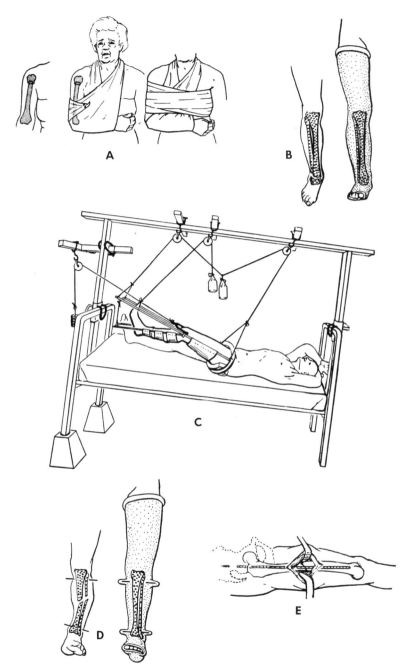

Figure 15–9 Five methods of management of fractures. *A*, No immobilization. *B*, Closed reduction and immobilization with plaster cast. *C*, Continuous balanced skeletal traction. *D*, External skeletal traction, Steinmann pins incorporated in a plaster cast. *E*, Open reduction and internal fixation with medullary nail. (From Rhoads, J. E., Allen, J. G., Harkins, H. N., and Moyer, C. A.: *Surgery, Principles and Practice.* 4th Edition. Philadelphia, J. B. Lippincott Co., 1970. Reprinted with permission.)

2. Continuous traction, usually skeletal traction, less commonly skin traction.

3. External skeletal fixation.

4. Open reduction and internal fixation.

5. No immobilization (perhaps a sling or a bandage).

CLOSED REDUCTION

If the position of the fragments is already satisfactory, reduction is not required, and immobilization is all that is necessary.

When the fracture fragments are displaced the essential preliminary step in reduction by manipulation is restoration of length of the broken bone. This is done by firm and steady traction and countertraction in the long axis of the limb. As a rule the distal fragment is replaced in apposition to the proximal. Rotary deformity should be corrected just before and angulation deformity just after apposition of the bone ends has been accomplished. Rotary deformity must be corrected completely. Angulation should always be corrected, particularly in fractures of the lower leg, forearm, or fingers. Considerable latitude is permissible in the correction of displacement. Complete apposition is not always necessary but should be sufficient to secure a stable reduction.

Closed reduction and immobilization are usually chosen when the contour of the fracture indicates that the reduction will be so stable that it will not be lost as long as good alignment is maintained by the immobilization. Under these circumstances, this is a conservative method of treatment involving a minimum risk of complications. It is the most common method of management for fractures of the extremities.

The most efficient external splint produces only relative immobilization of the fracture. It is a misconception to assume that when a limb is fixed in splints or circular plaster of paris casts the fracture fragments are completely immobilized. This is not true. The bone fragments and joints continue to move to some degree in response to their muscle motors, within a range roughly proportional to the thickness of flesh between the supposedly immobilized skeleton and the cast. Therefore, the surgeon must accept that what he clinically calls "external immobilization" provides only a relative immobility of the bone fragments.

The foregoing misconception is compatible with another common misconception — that total immobility of the fracture fragments is necessary to the process of bone repair. It is clear that movement, within certain limits, does not deter and may increase new bone formation. In clinical practice absolute immobility has seemed to be essential to the bone healing process only in a few specific fractures: notably, certain fractures of the femoral neck, scaphoid, and astragalus.

The disadvantages of external immobilization by plaster of paris casts are perpetuation of vascular stasis, interference with normal neuromuscular function, and restriction of joint motion. For these reasons it is advantageous for the patient to exercise muscles within the cast and mobilize joints beyond the splint or cast as soon and as completely as possible compatible with maintenance of reduction. When sufficient healing permits, the cast can be modified to permit additional muscle and joint function. These disadvantages can be ameliorated by intelligent use of this method of external immobilization.

CONTINUOUS TRACTION

Continuous traction is a means of maintenance of reduction when an oblique or comminuted fracture cannot be controlled by manipulative reduction and external immobilization. Continuous traction serves three purposes in the treatment of fractures: (1) reduction of pain and muscle spasm, (2) restoration of length, and (3) maintenance of length.

Reduction of pain and muscle spasm is important during the interval between admission of a patient and reduction of a long bone fracture. Release of spasm is especially important when the long muscles spanning a fracture have decreased the length of the bone. Spasm subsides steadily and often disappears as the muscles tire and stretch in submission to continuous traction. Whenever the reduction of a spiral, comminuted, or overriding transverse long bone fracture must be delayed for more than a short time, some form of temporary continuous traction should be used.

Restoration of length is an essential step preliminary to reduction. Continuous traction provides restoration of length. Full length should be achieved within the first 18 to 24 hours by addition of necessary weights, monitored at frequent intervals by x-ray, and then the weight reduced to the amount necessary to maintain length. Uncorrected overpull with distraction of fragments is an almost certain forerunner of delayed union or nonunion.

Maintenance of length is necessary to the integrity of reduction in most spiral and comminuted fractures. Whereas continuous traction provides maintenance of length it does not assure correction of rotation, angulation, and displacement. These corrections are made by adjustments in the traction apparatus to include the simultaneous use of devices such as slings, pads, and plaster of paris splints and casts, or by manipulative reduction within the apparatus.

It is a misconception that angulation and displacement deformities can always be corrected by traction alone. Persistence in this effort usually results in overpull with distraction of the fragments and a threat of delayed union or nonunion.

There are two methods of applying continuous traction to a long bone: (1) skin traction, and (2) skeletal traction.

Skin Traction: Skin traction is applied to an extremity by means of adhesive tape, adhesive moleskin, or nonadhesive foam rubber strips held in place by circular elastic bandages. Bony prominences are padded to avoid pressure sores. Circulatory impairment by tight circular bandages is known to occur and must be prevented. Traction is applied to a wooden or metal spreader just distal to the extremity.

Skin traction should be reserved for situations where not more than a few pounds of pulling force are required, and with few exceptions it is used as a temporary form of continuous traction. Prolonged use with over five pounds of pull soon causes skin blisters and blebs beneath the tape.

There are four main types of skin traction traditionally used:

1. *Forearm and arm traction* for treatment of fractures of the humerus, usually in infants. (See Fig. 17–13.)

2. *Bryant's traction* for treatment of fractures of the shaft of the femur in infants. (See Fig. 17–39.)

3. *Buck's traction* as a method of applying temporary skin traction to

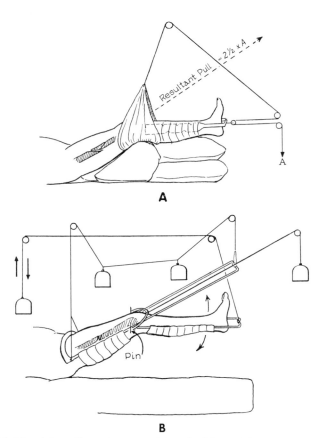

Figure 15–10 *A*, Russell traction. A useful method for stabilization of the lower extremity with a fracture of the femur when skeletal traction is contraindicated or undesirable. *B*, Skeletal balanced continuous traction. The lower extremity is suspended in the hammock formed by a half-ring splint and a Pearson low-leg attachment. Traction is applied through a pin transfixing the lower end of femur or the tuberosity of the tibia. When appropriate some knee motion can be maintained. (From McLaughlin, H. L.: *Trauma.* Philadelphia, W. B. Saunders Company, 1959.)

the lower extremity. Skin traction is applied to the leg with the extremity resting on a pillow. A cord is attached to a spreader distal to the extremity and passed through a pulley at the foot of the bed or stretcher. The pulling force is equal to the weight attached to the end of the cord (Fig. 15–6).

4. *Russell traction* as a method of applying traction on the fractured femur by a system of pulleys so arranged that the resultant of forces is a pull in the long axis of the femur. The thigh and leg are supported on pillows. Skin traction is applied to the leg and the spreader distal to the leg is equipped with a pulley.

The system is put into operation by a continuous length of cord which is first attached to a hammock supporting the knee. The cord is passed successively through an overhead pulley, through one pulley at the foot of the bed, back through the pulley attached to the spreader and finally through a second pulley at the foot of the bed. The force of pull on the femur is twice the weight suspended at the end of the cord (Figs. 15–10*A* and 17–41).

Skeletal Traction: Skeletal traction is applied directly to the bone involved or more often distal to the involved bone such as the tibial tubercle for fracture of the femur, the os calcis for fracture of the tibia, or the olecranon for fracture of the humerus. A Steinmann pin or Kirschner wire is drilled through the bone and a traction bow is applied to the pin or wire. If the wire is of small caliber, a traction bow is selected which also applies tension on the wire to make it rigid. Strict aseptic operating technique and environment are essential to avoid pin hole infection. A threaded wire lessens movement of the pin in the bone. Sliding of the pin may cause skin necrosis, and infection may result in osteomyelitis. A large pin may cause ring sequestrum formation. Proper technique of insertion and constant surveillance of the pin or wire lessens the incidence of these complications.

Balanced continuous traction for treatment of fractures of the femur or tibia is referred to as balanced suspension traction because the extremity is balanced or suspended in a system of splints such as a half-ring splint with Pearson leg attachment counterbalanced by weights (Fig. 15–10*B*). The suspension facilitates nursing care of the patient.

EXTERNAL SKELETAL FIXATION

External skeletal fixation or fixed skeletal traction-countertraction is a method of fracture management which employs Steinmann pins or Kirschner wires to transfix the bone fragments proximal and distal to the fracture. The projecting ends of these pins permit manipulation of the fragments and the length of the bone can be restored manually during reduction and maintained exactly thereafter by incorporating the projecting pins into a circular plaster of paris cast. Various mechanical pin holding devices have been designed to substitute for a cast in the treatment of fractures by external pin fixation. None are as safe, simple, or secure as plaster of paris (Fig. 15–9*D*).

The advantages of this method are fixed length and rigid fixation of the fragments. The disadvantages are overpull and infection. Overpull is avoidable and must be corrected. Infection is less likely if scrupulous sterile precautions are taken when the pins are inserted, if the pin hole sites are monitored, and if the pins are removed at the earliest possible date commensurate with early callus fixation of the fracture. By observing these tenets this method may prove most valuable.

OPEN REDUCTION AND INTERNAL FIXATION

Open reduction and internal fixation as a method of fracture management has many advantages and serious disadvantages. It consists of exposure of the fracture site whereby the fragments are brought into approximation under direct visualization. Usually some form of metal fixation (screws, plates, intramedullary nails, malleable stainless steel wire) is employed to maintain the reduction.

Open reduction and internal fixation affords the most exact reduction and offers many advantages; perfect apposition and alignment and full length are usually obtained. The excellent reduction predisposes to rapid union. It may provide the only means of reconstructing a disrupted joint at the shoulder, elbow, knee or ankle. Open reduction and internal fixation are absolute necessities in intracapsular fractures of the neck of the femur, intertrochanteric fractures of the femur, displaced fractures of the patella and olecranon, and irreducible fractures of the talus. It also may be a necessity in displaced fractures of the shaft of radius or ulna in the adult.

The disadvantages are chiefly infection, failure to achieve an anatomic reduction, and loss of fixation. These complications are a common cause of delayed union, nonunion, malunion, and sepsis.

Therefore, it must be stated that open reduction and internal fixation as a choice of method in the management of fractures should be limited to the surgeon of mature judgment who has explicit skills in the use of this method. The reader is referred to appropriate texts and training programs in accordance with his needs to acquire the prerequisite technical knowledge of evaluating the healing qualities of the skin, surgical exposures, the selection of the fixation equipment best suited to the mechanical problem, the limited holding power of mechanical fixation, and the amount of supplementary external fixation (plaster of paris) that may be required.

A great advantage of this method when it is properly used is the theoretical ideal of minimal casting of short duration to permit early restoration of muscle and joint function. This concept implies that open reduction and internal fixation are synonymous with "rigid fixation" achieved at operation. In other words, in planning open reduction the surgeon asks himself if he believes the configuration of the fracture, his available tools, and his personal skills can reasonably assure him that rigid internal fixation can be achieved. *If these postulates are uncertain or unobtaina-*

ble, *the indication for open operation should be reassessed and perhaps a different method chosen.*

Marked comminution of a fracture may defy rigid internal fixation. On the other hand, open reduction may be justified if it is the only way to accomplish reduction in those circumstances where perfect restoration of anatomy such as a joint surface is essential. Under such circumstances the fixation materials are used as an "internal suture," do not provide "rigid fixation" and external plaster of paris fixation is essential to the method. Only the operating surgeon can assess the stability or rigidity of his own operation, and on the basis of this evaluation the decision is made as to how much external fixation is necessary and when joint function can be started.

NO IMMOBILIZATION

The treatment of a fracture without immobilization is applicable to impacted fractures in which displacement will not occur with motion of the extremity. The position of the fragments is accepted, even though it may not be ideal. Immobilization is omitted in favor of early mobilization and this really is the keynote of the method. Actually, a sling or a bandage may be employed for a short period. These do not produce real immobilization but essentially provide some relief of pain during the first few days after injury.

This method should be employed in those fractures which do not require immobilization and in which early active exercise will lead to an earlier functional restoration of the part. It is particularly indicated in impacted fractures of the neck of the humerus and in undisplaced fractures of the radial head. It also is applicable in many chip fractures about the hand and the foot.

EARLY AFTERCARE OF FRACTURES

The first week after fracture reduction is a period of increasing swelling, during which the danger from loss of position and soft tissue complications is most pronounced. Immediately after reaction from anesthesia has occurred, the integrity of the circulation and peripheral nerves distal to the immobilizing dressing should be verified. Roentgenograms confirming the reduction should be taken.

The use of a circular plaster cast or any uncertainty concerning the circulatory status of the injured part requires that the patient be kept under close surveillance. This may necessitate hospitalization for several days or until the danger from circulatory embarrassment no longer exists. When plaster splints are applied, the gauze bandages used to bind them in place must be removed and replaced after the plaster has set. Otherwise the first bandages, wet by the plaster which they encircle, harden and may shrink and become the equivalent of a circular plaster.

No patient should be allowed out of sight, even overnight, without receiving specific instructions to return immediately at the first indication of white, blue, cold, or insensitive fingers or toes distal to the immobilizing dressing.

The patient should also be instructed to return if severe and intractable pain supervenes, for a well-reduced and immobilized fracture should not produce severe symptoms, and nonlocalized increasing pain usually signals increased tissue tension worthy of release.

A constant and localized burning pain usually is indicative of a pressure point under the plaster cast or a constrictive bandage which should be investigated and decompressed immediately, because once the over-compressed tissues commence to necrose, they also become relatively insensitive. A large and deep "pressure sore" may then develop silently and remain unrecognized until its telltale exudate seeps through and stains the plaster.

Advice concerning elevation of the injured part should be coupled with detailed instructions in finger or toe exercises to be carried out for short periods at frequent intervals. It should be explained in simple language that swelling constitutes the immediate danger; that the cause of swelling is accumulation of fluid which flows best downhill, and hence the rationale for elevation; that, with each motion of the fingers or toes, muscles pump some of this fluid back where it belongs; and that failure to reactivate these muscle pumps will retard the rate of recovery and jeopardize the final result.

It may justifiably be threatened that undue delay in muscle reactivation will allow the accumulated blood and fluid to clot and gel and will increase adhesions between moving structures that may require many months of tedious stretching exercises before motion can be regained.

This is the surgeon's opportunity to establish and explain his treatment. He should outline the projected plan of treatment, explain its rationale and objectives, delineate the patient's responsibilities and emphasize their importance, and establish a rapport ensuring mutual confidence and cooperation.

The patient should be re-examined the day after reduction and the immobilizing plaster splints or circular cast checked for comfort, efficiency, and absence of constriction or unwanted pressure. From time to time, until tissue swelling is past its peak, bandaged plaster splints may have to be rebandaged less tightly. A circular cast may require a longitudinal split and may need to be spread open for decompression of the tissues. As swelling recedes splints should be rebandaged more securely or a loose circular cast replaced for continued efficiency of fixation. The frequency of re-examination must be dictated by circumstances, and the injury never should be allowed to remain unchecked except for periods during which the surgeon is sure that all will remain in order.

PRINCIPLES OF TREATMENT OF OPEN FRACTURES

An open fracture is distinguished from its closed counterpart by a wound through which the fracture site communicates with the skin surface. This situation is attended by peculiar clinical implications unrelated to the size or cause of the break in the skin. Normal skin is host to a multitude of organisms, but it is also an impenetrable barrier against their entry into the deeper tissues. All fractures which communicate with a skin wound are contaminated by organisms. All must be considered to harbor incipient bone infection.

The size of the external wound may not bear a direct relation to the extent of tissue damage or the type and virulence of the organisms present in the wound. During the first few hours after injury (arbitrarily the first six hours) contamination is represented by the presence of organisms in the wound, but they are localized to the surface of the lacerated soft tissues and broken bone fragments and are enmeshed within the coagulating hematoma. Dead and devitalized tissues and hematoma constitute an ideal culture medium for the growth of all organisms and, if the external wound is an innocuous looking pin-point perforation of the skin, anaerobic growth in the deeper tissues may progress rapidly.

After the first few hours following injury, actual tissue invasion by organisms progresses inexorably. The status of the fracture area changes from contamination to infection with the rapidity dependent upon the extent of tissue death and the number and virulence of the organisms present in the wound.

During the contaminated phase, invasive infection can be prevented by excision of dead and devitalized tissues and wound lavage. The fracture can be reduced promptly. Following the onset of invasive infection, treatment consists of adequate surgical drainage in addition to debridement, and delay of fracture reduction may be necessary. The duration of the contaminated phase depends upon many variables and in the average open fracture is superseded by infection between 8 and 12 hours after injury. The "golden period" is the first 6 hours during which shock must be stabilized, infection prevented, and the fracture reduced.

WOUND MANAGEMENT

The objective of wound management is to prevent infection from occurring in a contaminated wound.

The skin of the wounded region is cleansed widely and as scrupulously as for a clean operation. The wound is covered with a sterile dressing so that the cleansing fluids do not run into the open wound. The surrounding skin is shaved. The damaged edges of the surface wound are excised mindful that skin is precious and essential to wound closure and only the crushed and devitalized skin edges should be removed. The skin incision must be long enough to lay open the full extent of the deep tissue lacerations. Similarly, all fascial envelopes must be opened widely enough for exposure of the depths of the wound from end to end. All dead and devitalized tissues must be removed. All foreign bodies, with the exception of certain imbedded or inaccessible missile fragments also need to be removed. Lacerated fascia and muscle may be widely excised. All bleeding points should be caught and ligated.

A muscle which does not bleed when cut or twitch when pinched with a forceps is dead and should be removed. Muscle which bleeds but does not twitch when pinched is alive but should be trimmed of all lacerated ends and separated fibers.

Essential structures—nerves, tendons, large blood vessels, and ligaments—should be cleansed mechanically; frayed areas should be trimmed economically, and the structures should be left in place.

Bone fragments completely free of soft parts may be removed if they are few and small. Large bone fragments, whether or not there are remaining soft part attachments, should be left in place. Bone is an essential structure. In general, it is better to err on the side of removing too little rather than too much. Dirty bone ends must be thoroughly cleansed, if necessary by a brush or a curette, removing the surface from which imbedded dirt cannot be removed.

The debrided wound cavity should be flushed clean by a mechanical lavage, from the depths outward, with copious amounts of warm saline. Lavage removes contaminating organisms and the many small separated particles of tissue which cannot be recognized, much less picked out.

Antibiotic agents do not prevent wound sepsis. They have no effect upon progressive tissue necrosis due to proteolytic enzymes or upon the decomposition of hematoma and dead tissue. Neither can they sterilize the dead tissue in a wound. These precursors of local infection must be eradicated by wound surgery. Antibiotic therapy should limit invasive infection and protect against septicemia. That it is commonly used from the start as a defense against infection does not alter these facts, but this practice has done considerable harm in encouraging a widespread misconception that modern wound surgery is less important and exacting for the prevention of local infection than it was in former years.

The inadequately excised wound is prone to sepsis with or without ancillary antibiotic therapy, and if a false sense of security has prompted closure of a wound, suppuration is apt to progress quietly under well-healed skin. Antibiotic protection will limit the spread of the infection, depress the systemic signs of suppuration and may save life; however, when a bag of pus finally becomes apparent several weeks after wounding, the limb may be in jeopardy.

The prevention of wound sepsis depends upon wound treatment; but control of infection depends upon adequate drainage supplemented by antibiotic therapy.

The attending physician must determine for each patient what prophylaxis for tetanus is required. Regardless of the active immunization status of the patient, meticulous surgical care, including removal of all devitalized tissue and foreign bodies, is to be provided immediately to all wounds. Such care is essential. Every patient should receive tetanus toxoid intramuscularly at the time of injury either as an initial immunizing dose or as a booster for previous immunization, unless he has received a booster or a full immunization series within the past 5 years. Whether to give human tetanus immune globulin for passive immunization must be decided for each patient. The character of the wound, the conditions under which it was incurred, and previous active immunization status must be considered. For complete details see page 37.

FRACTURE MANAGEMENT

The fracture fragments, which have been completely exposed in the course of wound treatment, should be reduced gently under direct vision. The type of fixation should be determined according to the mechanical problems of the injury. The safest method is a plaster cast or some form of traction.

If the wound is in satisfactory condition, the use of a metal implant to prevent the churning effect of moveable bone fragments which cannot be controlled by plaster of paris cast or traction is permissible and even desirable with one notable exception. Such an implant is contraindicated if it requires additional and extensive wound dissection which would open and expose clean fascial planes and tissues in a potentially contaminated wound. This statement implies that an "internal metal suture" such as a screw or two in an over-riding tibial fracture may do more good than harm, whereas an intramedullary rod in an open fracture of the femur may spread organisms throughout the femur and result in infection and disastrous sequelae. For this reason, the use of metal implants which entail extensive dissection and spreading of organisms thus predisposing to invasive infection is contraindicated as a primary method of fracture treatment. Once a clean, healed wound has been obtained, the indications for internal fixation are the same as for a closed fracture.

PRIMARY OR DELAYED PRIMARY WOUND CLOSURE

To close or not to close the incision is the final question requiring decision after wound and fracture treatment have been carried out. The dangers from sepsis in a wound that is closed are greater than in a wound left open. Therefore, primary closure is only permissible under ideal conditions. These include a lapse of only a few hours between injury and operation, minimal tissue damage, minimal contamination, adequate wound excision, good hemostasis, absence of dead space, and a skin incision which can be closed without tension.

Delayed primary wound closure is safer and advisable in the great majority of cases. At the conclusion of the operation the wound is left open. Between the third and sixth day after operation the wound is dressed under anesthesia. If sepsis is evident, the wound is already open and additional drainage can be provided as indicated. If the wound is healthy, delayed primary closure is performed by suture approximation of the skin edges. Delayed primary closure prior to the third day after operation is unsafe, and later than the sixth day is made difficult by tissue organization.

Whenever operation has been delayed more than 12 hours or tissue damage is severe or contamination extensive, the wound should not be closed primarily but should be left open and closed later or allowed to granulate pending revision or coverage by skin grafts at a later date.

Aftercare of an open fracture following wound healing should be similar to that for a closed fracture.

FRACTURE APHORISMS

1. The saving of life comes first; treat impending asphyxia, hemorrhage, shock and other life-endangering conditions before treating a fracture.
2. To minimize soft tissue damage and to avoid the conversion of a closed to an open fracture, "splint 'em where they lie."
3. Examine the injured part for signs of vascular and nerve injuries and record your findings.
4. Eliminate all unnecessary handling of the injured part. Disturb the patient as little as possible.
5. Never deliberately test for crepitus.
6. Make certain that the obvious fracture is the only fracture. There may be other fractures less apparent.
7. Do not be deceived by the absence of deformity and disability; in many cases of fracture, some ability to use the limb persists.
8. Treat every case of injury as a fracture until it is proved to be otherwise.
9. Obtain roentgenograms in at least two planes and examine them yourself.
10. Reduce the fracture with as little delay as possible. Do not wait for the swelling to go down.
11. Continued severe pain usually indicates circulatory constriction and requires immediate attention day or night.
12. In splitting a plaster cast, divide the plaster and the underlying padding to the last thread.
13. Make certain that continuous traction is checked frequently.
14. Immediately activate all joints that are not immobilized for treatment of the fracture.
15. Open fractures are contaminated wounds. Minimize the risk of

infection by adequate debridement, open drainage or closure of the wound as indicated, and immobilization.

16. The chief aim in the treatment of fractures of the upper extremity is to ensure the proper functioning of the hand. Shortening and some malalignment are often acceptable.

17. The chief aim in the treatment of fractures of the lower extremity is to ensure painless, stable weight bearing. Malalignment must be prevented, and full length is desirable.

18. Throughout the treatment of a fracture, focus attention on the patient as a whole as well as on the injured part.

Chapter 16

Fractures and Dislocations in Adults

FRACTURES AND DISLOCATIONS OF THE UPPER EXTREMITY

210

Smith's or reversed Colles' fracture
Barton's or marginal fractures
Fractures of the carpus
    Fractures of the navicular bone
Dislocations of the carpus
    Dislocation of the lunate
    Perilunar dislocation
    Midcarpal dislocation

Fractures and dislocations of the hand
Fractures and dislocations of the thumb including the first metacarpal
    Fracture of the base of the first metacarpal
    Bennett's fracture
    Fractures of the shaft of the first metacarpal
    Dislocation of the metacarpophalangeal joint
    Fractures of the phalanges of the thumb
Fractures of the finger metacarpals
    Fractures of the shafts
    Fractures of the necks of metacarpals
Fractures and dislocations of the phalanges of the fingers
    Dislocations of the metacarpophalangeal joints
    Dislocations of the proximal interphalangeal joint
    Fractures of the proximal phalanx
    Fractures of the middle phalanx
    Fractures of the distal phalanx
    Mallet or baseball finger (or fracture)
    Chip fractures

FRACTURES AND DISLOCATIONS ABOUT THE SHOULDER

Throughout the course of treatment of each of these injuries, edema of the hand must be avoided and active exercises of the figures must be carried out as much as possible to maintain the maximum function of the hand, which is the principal objective of the management of all injuries of the upper extremity. Pendulum exercises of the shoulder should be initiated as soon as practicable to maintain a normal range of motion in this joint (Fig. 16–1).

FRACTURES OF THE CLAVICLE

The clavicle acts as a strut for the shoulder so that it remains upward, outward, and backward in relation to the chest wall. With a fracture of the clavicle, the shoulder drops downward, forward, and inward (Fig. 16–2). Fractures of the clavicle may result from falls on the outstretched hand or the shoulder or from direct blows. The majority occur in the middle third.

Treatment: An entirely satisfactory method of holding a fracture of the clavicle in good reduction is yet to be devised. As a result, many methods have been tried and recommended. Each method attempts to hold the shoulder upward, outward, and backward, and to provide immobilization of the fracture. Each, therefore, is an application of the closed

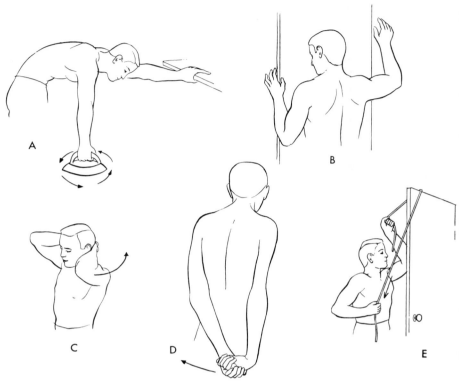

Figure 16–1 Mobilization of injured and painful shoulder.

A, Gravity-free pendulum exercises are more comfortable and efficient with a weight in the hand.

B, Crawling up the wall, assisted elevation; a strip of adhesive is placed on the wall to be marked in pencil as a record of the elevation attained each day.

C, Exercise for restoration of external rotation.

D, Exercise for restoration of internal rotation.

E, The normal extremity assists in elevation of the injured member. (From McLaughlin, *Trauma.* Philadelphia, W. B. Saunders, 1959.)

reduction and immobilization method. Open reduction and internal fixation, the only other method that might be considered, is rarely indicated. This method has resulted in a high incidence of complications, including many nonunions.

A simple and effective way to hold adequate reduction and provide immobilization is to use a figure-of-eight clavicular strap of one of the major splint manufacturers (Fig. 16–2). The strap requires adequate padding of both the anterior and posterior axillary folds on each side. A clavicular strap is applied easily about the shoulders and permits tightening or loosening as needed.

Other appliances for holding adequate reduction include a figure-of-eight plaster cast about the shoulders (Fig. 16–3), a T-splint (sometimes

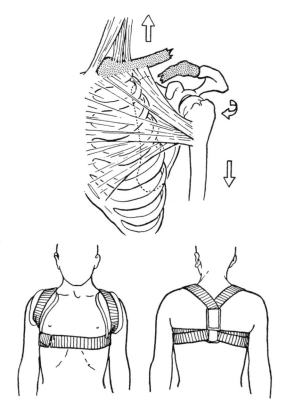

Figure 16–2 Fracture of the clavicle. *Top,* The shoulder drops forward, inward, and downward, resulting in over-riding of the fragments. *Bottom,* Immobilization by the standard clavicular strap which tends to hold the shoulder upward, backward, and outward. (From Rhodes, J. E., Allen, J. G., Harkins, H. N., and Moyer, C. A.: *Surgery, Principles and Practice.* 4th Edition. Philadelphia, J. B. Lippincott Co., 1970. Reprinted by permission.)

called a clavicular cross), and even a simple figure-of-eight soft roller bandage which can be fashioned from split 2-inch stockinet.

Solid union of the clavicle with an excellent functional result may be anticipated with any of the appliances, since nonunion of a fracture of the clavicle is uncommon. Union usually occurs, however, with some visible or palpable prominence at the fracture site.

Fractures of the clavicle must be splinted until union has occurred, which in adults usually requires 4 to 6 weeks and sometimes longer. Preferably strapping is maintained for 5 to 6 weeks, but during the last week or 10 days the patient may be given permission to remove it at home for bathing, after which it is reapplied.

FRACTURES OF THE SCAPULA

Fractures of the body of the scapula result infrequently from direct blows. Considerable comminution may occur. A heavy fall or blow on the point of the shoulder may cause a fracture of the neck of the scapula. The lateral fragment containing the glenoid is driven medially and often is impacted firmly into the body.

Treatment: Fractures of the body of the scapula require very little

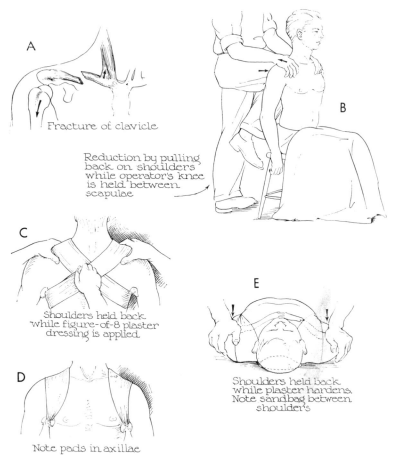

A, Fracture of clavicle

Reduction by pulling back on shoulders while operator's knee is held between scapulae

B

C

Shoulders held back while figure-of-8 plaster dressing is applied

E

D

Shoulders held back while plaster hardens. Note sandbag between shoulders

Note pads in axillae

Figure 16–3   Use of figure-of-eight plaster of Paris cast about the shoulders for fracture of the clavicle. *A*, Fracture of the middle third of the clavicle. *B*, The operator hyperextends the shoulders using his knee to support the trunk. *C*, Assistant applies a figure-of-eight plaster cast about the shoulders making certain that (*D*) the axillae are well padded. *E*, While the plaster is setting, the shoulders are held in hyperextension over a sandbag placed between the shoulder blades. (From Banks and Compere: *Pictorial Handbook of Fracture Treatment*, 5th Edition. Chicago, Yearbook Medical Publishers, 1963. Reprinted by permission.)

treatment. Pain may be alleviated by a sling or a sling and swathe holding the extremity to the chest. Pendulum exercises of the shoulder and exercises of all of the joints of the upper extremity should be initiated as soon as practicable.

Impacted fractures of the neck of the scapula also may be managed satisfactorily by a sling, with or without a swathe. Manual or skeletal lateral traction to disimpact the fracture is usually futile. Minimal immobilization and early active exercise of the shoulder lead to excellent results.

FRACTURES OF THE PROXIMAL END OF THE HUMERUS

Fractures of the proximal end of the humerus usually result from a fall on the outstretched hand or on the elbow. They are classified as either adduction or abduction fractures, depending upon whether the force causes the arm to go into adduction with lateral angulation or abduction with medial angulation. Either type may be firmly impacted or show minimal or severe comminution. While fractures of the upper humerus may occur at any age, usually they occur in the elderly.

Treatment: The majority of fractures, either of the anatomic or the surgical neck, are impacted (Fig. 16–4). For practical purposes, the position of the fragments should be accepted. An effort to disengage the fragments and improve their position is not recommended. Better and more prompt functional end-results will be obtained by accepting the position of impaction.

Impacted fractures of the upper humerus are managed by the no-im-

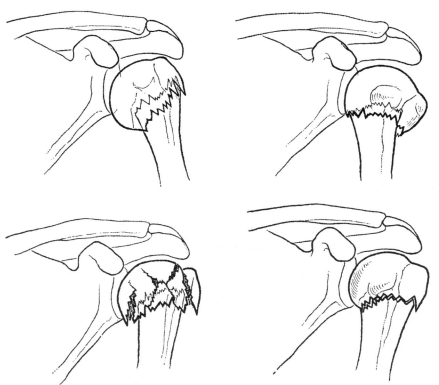

Figure 16–4   Varieties and contours of impacted fractures of the surgical neck of the humerus. (From DePalma: *The Management of Fractures and Dislocations — An Atlas,* 2nd Edition. Philadelphia, W. B. Saunders, 1970.)

mobilization method. Pain may be alleviated by supporting the extremity in a sling, perhaps supplemented by a swathe for a few days. Within less than a week, however, the swathe and, soon thereafter, the sling should be eliminated. Pendulum exercises in and out of the sling should be initiated within less than a week after injury and carried out energetically during the entire course of treatment. Under this regimen, the majority of patients will have partial use of the extremity within 2½ to 3 weeks after injury, but many months may elapse before a fuller range of motion in the shoulder is obtained. The patient, therefore, should not discontinue shoulder exercises merely because free use of the elbow, forearm, and hand has been obtained (Fig. 16–1).

Unimpacted fractures of the proximal end of the humerus in satisfactory position are managed almost as if they were firmly impacted. A sling and swathe are advisable and may be needed for 10 or 12 days after injury or until the head and shaft move as a unit. Thereafter, the bandage and the sling should be eliminated to permit active exercise as described for impacted fractures.

Displaced unimpacted fractures of the upper end of the humerus may require more aggressive treatment. Closed reduction with a longer period of immobilization or even continuous traction in some form may be necessary. The surgeon should be certain, however, that the amount of displacement warrants the application of either method. Excellent functional results may be obtained with minimal apposition and some alteration in alignment of the fragments.

Manipulative closed reduction almost always requires general anesthesia. Strong traction is applied at the flexed elbow against counter traction provided by an assistant pulling on a sheet looped through the axilla. The adducted proximal end of the distal fragment is forced laterally into apposition with the proximal fragment (Fig. 16–5). Strong steady traction often results in correction of the position of the proximal fragment.

Following satisfactory reduction of the fracture, immobilization using a sling and swathe to hold the extremity against the chest wall usually is adequate. The immobilizing dressing should remain in place for about 3 weeks. A sling may be necessary for an additional week. As soon as practicable, circumduction exercises of the shoulder should be initiated. Their intensity should be increased steadily as union of the fracture progresses.

If efforts at manipulative reduction are unsuccessful, continuous skeletal traction may be necessary, particularly in young adults. A wire is inserted through the olecranon and traction is made with the arm in forward flexion to 90 degrees and adduction with the elbow flexed to a right angle as illustrated in Figure 16–6. In some instances, the proximal fragment is abducted and externally rotated. In these, traction is made with the arm resting on the bed in abduction and external rotation as illustrated in Figure 16–13.

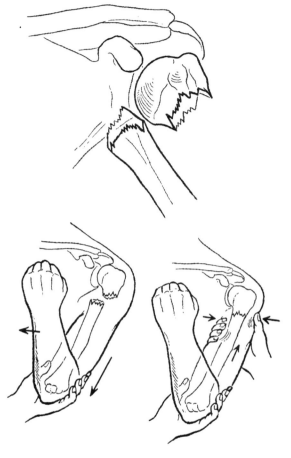

Figure 16–5 Displaced fracture of the proximal portion of the humerus and the maneuvers for its reduction. (From De-Palma.)

Some surgeons believe that the traction effect of a hanging cast or "collar-and-cuff" sling (Fig. 17–9) will lead to reduction of fractures of the proximal humerus because the tendon of the long head of the biceps rotates the proximal fragment into alignment. With either, manipulation may help in obtaining reduction.

FRACTURES OF THE GREATER TUBEROSITY

Isolated fractures of the greater tuberosity are sustained not infrequently, either from a fall on the point of the shoulder or when the humerus is forcibly abducted so that the greater tuberosity impinges on the acromion. Treatment depends upon the degree of displacement.

Undisplaced fractures require very little treatment. A sling may be employed for a few days for comfort, but early active exercise of the shoulder is indicated. If displacement does not result from the original trauma, it will not occur later. The postoperative regimen conforms to that for undisplaced fractures.

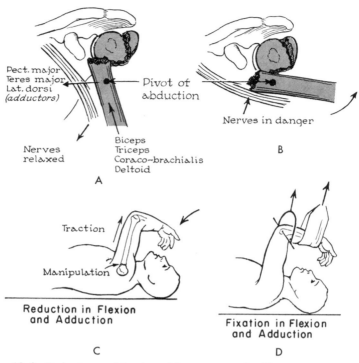

Figure 16–6   Reduction and fixation of fracture at neck of humerus.

A, The shaft fragment is pulled medialward by the adductor muscles. Shortening is produced by the long muscles of the arm. The pivot of shaft abduction is lowered from the humeral head to the level of the pectoral insertion.

B, Abduction tightens pectoral muscle, hinders reduction, and tilts the proximal end of the shaft fragment further into the axilla.

C, Reduction by overcoming shortening and manipulative correction of displacement should be done with the arm flexed and adducted for relaxation of the displacing muscles.

D, Fixation requires continued pectoral relaxation by continued flexion and adduction; humeral length is maintained by skeletal traction. (From McLaughlin.)

Minimally displaced fractures of the greater tuberosity usually should be managed as if no displacement had occurred. In those with upward displacement of more than 1 cm, open reduction and internal fixation of the fragment is usually indicated (see page 221).

DISLOCATIONS OF THE SHOULDER

Dislocation of the glenohumeral joint, the most common dislocation of a major joint, occurs from forced abduction and external rotation of the arm until the humeral head is levered downward out of the glenoid cavity. After it has torn through the inferior portion of the capsule of the shoulder joint, the head of the humerus may come to rest anteriorly beneath the coracoid process (subcoracoid dislocation, the most common), inferior to

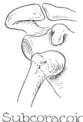 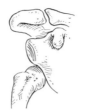 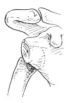

Subcoracoid   Subglenoid   Subspinous
dislocation   dislocation   dislocation(rare)

Figure 16-7   Position assumed by the head of the humerus in (left to right) subcoracoid, subglenoid, and subspinous (posterior) dislocation of the shoulder. (From Banks and Compere.)

the glenoid (subglenoid dislocation) or posteriorly (quite rare) behind the glenoid (posterior or subspinous dislocation) (Fig. 16-7).

Several salient diagnostic features characterize a subcoracoid or a subglenoid dislocation of the shoulder. The acromion is prominent and there is a visible and palpable absence of the subacromial fullness normally produced by the humeral head. The long axis of the arm points to the base of the neck. Pain is severe and little movement of the shoulder is possible. The displaced humeral head may be palpated deep to the pectoral mass. The elbow cannot be made to touch the side and the hand cannot be placed on the opposite shoulder unless there is an associated fracture of the humerus. The physical examination and the diagnosis are not complete until the neurologic and vascular status of the limb have been assessed.

While these signs often permit accurate clinical diagnosis and occasionally one may be tempted to perform a manipulative reduction without x-ray examination, good practice calls for a prereduction roentgenogram to confirm the diagnosis and to learn whether a complicating fracture of the greater tuberosity or other humeral injury is present. Occasionally, x-ray films will reveal the distressing complication of a displaced fracture of the neck of the humerus combined with dislocation of the humeral head. This complex injury is discussed later.

Treatment: Reduction of the dislocation at times may be accomplished without anesthesia or under the sedation of an opiate, but general anesthesia is preferable. The relaxation provided by general anesthesia usually makes reduction easy and minimizes the risk of the manipulations which might produce a fracture of the surgical neck of the humerus or further soft tissue damage.

Technique of Reduction: Dislocation of the shoulder may be reduced in several ways. All methods attempt to return the humeral head just inferior to the glenoid and then to cause it to re-enter the joint through the rent in the capsule. Each method offers advantages and disadvantages.

Straight traction without manipulation will reduce the majority of dislocated shoulders. Traction may be made at the wrist with the forearm extended or at the elbow with the forearm flexed. Counter-traction is provided by an assistant pulling on a folded sheet looped through the axilla. Traction is made first in the line of the position assumed by the arm (slight abduction). While traction is maintained, the arm is slightly adducted. If reduction is not obtained immediately, inward and outward rotation of the arm while traction is maintained may effect reduction.

If straight traction does not result in reduction, Kocher maneuvers may be used as illustrated in Figure 16–8. Fundamental maneuvers include traction on the flexed elbow with the arm first in slight abduction, then external rotation. Then the arm is adducted and finally rotated into full internal rotation, which should obtain reduction. During all the maneuvers, steady traction is maintained. Kocher maneuvers, while usually effective, are not without danger. The rotations, particularly, must be carried out without undue force lest the humerus be fractured through the surgical neck, a disheartening complication.

The Hippocratic maneuver, which is hazardous because the axillary vessels and nerves may be injured, is an alternative traction method. The shoeless heel of the surgeon is forced into the axilla for counter-traction, while straight traction on the extremity is applied at the wrist with the elbow extended. The pressure of the surgeon's heel against the humeral head is thought to aid in forcing it back into the joint.

Reduction may be obtained without anesthesia (perhaps with the usual

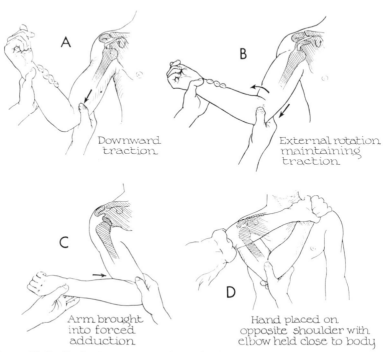

A   Downward
    traction

B   External rotation
    maintaining
    traction

C   Arm brought
    into forced
    adduction

D   Hand placed on
    opposite shoulder with
    elbow held close to body

Figure 16–8 Kocher's maneuvers for reduction of an anterior (subcoracoid or subglenoid) dislocation of the shoulder. (From Banks and Compere.)

dose of opiate) by using Stimson's method. The patient is placed facedown with the injured extremity hanging over the side of the table. This position is comfortable for the patient. A weight (8 to 10 pounds) is tied to the wrist for traction. Spasm of the shoulder muscles subsides as pain is relieved. After the extremity has been in traction for several minutes, reduction may occur spontaneously or after the shoulder has been gently rotated by the surgeon.

Postreduction Management: Authorities on dislocations of the shoulder do not agree on postoperative management. Some consider immobilization of the arm and shoulder to be of no value, while others insist on immobilization for some 6 weeks. A middle-of-the-road course is 3 to 4 weeks of immobilization in a sling and swathe. This course appears preferable for dislocations of the shoulder in patients under 40 year of age, in whom recurrent dislocation is the most common. For patients over 40 years of age, immobilization for 7 to 14 days is adequate. Recurrent dislocation in the latter decades of life is rare, and, therefore, all immobilization should be discontinued just as soon as comfort of the patient permits. Active pendulum exercises should be initiated early to prevent residual stiffness of the shoulder.

Complications of Dislocations of the Shoulder: These include fractures of the greater tuberosity, fractures of the surgical neck with displacement, damage to the axillary nerve, damage to the axillary vessels or accompanying nerve trunks, and recurrent dislocation of the shoulder (a delayed complication concerning which reference is made to standard textbooks on orthopaedic surgery).

FRACTURES OF THE GREATER TUBEROSITY OF THE HUMERUS: This complication of dislocated shoulders rarely occurs in young adults but does occur in 20 to 30 per cent of older patients. Reduction of the dislocation usually is accompanied by spontaneous anatomical reduction of the tuberosity fragment because the musculotendinous cuff and periosteal sleeve have remained intact. Treatment of the dislocation suffices for the fracture. Recurrent dislocation is a rare development when a fracture of the greater tuberosity has accompanied a dislocation of the shoulder.

When the fragment of greater tuberosity is not reduced concurrently with the dislocation, the fragment remains displaced superiorly which indicates that the musculotendinous cuff and the periosteal sleeve have been torn (Fig. 16–9). Operation is indicated to fix the fragment in accurate reduction and to repair the torn musculotendinous cuff. Postoperative management is the same as for dislocation of the shoulder without fracture.

FRACTURE-DISLOCATION OF THE SHOULDER: This complex lesion, which is rare in young adults, results from the same mechanisms which produce fractures of the upper humerus without dislocation, or dislocations of the shoulder without fracture. The fragment of head is extruded from the capsular cavity. It may consist of a single fragment essentially

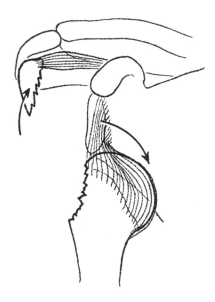

Figure 16–9 Anterior dislocation of the shoulder with a complicating fracture of the greater tubercle which is widely separated indicating a complete tear in the musculotendinous cuff. (From DePalma.)

devoid of soft part attachments. It may be comminuted with the greater and lesser tubercles as separate fragments.

Treatment often is exceedingly difficult. Occasionally when some continuity of the periosteal sleeve is maintained, reduction may be achieved by steady traction on the extremity and direct pressure on the displaced humeral head. When the displaced humeral head has no soft tissue attachments, efforts at closed reduction are almost always unsuccessful and operative reduction is indicated. Even at operation, reduction is often difficult. The postoperative regimen is comparable with that described for displaced fractures of the surgical neck which have been reduced by manipulation (see page 216).

The results of both open and closed reductions of fracture-dislocations of the shoulder are poor. The incidence of late avascular necrosis of the humeral head is high regardless of the method of reduction. Operative replacement of the humeral head by a prosthesis merits consideration by experienced surgeons as a primary treatment when a single head fragment devoid of soft tissue attachments has been dislocated. If the lesser tubercle has remained attached to the head, however, the humeral head should always be preserved as it may not undergo avascular necrosis.

INJURY TO BLOOD VESSELS OR NERVES: Damage to the axillary nerve by the humeral head as it leaves the shoulder joint is a rather frequent complication, occurring in about 15 per cent of dislocations. The nerve injury causes anesthesia in the sensory distribution of the axillary nerve and paralysis of the deltoid muscle. Fortunately, the prognosis is usually good. The nerve is usually only bruised and not torn, so recovery is spontaneous.

Occasionally, signs of trauma to the axillary vessels and large nerve trunks are present. Usually nerves are merely bruised and not torn, so motor or sensory nerve deficits may be expected to disappear spontaneously. If signs of impaired arterial flow are present, immediate operation to explore and repair the axillary artery is indicated.

ACROMIOCLAVICULAR DISLOCATIONS

Acromioclavicular separations or dislocations result from falls on the point of the shoulder. They may be either complete or incomplete. Complete lesions are described as complete separations or dislocations. Incomplete lesions are called subluxations or incomplete dislocations.

The stability of the acromioclavicular joint depends upon the strong coracoclavicular and the acromioclavicular ligaments. In complete dislocations, both are torn so that the outer end of the clavicle goes upward and backward. In incomplete dislocations or subluxations, the acromioclavicular ligaments are torn to some degree but the coracoclavicular ligament is not torn significantly.

Treatment: Subluxations or incomplete dislocations require very little treatment. An attempt may be made to stabilize the outer end of the clavicle with adhesive strapping over a felt pad applied over the outer end of the clavicle and a sling applied to lift the arm and shoulder. These procedures probably are of little benefit, but they may minimize pain about the injured joint. Certainly, prolonged immobilization is not necessary. The prognosis is good, although the outer end of the calvicle may remain somewhat prominent and perhaps a bit loose. These injuries should be undertreated rather than overtreated.

Complete dislocations (Fig. 16–10) usually require operative manage-

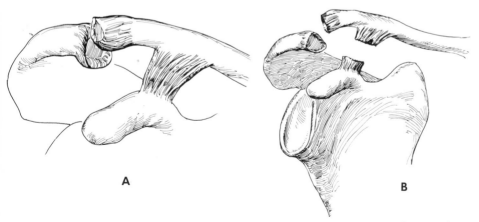

A   **B**

Figure 16–10   *A*, Incomplete subluxation of the acromioclavicular joint. The acromioclavicular ligaments are torn but the corococlavicular ligament remains intact. *B*, A complete dislocation of the acromioclavicular joint. All supporting ligaments have been disrupted leading to wide separation between the clavicle and acromion. (Modified from Davis: *Christopher's Textbook of Surgery.* 9th Edition. Philadelphia, W. B. Saunders, 1968.)

ment. Although many cumbersome pieces of apparatus and methods of immobilization have been described for nonoperative management of these injuries, none is likely to be effective. All are exceedingly uncomfortable. With open reduction, chips of bone and cartilage may be removed from the acromioclavicular joint and tags of torn ligament released and sutured. Stabilizing internal fixation must be employed. Two pins may be inserted through the acromion and down the medullary canal of the clavicle. The pins are removed after healing about 6 weeks later. A lag screw which passes through the clavicle into the coracoid process may be used. With good fixation, only a sling is necessary. Early pendulum exercises may be initiated. The lag screw should be removed about 6 or 8 weeks after it is inserted. With early operative stabilization of complete dislocations of the acromioclavicular joint, the result should be a normal or near normal shoulder.

FRACTURES OF THE SHAFT OF THE HUMERUS

The humeral shaft extends from about 2 inches below the shoulder to about 2 inches above the elbow. The blood supply of the shaft is not as good as that near the shoulder and elbow. The radial nerve is in close contact as it coils around the humeral shaft in the musculoskeletal groove and is susceptible to injury when the bone is fractured.

Fractures of the humeral shaft may be caused by a direct blow, excessive torsion, or undue leverage on the arm when the shoulder is relatively fixed. They may be transverse, spiral, oblique, or comminuted.

Several strong muscles or muscle groups may cause displacement and angulation of fractures of the humeral shaft. The pectoralis major muscle may adduct and the deltoid muscle may abduct the fragments to which they attach (Fig. 16–11). The forearm muscles arising from the medial and the lateral condyles may cause angulation of the lower fragment in fractures of the lower shaft.

TREATMENT

The majority of fractures of the shaft of the humerus respond satisfactorily to a **hanging cast** (Fig. 16–12). This method is not closed reduction and immobilization but continuous traction. The hanging cast is applied with the elbow flexed to a right angle and extends from the level of the humeral fracture (not above it) to the midpart of the hand. The weight of the cast as it hangs provides continuous traction which leads to relaxation of the several muscle groups affecting the fragments and usually produces adequate apposition and satisfactory alignment. Obviously, the patient must sit or stand for the traction to be most effective. However, traction may be provided when the patient is recumbent by means of a weight on the end of a rope tied to a loop at the elbow and passing over a pulley at the foot of the bed.

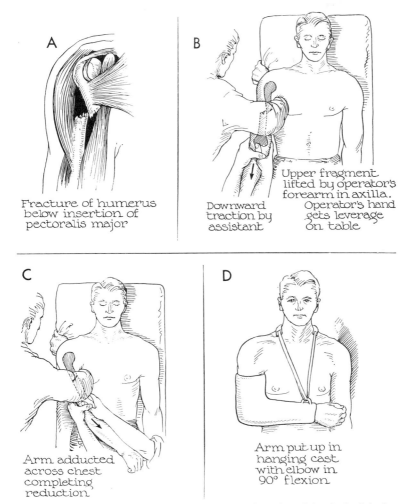

A

Fracture of humerus
below insertion of
pectoralis major

B

Downward
traction by
assistant

Upper fragment
lifted by operator's
forearm in axilla.
Operator's hand
gets leverage
on table

C

Arm adducted
across chest
completing
reduction

D

Arm put up in
hanging cast
with elbow in
90° flexion

Figure 16–11 *A*, Displaced fracture of the proximal portion of the shaft of the humerus.
B, Manipulative maneuvers for reduction. *C*, Reduction is completed as the arm is adducted
across the chest. *D*, Reduction is maintained in a hanging cast with the elbow flexed to 90
degrees. (From Banks and Compere.)

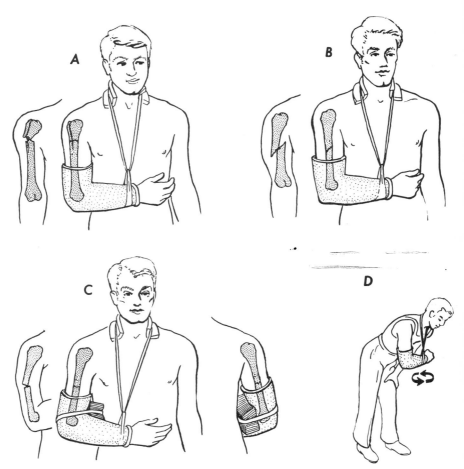

Figure 16–12 Treatment of fractures of the shaft of the humerus with a hanging cast. *A*, An angulated fracture of the proximal portion of the shaft which is corrected by the traction provided by a hanging cast. *B*, Oblique fracture of the middle third of the shaft with considerable displacement which is corrected by the traction provided by a hanging cast. *C*, Fracture of the middle third of the shaft of the humerus in a hanging cast. Lateral angulation is corrected by large pad placed on the inner side of the cast at the elbow. *D*, Circumduction exercises of the shoulder should be carried out diligently to avoid restriction of motion in that joint. (From Rhodes, Allen, Harkins, and Moyer.)

A hanging cast should be applied with the extremity held as much as possible in the position in which it will hang later when the patient sits or stands. Hanging casts applied with the arm in the hanging position are always more comfortable. Usually anesthesia is not required as the hanging position may be expected to provide sufficient relief from pain. The cast must not be heavy enough to distract the fragments. A loop sling is passed through a loop of plaster or wire at the wrist and tied around the neck. Another loop at the elbow will facilitate traction during periods of recumbency as described above.

Check **roentgenograms** should be made at intervals of 4 and 7 days during the first few weeks to be certain that the fragments remain in good reduction. Anterior or posterior angulation at the fracture site indicates that the level of the wrist should be raised or lowered by changing the length of the sling about the neck. Occasionally, medial or lateral angulation may be corrected by moving the wrist loop inward or outward or by pads of sponge rubber or felt taped on the inner side of the upper end of the cast or at the inner side of the elbow as indicated (Fig. 16–12C). Sometimes angulation of fractures at the junction of the middle and lower thirds may be corrected by changing the cast and providing more pronation or supination of the forearm. Occasionally distraction of the fragments may necessitate substitution of a shoulder spica for the hanging cast. Some surgeons abhor the hanging cast for fractures of the shaft of the humerus and prefer a mere collar-and-cuff sling which also is a traction method.

As a rule, **gentle swinging exercises** of the shoulder should be instituted within a few days (Fig. 16–12D). If the patient leans well forward while the extremity remains suspended by the loop sling, the alignment of the fracture is not disturbed. Shoulder exercises during the period of healing is a distinct advantage of the hanging cast. Other methods mentioned below do not permit these exercises and often result in loss of motion in the shoulder joint.

Other methods of treatment for fractures of the humeral shaft include a sling and swathe, a shoulder spica cast, skeletal traction with the arm abducted from the side and with the forearm suspended from above (Fig. 16–13), and open reduction and internal fixation. The **sling and swathe** are applicable when the fragments are minimally displaced and assume good alignment when the arm is placed against the chest wall. About the

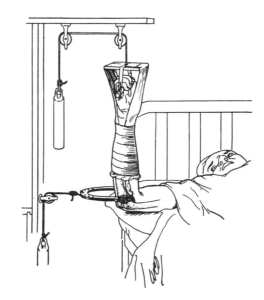

Figure 16–13 Continuous balanced skeletal traction for fractures of the shaft of the humerus. (From Davis.)

only indication for a **shoulder spica cast** is when distraction of the fragments follows traction in a hanging cast or collar-and-cuff sling. When other injuries or diseases confine the patient to bed, **skeletal traction** may be indicated.

Open reduction and internal fixation occasionally are advisable when other methods have not resulted in adequate reduction. These procedures, however, do not insure a united fracture as they have been shown to carry a high incidence of nonunion. When muscle is interposed between fragment ends and when displacement and deformity cannot be overcome, open reduction is called for. In fractures of the humeral shaft complicated by signs and symptoms of a radial nerve paralysis, early open reduction may be indicated to make certain that the nerve is free from impingement by the fragments although the prognosis for spontaneous recovery of nerve function is good without operative intervention.

When a hanging cast is used, it is left in place until sufficient clinical and x-ray evidence of union make traction no longer necessary. Then a sling and swathe or collar-and-cuff sling may be substituted until union is solid. Healing of fractures of the humeral shaft usually requires from 8 to 12 weeks. When skeletal traction in recumbency is used, it is continued until the patient is ambulatory and then one of the other methods is substituted. When internal fixation is employed, a sling and swathe or a light hanging cast is advisable until the fracture is united.

NERVE INJURIES

The radial nerve in the musculospiral groove is particularly susceptible to injury by fragments of the humerus. Rarely, the median or ulnar nerve may be injured. As in all extremity injuries, at the first examination, the physician must determine whether a deficit in the sensory and motor function of the major peripheral nerve trunks is present. This is easily done by observing the various movements of the fingers and thumb and by testing for sensation of the hand. If signs of nerve paralysis are present when the patient is first seen, open reduction and internal fixation of the fracture may be worthwhile.

The function of the major peripheral nerves, especially of the radial nerve, must be verified again after the extremity has been placed in a hanging cast or skeletal traction, or has been operated upon. Signs indicating nerve damage suggest trauma to the nerve during manipulation of the fragments.

FRACTURES AND DISLOCATIONS ABOUT THE ELBOW

COMPLICATIONS

Severe early complications may be associated with fractures or dislocations in the region of the elbow. The anatomical relationships place muscles over the front of the joint, with a complete envelope of nonelastic fascia surrounding the entire area. When a displaced fracture occurs, periosteum and muscles are torn. Bleeding ensues which may lead to pressure beneath the fascial sleeve, first upon the veins and then the arteries and may shut off the circulation to and from the forearm and hand. As extreme swelling develops, the pulse becomes weak at the wrist, the hand becomes cool and pale, and all motor and sensory function is impaired or lost. If this situation is not relieved promptly, Volkmann's ischemic paralysis develops. One should be aware of the four P's: *pain, pallor, pulselessness,* and *paralysis.* When these findings persist, the process becomes irreversible (see page 349).

Nerve injuries also may occur with dislocations or fractures about the elbow, or they may occur during reduction or subsequent treatment. In closed injuries, the nerve injury usually is a contusion or stretching, but a nerve may be caught between bone fragments. It is therefore imperative that the function of the three nerves (radial, median, and ulnar) be tested for both motor and sensory deficits at the initial examination and again after reduction has been accomplished. Accurate records must be kept of the results of each testing.

FRACTURES OF THE LOWER END OF THE HUMERUS

Transverse Supracondylar Fractures: These are not common fractures in adults. Usually, mild posterior displacement of the distal fragment occurs, perhaps with slight medial or lateral shift. Posterior displacement in adults is rarely as severe as in children. Accurate reduction is not essential. Frequently applying a posterior plaster slab and a sling for about 3 or 4 weeks will suffice. In that time, the fracture becomes "stuck" so that gentle active exercises may be instituted without fear of further displacement, particularly if a sling is used for an additional week to guard against full extension.

T- or Y-shaped Fractures of the Lower Humerus (Intercondylar or Dicondylar):   These fractures result from a blow or a fall directly on the elbow. The trauma causes the olecranon to wedge the two condyles apart and away from the shaft of the humerus. Marked displacement is common with the condylar fragments widely separated and often tilted downward at different angles. Satisfactory motion in the joint cannot be expected unless the fragments are adequately reduced.

If the fragments are of substantial size and particularly if the patient is young or middle-aged, open reduction and internal fixation with screws or small pins may be required (Fig. 16–14). Stable fixation of the fragments in good position will permit early active exercises which are essential for satisfactory elbow function. If the patient is elderly or the fracture is so badly comminuted that adequate reduction and fixation are impossible even with operation, continuous traction using a Kirschner wire through the ole-

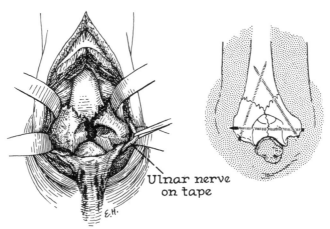

Ulnar nerve
on tape

Figure 16–14 Displaced supracondylar T- or Y-fracture of the humerus as visualized at open reduction. The precisely reduced fracture is maintained by internal fixation with multiple pins. (From Hampton and Fitts: *Open Reduction of Common Fractures.* New York, Grune and Stratton, 1959. Reprinted by permission.)

cranon with the arm elevated anteriorly may be preferable. Traction tends to pull the fragments into better position, and gentle active exercises may be started with the arm in traction. It is inadvisable to keep some elderly patients on their backs in traction for 3 or 4 weeks for fear of pneumonia or other complications. In such instances, the position of the fragments may be ignored and the patient allowed up with the arm in a sling, or in a hanging cast for 2 or 3 weeks (Fig. 16–15). Active exercises should be started as soon as practicable. Often a patient may recover satisfactory elbow function without reduction of these fractures.

Fractures of the Medial or Lateral Condyle: In adults, fractures of the medial condyle are rare; those of the lateral condyle are more common. Undisplaced fractures require only a plaster cast for a few weeks. If adequate closed reduction of displaced fractures of either condyle cannot be obtained readily, open reduction and internal fixation with two or more screws or Kirschner wires is advisable. Postoperatively, a sling for immobilization may be adequate. A posterior plaster splint may be used as a supplement to the sling. Active exercises after a week to 10 days are permitted commensurate with the stability of the internal fixation.

Fractures of the Capitellum: These are uncommon but serious fractures. The capitellar fragment is usually displaced proximally or is rotated 90 degrees forward (Fig. 16–16). Unless this fragment is removed or replaced, elbow motion will be poor. A capitellar fracture involves the anterior half of the capitellum and, therefore, is covered with articular cartilage. Frequently the line of fracture extends medially into the lateral aspect of the trochlear process.

The fragment of capitellum usually should be removed at operation because it no longer has soft tissue attachment or blood supply, and even if

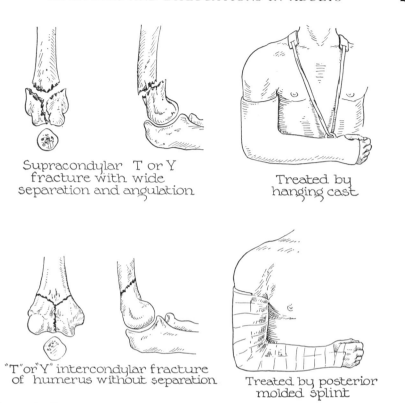

Supracondylar T or Y
fracture with wide
separation and angulation

Treated by
hanging cast

"T" or "Y" intercondylar fracture
of humerus without separation

Treated by posterior
molded splint

Figure 16–15 Supracondylar T- or Y-fracture of the humerus reduced by the traction provided by hanging cast, and similar fracture without separation immobilized by a posterior molded plaster splint to be supported by sling. (From Bands and Compere.)

reduced, it is likely to undergo avascular necrosis. Further difficulty with the elbow will result. If the fragment is so large that removal is certain to leave an unstable elbow, it may be reduced and fixed in position at operation in an effort to achieve a good functional result, even though the prognosis is not good.

Fractures of the Medial Epicondyle: Fractures of the medial epicondyle in the adult are rare. Generally they occur from a direct blow on

Figure 16–16 *A*, Capitellar fragment displaced proximally. *B*, Capitellar fragment rotated 90 degrees forward.

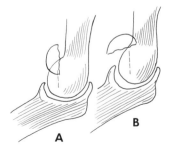

the inner side of the elbow. Unless the fragment is widely displaced, the best treatment is support of the extremity in a sling for a week to 10 days. If the fragment is widely displaced, operative fixation in good position will re-anchor the origin of the flexor muscles of the forearm.

FRACTURES OF THE OLECRANON

These fractures result from falls or blows on the back of the elbow. They may be undisplaced or separated and displaced. In undisplaced fractures, extensor power of the elbow is not lost. The joint becomes filled with blood and may be quite painful. The best treatment is aspiration of the he-marthrosis to relieve pain, and immobilization of the elbow at 90 degrees 7 to 10 days in a sling, perhaps supplemented by a posterior molded plaster splint. Thereafter, the sling should be removed several times daily for warm soaks and mild active exercise of the elbow. Full return of function may be anticipated.

When fractures are separated, extensor power of the elbow is lost. The fascial expansions of the triceps tendon are torn on one or both sides. Operation is necessary, therefore, to replace and fix the fragment and to repair the torn triceps expansions. The bony fragment is fixed internally, either with a 3- to 3½-inch wood screw, a lag screw, or a loop of large cali-ber wire. The torn triceps expansions may be repaired with any suture material. If the proximal fragment is severely comminuted, excision is acceptable. Then, the triceps tendon is attached to the proximal end of the distal ulnar fragment and the torn expansion is repaired. Postoperatively, a sling will suffice for immobilization. Minimal immobilization permits con-trolled early exercise.

FRACTURES OF THE HEAD AND NECK OF THE RADIUS

Fractures of the radial head are of three categories: undisplaced, displaced single fragment, and comminuted fractures (Fig. 16–17).

An undisplaced fracture may be a mere crack (chisel-type), so that diagnosis on the initial x-ray films may be difficult. Clinically, a fracture of the radial head may be suspected because the joint is distended with blood, producing considerable pain. Treatment is aspiration of the elbow joint and complete arm rest in a sling for about 48 hours followed by warm soaks and active exercises. Roentgenograms made 2 to 3 weeks later may demon-strate the fracture line.

When a single fragment of the radial head is displaced (Fig. 16–17B), the entire radial head usually should be excised. In selected instances when the line of fracture is away from the articulation with the radial notch of the ulna, excision of the fragment may give good results. Dis-placed fragments should not be left loose in the joint because they would interfere with joint motion and cause persistent pain. When several loose fragments are present, the injury should be managed as a comminuted fracture.

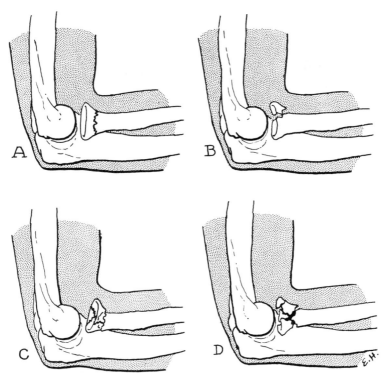

Figure 16–17 Varieties of fractures of the head of the radius. *A*, Undisplaced fracture that should be treated by mobilization rather than by immobilization. *B*, Displaced marginal fracture involving less than one-third of the articular surface for which early excision is usually indicated. *C*, Comminuted fracture of the radial head with minimal displacement for which complete excision of the radial head is indicated. *D*, Severely comminuted displaced fracture of the radial head for which excision of all of the fragments is indicated (From Hampton and Fitts.)

In comminuted fractures (Fig. 16–17*C* and *D*), the entire radial head should be excised within the first 24 to 48 hours following injury. The operation is performed through a posterolateral incision, entering the joint anterior to the anconeus muscle. The hematoma in the joint is evacuated and the entire comminuted radial head is removed. A bulky dressing about the elbow and a sling are adequate for postoperative immobilization. Active motion should be started within 48 to 72 hours after operation. After the wound is healed, soaks in warm water for brief periods four to five times daily along with active exercises are advantageous.

MONTEGGIA OR "PARRY" FRACTURE DISLOCATIONS

These are a combination of two injuries: a fracture of the ulnar shaft and a dislocation of the head of the radius (Fig. 16–18). The ulnar fracture may be just distal to the coronoid process or in the upper or middle third of the shaft. If angulation or over-riding is present, the ulna in effect

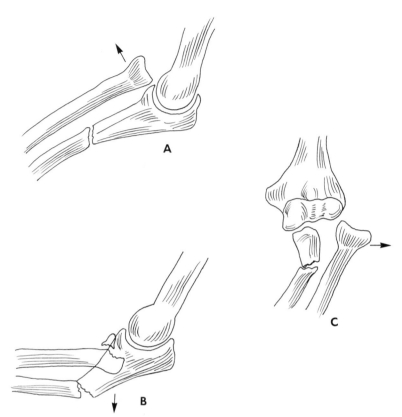

Figure 16–18   Varieties of Monteggia fractures. *A*, Fracture of ulna with apex of ulnar angulation forward and anterior dislocation of radial head. *B*, Fracture of ulna with apex of ulnar angulation posterior and posterior dislocation of radial head. Note fracture of radial head. *C*, Uncommon lateral dislocation of radial head.

is shortened. Consequently the radial head dislocates, always in the direction of the apex of the angular deformity of the ulna. Usually this is anteriorly but may be posteriorly, or even laterally. When the radial head subluxes posteriorly, a fracture of the anterior lip of the radial head is common.

When a fracture of the ulna is suspected, a mere x-ray examination of the forearm is not enough. The elbow joint must be included in order to ascertain the position of the radial head. A dislocation of the radial head must be recognized and reduced or marked impairment of elbow function will result (Figs. 17–30 and 17–31).

The fracture of the ulna is often oblique or comminuted with over-riding of the fragments. Therefore, even good closed reductions are unlikely to hold long enough for the fracture to heal or to prevent redislocation of the radial head. The preferable treatment is open reduction and rigid fixation of the ulnar fracture. Internal fixation is achieved either with a Rush-type intramedullary pin or with a plate and screws. Reduction of the ulna usually leads to reduction of the head of the radius. If the dislocated radial head has pulled out from beneath an intact orbicular ligament, the ligament must be divided, the radial head replaced, and the ligament repaired. If there is a fracture of the dislocated radial head, probably the entire head should be removed. The Boyd posterolateral approach is excellent for the operation, since it allows access not only to the fracture of the ulna, but also to the dislocated or fractured radial head. Operations for Monteggia fracture-dislocations should not be undertaken lightly. They are procedures for experts.

DISLOCATIONS OF THE ELBOW

Dislocation occurs from a fall on the outstretched hand with the elbow extended. The upper radius and ulna usually are displaced posteriorly and slightly laterally. A straight lateral dislocation is less common. Anterior dislocations do not occur without an accompanying fracture of the olecranon.

An obvious deformity at the elbow is apparent early, but later swelling may obliterate the deformity. Circulation and nerve function should be checked and recorded before reduction is attempted. Roentgenograms should be taken to rule out fractures, particularly of the radial head.

Treatment involves reduction of the dislocation as soon as possible (Fig. 16–19). This may be accomplished by applying steady traction at the wrist while countertraction to the arm is provided by an assistant. After traction has led to some relaxation, the forearm is levered forward and, if needed, medially. If reduction is not complete, it is impossible to flex the elbow freely. Occasionally reduction can be achieved without anesthesia but, as a rule, general anesthesia is necessary. Roentgenograms should be made immediately to verify reduction. The elbow is immobilized for 7 to 10 days at about 90 degrees in a posterior molded splint and a sling. Thereafter, only a sling is required. Flexion may be allowed freely but only limited extension should be permitted until at least 3 weeks after injury. Warm soaks and active exercises should be carried out at least four or five times daily, even during the period when the elbow is kept in the sling. Several months are required before full elbow motion is recovered. Under no circumstances, however, should passive manipulation be carried out in an effort to increase the range of motion.

FRACTURES OF THE SHAFTS OF THE BONES OF THE FOREARM

FRACTURES OF THE SHAFTS OF BOTH BONES OF THE FOREARM

In this injury in adults the fragments are usually displaced and overriding. Some comminution of one or both fractures is common, making accurate reduction difficult.

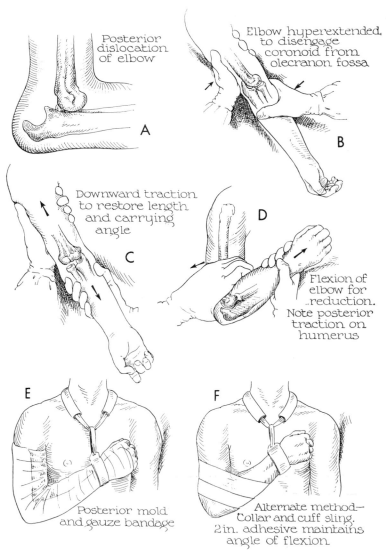

Figure 16–19   Posterior dislocation of the elbow and the maneuvers for reduction and immobilization. (From Banks and Compere.)

Efforts at closed reduction and immobilization are successful in a few instances if the fractures are transverse so that a stable reduction under general anesthesia is possible (Fig. 16–20). The "board splint method" supplemented by the long-arm plaster cast may be highly advantageous (Fig. 16–21).

Open reduction and internal fixation, however, are often necessary. Operative intervention is often selected primarily by experienced fracture surgeons as it affords accurate stabilized reduction of the fragments. Intramedullary pins or plates and screws may be used. Either technique insures that reduction will not be lost during cast changes. The cast applied after the operation must extend above the elbow. Nonunion of these fractures is not uncommon; therefore, supplementary bone grafting at the time of open reduction and internal fixation is worthwhile.

Fractures of the bones of the forearm in adults do not unite rapidly. Immobilization must be maintained until the fragments are united which may require 12 to 16 weeks. With stable internal fixation, immobilization may be shorter.

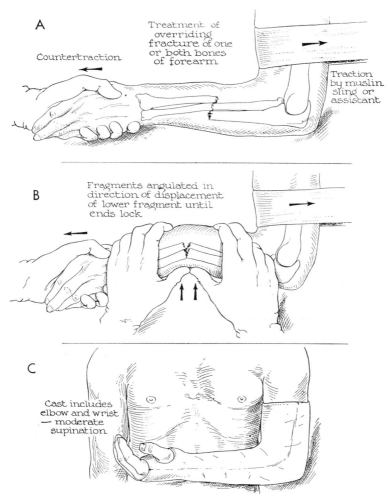

Figure 16-20   Closed reduction of transverse fractures of the middle part of the shafts of the bones of the forearm and immobilization in long-arm plaster cast with the forearm in supination. (From Banks and Compere.)

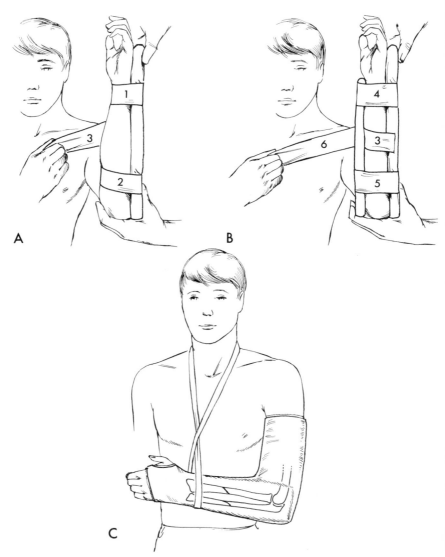

Figure 16–21 Two-board method plus a plaster cast for fractures of the shaft of both bones of the forearm. With the forearm supported so that the fragments of each bone of the forearm are in good alignment, a long board *slightly wider* than the forearm itself is applied to the dorsal surface from the elbow to the metacarpophalangeal joints with 3 strips of adhesive tape. Then, a short board of the same width is applied to the volar surface from the elbow to the wrist with 3 additional strips of adhesive tape applied at the same point on the forearm as the first 3. Finally, a long arm plaster cast is applied from well above the elbow to the knuckles. The boards aid in maintaining good alignment of the fragments while the cast is being applied. The compression of the soft parts provided by the boards serves to compress soft parts between the bones and thereby help maintain the interosseous space. Because *the boards are wider than the forearm itself* and are applied individually, circulation is not embarrassed. The 2-board method may be a valuable aid in proper management of fractures of the shaft of both bones of the forearm. (From Rhodes, Allen, Harkins, and Moyer.)

FRACTURES OF THE SHAFT OF THE RADIUS ALONE

These injuries are common at the junction of the middle and lower thirds of the shaft. The pronator quadratus muscle in the lower third of the forearm usually pulls the distal fragment of the radius toward the ulna, a displacement difficult to overcome by closed reduction. Full radial length must be restored to prevent subluxation of the ulna at the wrist.

Efforts at closed reduction are worthwhile if a fracture of the radius is transverse or nearly transverse. Stable reduction may be achieved and maintained in a long-arm plaster cast. A plaster cast extending only to the elbow does *not* provide sufficient immobilization and is condemned for any fracture proximal to the level of Colles' fracture (see page 244).

In many fractures of the radial shaft, the fracture line is oblique, so that a stable closed reduction cannot be achieved. Therefore, open reduction and internal fixation by means of an intramedullary pin or a plate and screws frequently are indicated. Because this fracture is a rather common site of nonunion, primary bone grafting, supplementing internal fixation, is advantageous.

FRACTURE OF THE SHAFT OF THE ULNA ALONE

This injury usually results from a direct blow on the forearm. If the force causes significant angulation of the ulnar fragments, the head of the radius becomes dislocated (a Monteggia fracture). When a fracture of the ulna angulates or over-rides, the radius is either broken or dislocated.

Fractures of the shaft of the ulna without a complicating fracture or dislocation of the radius are usually undisplaced or minimally displaced. The extremity is immobilized in a plaster cast extending from the upper arm to the proximal palmar crease of the hand with the elbow at 90 degrees and the forearm in midpronation. These fractures are prone to slow union. Immobilization must be continued until the fracture unites which usually requires 8 to 16 weeks. Nonunion of fractures of the ulnar shaft is not rare.

FRACTURES AND DISLOCATIONS ABOUT THE WRIST

FRACTURES OF THE DISTAL END OF THE RADIUS

Fractures of the distal end of the radius are the most common fractures of the upper extremity and probably are the most common fractures in the body. They may be associated with a fracture of the ulnar styloid or distal end of the ulnar shaft. Even if a fracture of the ulna is not present, the ulnar collateral ligament probably is injured. Appropriate treatment of the fracture of the radius suffices for any injury to the distal ulna.

Three eponyms are commonly used to denote fractures of the distal radius, two according to the direction of displacement of the distal fragment, the third according to the location and direction of the fracture line (Fig. 16–22).

Colles' fracture is used when the distal fragment is displaced dorsally. Smith's or reversed Colles' fracture (much less common than Colles') is used when the distal fragment is displaced toward the volar surface of the wrist. Barton's or marginal fracture denotes a longitudinal fracture involving the dorsal or volar margin of the distal radius.

Colles' fracture and Barton's fracture involving the dorsal margin of the distal radius are hyperextension injuries resulting from falls on the outstretched hand. Smith's (reversed Colles') fracture and Barton's fracture involving the volar margin of the distal radius are hyperflexion injuries resulting from a fall onto the dorsum of the hand. In each, any degree of displacement may occur. In Colles' and Smith's fractures, impaction of the distal into the proximal fragment is common. The distal fragment, however, may be severely comminuted with each fragment displaced and lines of fracture disturbing the articular surface. In Barton's fracture, displacement usually is absent or is minimal.

Treatment: Closed reduction by manipulation is the method of choice in practically all displaced fractures of the distal radius.

The objectives of reduction are the restoration of full radial length and the anatomical inclinations of the distal articular surface. The fundamental maneuvers for closed reduction are strong traction against equally strong counter-traction applied at the flexed elbow, combined with pressure or manipulation of the distal fragment until the fracture is reduced.

Anesthesia, either local or general, almost always must be employed. Any effort at closed reduction without anesthesia in adults is likely to lead to the acceptance of inadequate reduction because of painful resistance by the patient. Local anesthesia (about 10 to 15 cc of 1 per cent procaine) in-

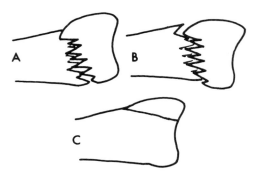

Figure 16–22   *A*, Colles' fracture; *B*, Smith's fracture; *C*, Barton's fracture.

jected from the dorsum into the hematoma about the fracture is highly satisfactory when fractures are treated within a few hours after injury. A few cc of procaine injected about the distal end of the ulna makes the local anesthesia more effective. Local anesthesia is less likely to be effective when the fracture is being treated 12 or more hours after injury because the blood about the fracture is clotted and the procaine diffuses poorly. General anesthesia may be used with proper precautions against aspiration of regurgitated gastric contents.

Knowledge of the normal anatomical relationships of the distal ends of the bones of the forearm is important in determining when a satisfactory reduction has been achieved. Normally, the tip of the styloid process of the radius extends about 1 cm distal to the styloid of the ulna. The distal articular surface of the radius is inclined toward the ulnar side of the hand at an angle of 25 to 30 degrees. The distal articular surface of the radius also inclines toward the palmar surface of the hand at an angle of 10 to 15 degrees. Unless full length and the inclinations of the distal articular surface of the radius have been restored, complete reduction of a fracture of the distal radius has not been achieved (Fig. 16–23).

Colles' Fracture: A Colles' fracture occurs principally in the middle and later decades of life. The distal fragment may remain in position or be displaced. In a typical displaced Colles' fracture, all of the relationships of the distal articular surface are distorted. The distal fragment is driven dorsally and into radial deviation so that the articular surface inclines dorsally and radially. The distal fragment may be impacted into the proximal fragment with crushing of the cancellus bone, or it may be severely comminuted. The characteristic displacements produce a "silver-fork deformity" so-called because the hump on the dorsum of the wrist is analogous to the hump of a table fork. Radial deviation of the distal fragment results in increased prominence of the distal end of the ulna.

Figure 16–23   A, Colles' fracture with radial and dorsal displacement of the distal fragment. *B*, Following reduction, the normal inclinations of the articular surface of the radius have been restored and the styloid of the radius extends well beyond the styloid of ulna. (From Rhodes, Allen, Harkins, and Moyer.)

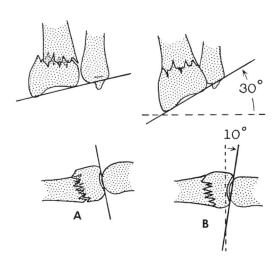

Colles' fracture should be reduced soon after injury. Closed reduction, as previously outlined, is based upon a combination of traction and manipulation. In the usual closed reduction, the surgeon grasps the hand of the injured wrist in a handshake manner and applies traction while countertraction is provided by an assistant holding the lower arm just above the flexed elbow (Fig. 16–24). As the surgeon makes strong traction with one hand, pressure is applied against the dorsal surface of the distal fragment with the other thumb so as to force it into reduction. The hand is pulled toward palmar flexion and full ulnar deviation with the forearm in pronation. Reduction will have been obtained when the normal contour of the

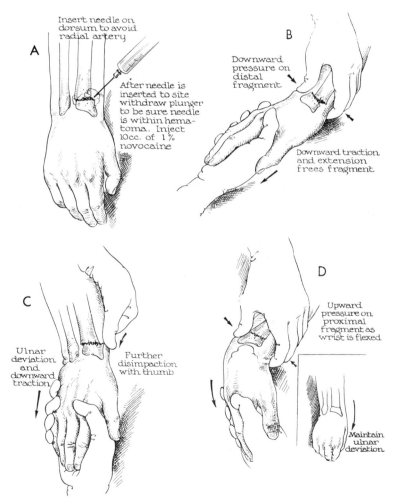

Figure 16–24   Closed reduction of Colles' fracture under local anesthesia. (From Banks and Compere.)

wrist is restored and the tip of the styloid process of the radius extends 1 cm distal to that of the ulna.

Traction and manipulation for closed reduction may be applied in another way. Strong and steady traction is applied to the hand for several minutes against equally strong counter-traction. Strong pull on Japanese finger traps applied to the fingers is an alternate method of obtaining traction (Fig. 17–35) and makes application of plaster easier than when the hand is held by an assistant. After the fragments have become distracted as a result of traction, the distal fragment of the radius is molded into reduction.

The wrist is immobilized with the hand in moderate palmar flexion and full ulnar deviation with the forearm in pronation by a lightly padded plaster cast or anterior and posterior molded plaster splints (Fig. 16–25). Full palmar flexion, the so-called Cotton-Loder position, is to be avoided. Any advantage to be gained in maintaining better reduction of a difficult fracture is far over-shadowed by the hazards of edema and stiffness of the fingers, which cannot be exercised in this position, and of permanent restriction of motion in the wrist. The cast or splints extend distally only to the proximal transverse palmar crease and to just proximal to the metacarpal heads on the dorsum of the hand so that full motion of the fingers is possible. Ordinarily, the plaster is extended proximally to just below the elbow although in comminuted fractures there is reason to extend the plaster to the upper arm with the elbow at 90 degrees. In undisplaced fractures, the hand is immobilized in the neutral position of slight dorsal flexion and ulnar deviation.

Roentgenograms should be made as soon as the plaster has set while anesthesia is still effective to be certain that adequate reduction has been achieved. If the reduction is not satisfactory, the plaster is removed immediately and closed reduction is again attempted. While perfect reduction cannot always be obtained, certainly only the best possible reduction should be accepted.

Reduction will not always be maintained even in a snug fitting cast, especially if the distal fragment is badly comminuted. As swelling subsides, immobilization becomes incomplete and redisplacement of fragments may occur. Telescoping of fragments often occurs particularly in the aged. It is advisable, therefore, to obtain roentgenograms about the fifth postreduction day and again about the tenth day. If some slipping of fragments has occurred, another reduction and a new cast may be indicated if the surgeon believes he can obtain and maintain an improved position.

During postreduction management, chief objectives are to maintain a full range of motion of the fingers and the shoulder. Edema of the fingers must be controlled as much as possible. Measures to accomplish this include real elevation of the hand almost constantly for a few days with strenuous active exercises of the fingers. In some instances, a pressure dressing may be kept about the fingers with an elastic bandage over sheet

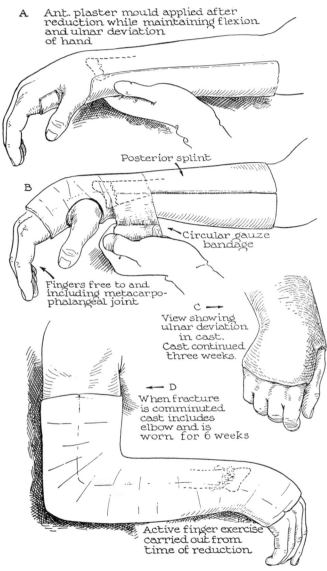

A   Ant. plaster mould applied after reduction while maintaining flexion and ulnar deviation of hand

Posterior splint

B

Circular gauze bandage

Fingers free to and including metacarpophalangeal joint

C →
View showing ulnar deviation in cast. Cast continued three weeks.

← D
When fracture is comminuted cast includes elbow and is worn for 6 weeks

Active finger exercise carried out from time of reduction

Figure 16–25 Postreduction immobilization of reduced Colles' fractures utilizing anterior and posterior splints (a plaster cast extending to the elbow or a plaster cast extending well above the elbow may be used). Note that the hand is in mild palmar flexion and ulnar deviation and is in full pronation. (From Banks and Compere.)

cotton for several days. When this is used, small strips of felt with holes cut out for the knuckles should be placed between the fingers. Throughout the period of immobilization, the patient must be encouraged to carry out a full range of forceful motion of the fingers. Similarly, the patient must repeatedly (every hour on the hour) put the shoulder through a full range of motions, including full overhead reach and full internal and external rotation. Loss of motion in the shoulder joint following fractures of the distal end of the radius is a preventable complication; yet, it is too frequently observed because exercises of the shoulder have been neglected.

Immobilization of the wrist is maintained until union of the fracture has occurred. In adults, fractures which required reduction should be immobilized about 6 weeks. In some elderly patients it is advisable to change the cast after 3 weeks in order to bring the hand out of even moderate palmar flexion into the neutral position or into slight dorsal flexion. No force should be used in obtaining this corrected position as displacement of the distal fragment might occur.

Smith's or Reversed Colles' Fracture: The volarward inclination of the articular surface is increased in Smith's fracture, but deformity is usually less pronounced than with a Colles' fracture. Some degree of comminution frequently is present.

The maneuvers for manipulative reduction are somewhat the reverse of those for Colles' fracture, although traction is necessary. With the forearm in supination, the hand is brought into mild hyperextension and the distal fragment is forced backward with the thumb. Immobilization is provided by a plaster cast or anterior and posterior molded plaster splints which hold the hand in mild hyperextension, usually with the forearm in supination. The postreduction management is comparable to that outlined for Colles' fractures.

Barton's or Marginal Fractures: Barton's fractures usually involve only a small portion of the articular surface, but because they involve the articular surface, accurate reduction is essential. Direct pressure on the fragment under local anesthesia usually forces it into satisfactory position.

Immobilization should be provided for about 4 weeks by a plaster cast in which the hand is held in the neutral or slightly dorsal flexed position. Persistent exercise of the fingers and shoulder throughout the period of postreduction management is as important as in other fractures about the distal end of the radius.

FRACTURES OF THE CARPUS

The most important fracture of the carpus is a fracture of the navicular bone. Fractures involving the other carpal bones are usually mere chips or undisplaced cracks requiring, at the most, only a few weeks immobilization in a plaster cast with the wrist in the functional position. Fractures of the navicular bone, by far the most common fractures of the carpus, deserve special consideration.

Fractures of the Navicular Bone: These injuries, like Colles' fractures, result from falls on the outstretched hand. They occur usually in young adult males whose strong musculature seems to prevent extreme dorsal flexion, thereby causing the navicular rather than the lower radius to receive the force of impact.

The navicular, the longest of the carpal bones and the only one not cuboidal in shape, has a precarious blood supply. The major blood supply comes from a small artery which enters the distal portion of the bone. When a fracture is sustained across the waist or proximal pole of the navicular, most of the blood supply of the proximal fragment may be destroyed. The result may be avascular necrosis of that fragment.

The diagnosis of a fracture of the navicular bone is not always easy. Clinically, the patient complains of pain in the wrist, and some swelling is present, perhaps because of hemarthrosis of the wrist joint. Tenderness in the anatomical snuff-box is usually severe. With such a clinical picture, an oblique view of the wrist in addition to the routine anteroposterior and lateral views is mandatory, since a fracture of the navicular often can be visualized only in an oblique view. Because a fracture of the navicular bone is easily overlooked, three views of the region should be routine in every injured wrist.

A significant sprain of the wrist is an exceedingly rare injury. Careful x-ray examination in three views will usually disclose either a fracture of the navicular or the distal radius. Certainly, a sprain of the wrist which is not completely asymptomatic in 10 days is likely to be a fracture of the navicular. A fracture of the navicular may not be disclosed on x-ray films made soon after injury and, yet, repeat films 10 to 14 days later will show a fracture. The fracture line becomes visible as a result of absorption about it. There should be no hesitancy, therefore, in repeating x-ray films after 10 to 14 days if the patient's symptoms have not been completely relieved. If a diagnosis of a sprain is made originally, good practice calls for plaster immobilization for 10 to 14 days so that an unrecognized navicular fracture will be immobilized. Repeat roentgenograms are made after the cast is removed.

Treatment: As a rule, the fragments are in good position and reduction is not necessary. If the fragments of a fracture of the navicular are displaced, there is or has been an associated dislocation of another carpal bone.

The overwhelming majority of the fractures of the navicular will unite if they are adequately immobilized long enough. Immobilization is established with a plaster cast which extends from just below the elbow to the proximal palmar crease and to the interphalangeal joint of the thumb with the hand in dorsal flexion and radial deviation (Fig. 16–26). This position of the hand is important as it tends to approximate the fragments more closely. Some orthopedic surgeons in recent years have extended the cast to above the elbow for better immobilization. Immobilization must be provided until the fracture has united as shown by roentgenograms. Usually

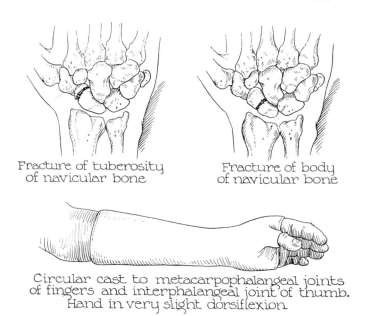

Fracture of tuberosity
of navicular bone

Fracture of body
of navicular bone

Circular cast to metacarpophalangeal joints
of fingers and interphalangeal joint of thumb.
Hand in very slight dorsiflexion

Figure 16–26 Fractures of the tubercle and waste of the carpal scaphoid and a plaster cast for immobilization of such injuries. Note that the cast extends to the interphalangeal joint of the thumb. (From Banks and Compere.)

immobilization for at least 3 months is required. At times 6 to 9 months or even a year may elapse before the fragments have united. Watson-Jones has emphasized that all navicular fractures will unite if the immobilization is continuous and sufficiently prolonged and that failure of union is the result of delay in providing immobilization or its removal before union has occurred. Usually, the cast should be removed every 6 weeks, new roentgenograms made, and a new cast applied until immobilization may be eliminated.

An outstanding complication of fractures of the navicular is avascular necrosis, usually of the proximal fragment. In spite of this, union of the fracture can occur with prolonged immobilization, and the blood supply to the avascular fragment may be re-established so that the dead bone will be replaced by living bone. Immobilization should be continued until the revascularizing process is well established.

With nonunion of the carpal scaphoid, with or without avascular necrosis of the proximal fragment, traumatic arthritis of the wrist joint may develop as an early or a late complication. Once traumatic arthritis has developed, operative fusion of the wrist joint in the position of function may be necessary to obtain a painless stable wrist.

DISLOCATIONS OF THE CARPUS

Each of the dislocations about the wrist results from forced hyperextension of the hand from a fall on the outstretched hand or when the hyperextended hand is jammed against a wall to guard against impact. A miscalcuated "stiff-arm" in football could cause a dislocation of the carpus.

Clinically it can be determined that a significant wrist injury has been received, but exact diagnosis is made only on x-ray examination. Anteroposterior and lateral views usually are sufficient but oblique views may be helpful. Films of the normal uninjured wrist for comparison aid in establishing the diagnosis.

Dislocation of the Lunate: The dorsal ligamentous attachments of the lunate are torn as the bone is dislocated. It is then rotated and extruded anteriorly to a point deep to the flexor tendons and the volar carpal ligament. Its only remaining ligamentous attachment is to the anterior lip of the radius. Median nerve hypesthesia and impaired finger flexion may occur as a result of impingement of the dislocated bone on the nerve and tendons.

In the lateral roentgenogram, the lunate does not articulate with the radius and is displaced anteriorly. The capitate appears to articulate with the radius. In the anteroposterior view, rather than round, the lunate appears elongated and square or rectangular.

Under general anesthesia, closed reduction should be attempted as promptly as possible (Fig. 16–27). While one assistant provides countertraction, another makes strong traction on the hand to open the space for the lunate and on instruction hyperextends the hand at the wrist. The surgeon applies pressure with his thumbs to force the lunate into reduction and then the hand is quickly pulled into palmar flexion by the assistant.

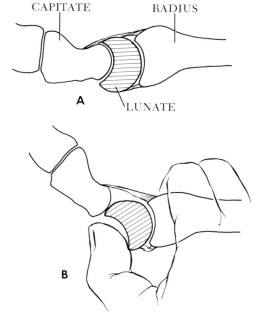

CAPITATE   RADIUS

A

LUNATE

B

Figure 16–27   *A*, Drawing to show the ligamentous attachments of the lunate bone which is almost entirely covered by articular cartilage. *B*, Maneuver for reduction of dislocation of the lunate which includes traction on the hand, dorsiflexion of the hand, and direct pressure on the lunate with the thumb. (From Davis.)

When the lunate is reduced, the wrist assumes a more normal appearance and can be moved easily through practically a full range of motion. Reduction should be immediately confirmed by x-ray examination before application of the cast. A forearm and hand cast which holds the hand in slight palmar flexion should be provided for about 3 weeks.

If efforts at closed reduction are not successful, either open reduction or excision of the lunate is indicated. Opinions vary as to the most desirable operative procedure. Following open reduction, there is a high incidence of avascular necrosis of the lunate, probably secondary in part to the operative destruction of blood supply to the bone. On the other hand, excision of the bone usually produces a weak wrist.

Perilunar Dislocation: In this injury, instead of forward displacement of the lunate as the hand is forcibly hyperextended, the lunate remains in normal relationship with the radius but the remaining carpus with the hand are displaced backward. The scaphoid may be fractured. If so, its proximal fragment usually remains behind in the joint with the lunate.

Closed reduction under anesthesia is usually possible by strong traction and manipulation against counter-traction. Immobilization by a plaster cast with the hand in slight palmar flexion is provided for 3 to 4 weeks, although if the navicular has been fractured, much longer immobilization is indicated. At the end of 3 to 4 weeks, a more conventional position of the immobilized hand for a fracture of the navicular should be provided (see page 246).

Perilunar dislocation at the wrist is a serious injury and some permanent restriction of motion is to be anticipated.

Midcarpal Dislocation: As the hand is forcibly hyperextended, the distal row of carpal bones may be dislocated dorsally on the proximal row. The correct diagnosis is frequently missed, because the relationship of the carpus is not closely observed on the lateral view. This is a serious injury which can result in severe permanent limitation of function of the hand particularly if it is not reduced promptly.

Closed reduction under anesthesia is usually feasible, especially if it is attempted soon after injury. Reduction is best maintained by immobilization in a plaster cast with the hand in slight palmar flexion for a period of 3 or 4 weeks. If efforts at closed reduction are unsuccessful, early open reduction is indicated.

FRACTURES AND DISLOCATIONS OF THE HAND

Fractures and dislocations of the various components of the hand often result in significant permanent disability not only because the injury frequently traumatizes the intricate mechanisms which provide smooth gliding joints and tendons but also because basic principles of the management of hand injuries often are violated.

The basic objectives of management of these injuries are the maintenance of function of uninjured parts and the maximum return of function of fractured or dislocated parts. The principles under which these injuries should be treated call for the injured parts to be restored promptly to as near their normal relationships as is possible, with splinting in the position of function. **Overzealous efforts to salvage badly injured digits must not be allowed to prejudice eventual function of those digits that were not injured.**

Splinting of the hand or even parts of it in the position of function often starts with immobilization of the wrist in slight dorsal flexion. The finger or fingers are held in moderate flexion at each joint and the thumb usually in slight opposition. A hand grasping a baseball assumes the position of function.

In only a few fractures or dislocations of the hand should the entire hand be immobilized. Preferably only injured digits, or, at times, uninjured digits contiguous with fractures of the metacarpals should be splinted. Uninjured digits usually should remain unsplinted to permit diligent active exercises. Splinting for fractures or dislocations of the hand should be eliminated at the earliest practical time which will vary according to the specific injury or injuries. Splinting longer than is necessary is a common cause of permanent restriction of motion particularly in the joints of the fingers.

Of course, any combination of skeletal injuries may occur simultaneously and present a complex problem. Moreover, closed or open skeletal injuries may be associated with extensive tendon and nerve injuries. Extensive open wounds, perhaps with loss of skin, may further complicate the problem and plans for surgical repair of the hand. Reference is made to Chapter 20 in which principles of surgery for injuries to various components of the hand are well enunciated. The following discussion of the various common skeletal injuries of the hand covers closed injuries. The same methods recommended for closed fractures and dislocations are applicable in general to open fractures but the choice of a method to hold them in reduction may be affected by the presence of an open wound or by associated soft part injuries. Certainly a healed fracture of a digit in good position is likely to be insignificant if the digit is without adequate tendon function or joint motion. In some injuries, the desirable method for the skeletal injuries must be bypassed for a less effective method in order to facilitate the optimal repair of soft part injuries.

FRACTURES AND DISLOCATIONS OF THE THUMB INCLUDING THE FIRST METACARPAL

Injuries to the thumb usually occur as a result of a fall or a blow on the tip, although trauma at any point on the thumb which forces any part beyond its normal range of movement may result in a fracture or dislocation or a combination of both. Injuries to the thumb, an exceedingly important part of the hand, often cause considerable temporary disability and, at times, significant permanent disability.

Fracture of the Base of the First Metacarpal: Undisplaced fractures require only about 4 weeks in a plaster cast which incorporates the entire thumb, the base of the hand, and the forearm. Displaced fractures require accurate reduction which often can be achieved by manipulation under local or general anesthesia and maintained by a cast. In some fractures, particularly those quite comminuted, traction with a "banjo" arrangement incorporated in the cast (Fig. 16–28) may be advisable for 3 or 4 weeks.

Bennett's fracture is a fracture–partial dislocation or subluxation of the base of the first metacarpal which can lead to considerable restriction of motion in the carpometacarpal joint. This joint provides the great range of motion of the thumb. The injury requires precise reduction for an acceptable result.

At times, Bennett's fracture can be reduced adequately by closed manipulation and held in a plaster cast. In some instances continuous traction in a "banjo" cast shown in Figure 16–29 gives a good reduction. Many of these injuries, however, require internal fixation for reduction and stabilization. Internal fixation with small pins may be provided at an open operation or, at times, by percutaneous pinning, while the fracture is held reduced by an assistant (Fig. 16–30). With open reduction and internal fixation, the pins are cut short to remain permanently. With percutaneous pinning, the pins remain projecting through the skin. They are protected with a sterile dressing and are pulled out easily after sufficient healing of the fracture has occurred.

Fractures to the Shaft of the First Metacarpal: Undisplaced fractures and those that can be reduced by manipulation under local or general anesthesia require only a plaster cast comparable with that used for fractures of the base of the metacarpal. About 4 weeks of immobilization will usually suffice for healing. An oblique or severely comminuted fracture may need continuous traction as shown in Figure 16–29 for Bennett's fracture.

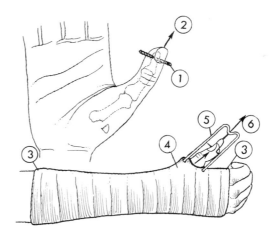

Figure 16–28 Banjo traction for fracture of base of first metacarpal. (1) A pin is passed through the bone or through tissue of the distal phalanx. (2) While manual traction is applied to the thumb, a plaster cast is applied to the hand and forearm. (3) The cast is molded well at the base of the first metacarpal. (4) A loop of strong wire is incorporated in the cast. (5) Continuous rubber-band traction is established from the pin through the distal phalanx to the "banjo" loop of wire (6). (From DePalma.)

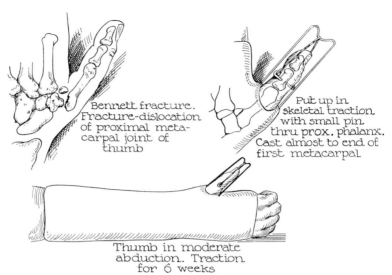

Figure 16–29 Continuous rubber-band skeletal traction in a plaster cast for Bennett's fracture using a pin through the proximal phalanx. The tissue of the web of the hand and over the base of the thumb must be well padded. (From Banks and Compere.)

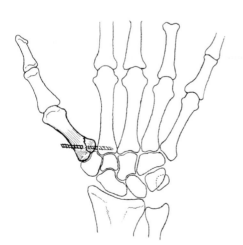

Figure 16–30 Percutaneous (or open) pinning to stabilize a Bennett's fracture in good reduction. (From DePalma.)

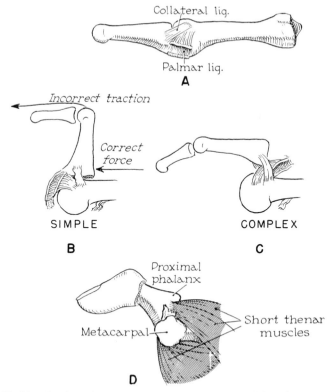

Figure 16–31   Simple and complex metacarpophalangeal dislocation.

A, The volar aspect of a metacarpophalangeal joint capsule is reinforced with a palmar ligament or fibrocartilage.

B, In a simple dislocation the phalanx is hyperextended and the palmar ligament hangs like a curtain over the metacarpal head. Traction may pivot the phalanx on the intact collateral ligaments and interpose the palmar ligament between the bones. The phalanx should be pushed into place.

C, The finger is not hyperextended on, but more nearly parallel to, the metacarpal in a complex dislocation. The volar joint capsule and palmar ligament are interposed, and usually prevent reduction by manipulation.

D, In the metacarpophalangeal joint of the thumb the short thenar muscles augment the pivot force predisposing to complex dislocation. (From McLaughlin.)

Dislocations of the Metacarpophalangeal Joint: The metacarpophalangeal joint differs from the interphalangeal joint not only in size but also in the manner in which the tough palmar ligament is incorporated into the volar capsule. Dislocation is produced by hyperextension which may cause the proximal end of the phalanx to displace onto the dorsum of the metacarpal. Reduction is achieved by pressure on the base of the displaced phalanx which is pushed into place (Fig. 16–31*B*). Traction is contraindicated because a tongue of avulsed palmar ligament may be dragged into the joint and become interposed between the phalanx and the metacarpal, necessitating open reduction (Fig. 16–31*C*).

A complex dislocation occurs when the head of the first metacarpal is buttonholed through a rent in the capsule and is entrapped by the "noose" of joint capsule, short thenar muscles, and the interposed palmar ligament. Attempts at reduction by traction merely tighten the "noose." Under these circumstances, the thumb is usually found parallel to the metacarpal rather than hyperextended on it (Fig. 16–31*C* and *D*). When reduction is not achieved by hyperextending the thumb and pushing on the base of the phalanx, open reduction is necessary.

Following closed or open reduction, a plaster cast as described for fractures of the first metacarpal is indicated for 10 to 14 days. Thereafter, the thumb should be protected from reinjury for several weeks.

Fractures of the Phalanges of the Thumb: Undisplaced fractures of the proximal phalanx require the use of splints or a cast for 3 or 4 weeks. Displaced fractures may be reduced by manipulation or continuous traction in a "banjo" cast (Fig. 16–28). Fractures of the proximal phalanx involving the articular surface of the metacarpophalangeal joint tend to cause permanent restriction of the normally small range of motion in this joint. Therefore, the best possible reduction should be achieved.

Fractures of the distal phalanx are painful but usually inconsequential injuries. The majority require only a dressing for protection although occasionally the amount of displacement warrants closed reduction, which is maintained by a protective splint over the flexor surface of the phalanges. Immobilization of the carpometacarpal and metacarpophalangeal joints ordinarily is not necessary.

FRACTURES OF THE FINGER METACARPALS

Fractures of the Shafts.   Fractures of the metacarpal shafts in adequate apposition and good alignment and those which can be reduced by manipulation need only to be immobilized for about 4 weeks. Rotational deformity must be avoided since it would result in finger overlap when the digit is flexed, a very distressing functional result. Proper rotation may be assessed by a simple guideline. When each digit is flexed so as to make a soft fist, the tip of each finger must point toward the tuberosity of the carpal navicular (Fig. 16–32). Although restoration of normal length is desirable, efforts to achieve full length should not be allowed to prejudice function of contiguous fingers.

A plaster cast over the forearm and hand, extending just proximal to the metacarpophalangeal joints, provides adequate immobilization for many metacarpal fractures. For others, the finger or fingers contiguous to the broken bone(s) must be splinted on a metal splint incorporated in the cast (Fig. 16–33). When fingers are splinted there should always be moderate flexion at each joint. They should never be splinted in extension. A splinted finger should be mobilized for exercises as soon as enough union of the metacarpal permits. Usually 2 or 3 weeks of immobilization will suffice.

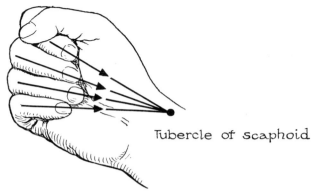

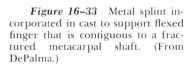

Tubercle of scaphoid

Figure 16–32 Axes of the flexed fingers do not correspond to those of the metacarpal or forearm bones but converge on the tubercle of the scaphoid. Finger splinting in flexion should be in this direction. (From McLaughlin.)

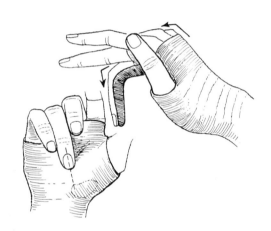

Figure 16–33 Metal splint incorporated in cast to support flexed finger that is contiguous to a fractured metacarpal shaft. (From DePalma.)

Continuous traction on flexed fingers has been used by some surgeons in an effort to achieve healing of metacarpal fractures in full length. At times such treatment has been effective, but often it has led to restricted finger motion and, moreover, frequently has not produced improved position of the fracture. Continuous traction for metacarpal fractures is of doubtful value.

In highly selected injuries, open reduction and intramedullary pinning of metacarpal fractures (Fig. 16–34) may be indicated to assure precise reduction and to maintain excellent alignment. Open reduction and internal fixation, however, should be reserved for those fractures in which operation may be expected to give a better functional result than would be obtained by nonoperative methods.

Fractures of the Necks of Metacarpals: These fractures may involve any of the metacarpals, but those of the fifth are the most common. They

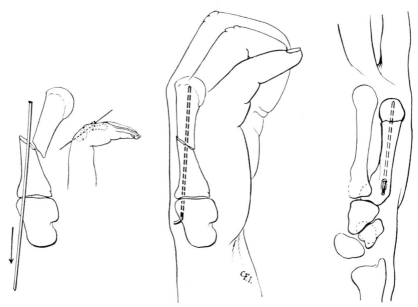

Figure 16–34　Fracture of a metacarpal shaft stabilized in reduction by an intramedullary pin. (From Milford, Lee: The hand. *In* Crenshaw, A. H. (ed.): Campbell s Operative Orthopaedics, 5th edition. St. Louis, The C. V. Mosby Company, 1971. Reprinted by permission.)

occur frequently during fist fights and are sometimes called "fist-fight fractures." They may occur any time the proximal knuckle of a finger forcibly strikes a solid object when the fingers are tightly flexed.

Many fractures of the neck of metacarpals are impacted tightly. When fragments are impacted in mild to moderate angulation, the position often may be accepted. Only a compression dressing and sling are used for a few days for comfort. Active exercises of the joints of the contiguous finger are initiated promptly. Fractures impacted in severe angulation and angulated unimpacted fractures require more aggressive treatment. Under local or general anesthesia, the impaction must be broken up by forceful manipulation, converting the fracture to an unimpacted status. Unimpacted fractures must be reduced — angulation particularly must be corrected — and held reduced for several weeks by appropriate splinting immobilizing the injured portion of the hand and the contiguous finger. Splinting of the finger in extension is contraindicated. In contrast, the finger must be splinted in flexion, with the proximal joint often at 90 degrees. Figure 16–35 shows an excellent way to achieve and hold reduction of a fracture of a metacarpal neck. While the plaster cast is setting, firm but not excessive pressure should be made downward on the proximal fragment and upward on the flexed middle joint. Excessive pressure at the flexed middle joint can result in necrosis of the skin and even of the underlying portion of the extensor tendon, a complication which certainly would lead to marked impairment of function of the finger.

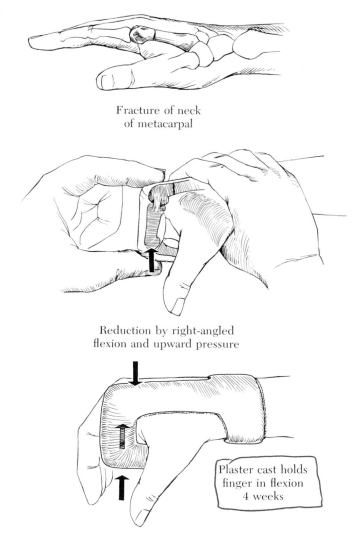

Fracture of neck
of metacarpal

Reduction by right-angled
flexion and upward pressure

Plaster cast holds
finger in flexion
4 weeks

Figure 16–35 Reduction and plaster immobilization for angulated fracture of the neck of the index (or fifth) metacarpal. (Modified from Banks and Compere.)

FRACTURES AND DISLOCATIONS OF THE PHALANGES OF THE FINGERS

Dislocations of the Metacarpophalangeal Joints: Dislocation of the metacarpophalangeal joint commonly involves the index finger, although occasionally dislocation of another finger may be seen. Ordinarily reduction is not difficult and often may be achieved without anesthesia. The proximal end of the displaced phalanx should be pushed into reduction (Fig. 16–31). Redislocation is very unlikely to occur; therefore, simple splinting or a compression dressing for a few days will suffice.

Occasionally, however, an anteriorly displaced head of the metacarpal will be trapped by the joint capsule or the tendon of the flexor of the finger (Fig. 16–36). Manipulative reduction in this situation may be unsuccessful. If so, open operation is necessary to free the metacarpal head from entrapment; afterwards reduction of the dislocation is easy. After operation, splinting of the finger in moderate flexion for 2 to 3 weeks is advisable.

Dislocations of the Proximal Interphalangeal Joint: Chip fractures of various sizes may be associated with these injuries. Dislocations uncomplicated by fractures usually can be reduced easily by strong manual traction, often without anesthesia. The finger should be splinted with each joint in moderate flexion for 1 to 2 weeks. Thereafter, active exercise is likely to restore most or all of the motion in this joint.

A dislocation complicated by a fracture of one of the involved phalanges may present a very complex problem. When the fracture is merely a chip of insufficient size to make the joint unstable and does not lead to subluxation, the fracture may be ignored. In many instances, however, the fracture involves a significant part of the articular surface so that reduction of the dislocation and the fracture are not maintained. Because incomplete reduction is certain to lead to marked restriction of motion (the joint of the finger which has the greatest range of motion), every effort must be made to achieve the best possible reduction.

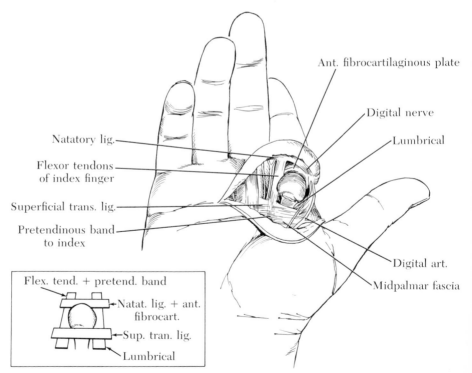

Figure 16–36   Entrapped dislocated index metacarpal head. (from Kaplan, E. B.: J. Bone & Joint Surg., 39A:1081, 1957.)

In some instances adequate reduction of both the fracture and the subluxation may be obtained by continuous traction on the finger. To institute traction, a plaster cast is applied over the forearm, wrist, and hand and a splint is incorporated into the cast. The splint must be designed to permit moderate flexion of each of the joints of the finger and to provide for an attachment of rubber-band traction from a wire or small pin inserted through the middle phalanx or the tough tissue of the distal portion of the distal phalanx. An arrangement which permits some active motion of the proximal interphalangeal joint while the finger is in traction is preferable. Even if continuous traction for 2½ to 3 weeks gives good reduction of the fracture and dislocation at the middle joint, rather marked impairment of function of this joint is to be anticipated.

In some instances, reduction of the fracture and the dislocation can be maintained only by internal fixation at open operation. Operative management of these injuries requires precise skill and experience.

Fractures of the Phalanges

FRACTURES OF THE PROXIMAL PHALANX: These fractures may lead to considerable loss of motion in the interphalangeal joints, particularly in the proximal interphalangeal joint. This occurs from loss of elasticity of the ligaments about the proximal interphalangeal joint and of the gliding mechanisms of the flexor and extensor tendons which are in close contact with the proximal phalanx. (See Chapter 20.)

Undisplaced fractures of the proximal phalanx require about 3 weeks of simple splinting that immobilizes all three joints of the finger in moderate flexion.

Displaced fractures of the proximal phalanx are usually angulated anteriorly (Fig. 16–37) and many are in poor apposition. Reduction by manipulation under good local or general anesthesia may be obtained at times. Good apposition and excellent alignment without rotational deformity are crucial. The entire finger must be immobilized in considerable flexion especially in the middle joint. Special precaution is necessary to insure that the tip of the flexed finger points toward the carpal navicular as a safeguard against malrotation and finger overlap (Fig. 16–32).

A plaster cast holding the wrist in slight dorsal flexion and incorporating a metal splint for the injured finger provides excellent immobilization. The finger portion of the cast may be constructed with plaster of Paris (Fig. 16–37). Usually 3 weeks of immobilization will suffice for enough union of the fracture to permit active exercises. The patient should protect the finger from reinjury for several additional weeks.

FRACTURES OF THE MIDDLE PHALANX: Fractures in this portion of the finger, especially those close to the middle joint, often cause permanent loss of motion in that joint. In many instances, loss of flexion in the distal joint occurs because of tendon fixation at the fracture site.

Undisplaced fractures of the middle phalanx require about 3 weeks of simple splinting that holds the middle and distal joints in some flexion. Immobilization of the metacarpophalangeal joint is not necessary.

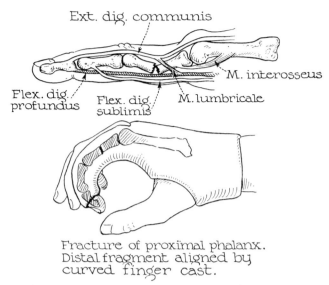

Ext. dig. communis

M. interosseus

Flex. dig. profundus   Flex. dig. sublimis   M. lumbricale

Fracture of proximal phalanx.
Distal fragment aligned by
curved finger cast.

Figure 16–37   Fracture of proximal phalanx of the index finger with palmar angulation; reduction and plaster cast immobilization. (From Banks and Compere: 2nd Edition, 1947.)

Displaced fractures must be reduced into adequate apposition and excellent alignment without rotational deformity. Fractures in the middle phalanx may be angulated dorsally or toward the palm (Fig. 16–38). Correction of the angulation in either direction by manipulation usually is not difficult. Precautions against malrotation are necessary. Splinting of fractures angulated palmarward should immobilize the three joints of the injured finger in moderate flexion; for those angulated dorsally, the middle and distal joints must be in extension. These fractures usually unite sufficiently within 3 weeks to permit the elimination of the splint and initiation of exercises.

FRACTURES OF THE DISTAL PHALANX: Fractures in this portion of the finger usually remain in adequate reduction even though they are severely comminuted. Rarely, a fracture across the middle of the phalanx is severely angulated. Ordinarily this angulation can be corrected easily by manipulation under digital block anesthesia. Because there are no tendon attachments to displace the fragments, splinting is not necessary. On the other hand, these are painful injuries, and some splinting to protect the end of the finger from bumps and pressures contributes significantly to the comfort of the patient. A splint applied to the finger for fractures of the distal phalanx should extend only to the midportion of the middle phalanx to allow active exercise of the proximal and middle joints.

MALLET OR BASEBALL FINGER (OR FRACTURE):   This injury is caused by a sharp blow on the end of the finger such as that sustained when the finger is struck by a baseball, hence the name by which it is often called. At times the injury is an avulsion of the extensor tendon from the distal phalanx so that x-ray films are negative. In other instances, a small fragment of the

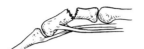

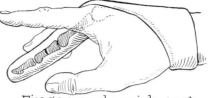

Fracture of middle
phalanx proximal
to insertion of flexor
dig. sublimis tendon.

Finger and wrist cast.
Prox. joint in flexion.

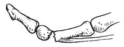

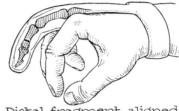

Fracture of middle
phalanx distal to
insertion of flexor
dig. sublimis tendon.

Distal fragment aligned
by mild flexion.

Figure 16–38 Fracture of middle phalanx of long finger with dorsal angulation, and another with palmar angulation; reduction and plaster splinting for each. (From Banks and Compere: 2nd Edition, 1947.)

dorsal and proximal portion of the distal phalanx, including some of the articular surface, is broken off (Fig. 16–39). Some authors consider that the injury results from forced hyperflexion of the phalanx. Others, particularly when a small fracture is present, consider the injury to be caused by hyperextension of the distal phalanx which jams the portion that breaks off against the middle phalanx. It seems likely that the latter explanation is correct when a fracture is present, and possibly hyperflexion is the cause of a tendon avulsion.

Either a tendon avulsion or a fracture cause considerable pain and tenderness over the dorsum of the distal joint and loss of the ability to extend

Extensor tendon

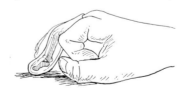

Avulsion (baseball)
fracture of distal
phalanx

Skin-tight plaster cast.
Distal phalanx hyperextended.
Middle and proximal
phalanges flexed

Figure 16–39 Baseball or mallet finger treated by plaster immobilization holding the middle joint in almost 45 degrees of flexion and the distal phalanx in hypertension. (From Banks and Compere.)

the distal phalanx completely. The distal phalanx remains in a "dropped" position, hence the term mallet finger.

Treatment may be either simple splinting or, in selected instances, operation to reattach the extensor tendon to the distal phalanx or fix the fragment in perfect position to restore extensor power. The physician should keep in mind that excellent functional results are likely to be obtained by simple measures even though some dropping of the distal phalanx may persist permanently.

Simple splinting consists of a short splint which does not immobilize the middle joint but holds the distal phalanx in extension. Splinting should be maintained for 5 or 6 weeks, and, thereafter, use of the short splint at night for several weeks may contribute to a more satisfactory result. Ideally, the finger should be splinted with the middle joint in about 45 degrees of flexion and the distal joint hyperextended as shown in Figure 16–39 which illustrates the use of a small plaster splint. Stock splints are available for holding the middle and distal joints of the injured finger in the desired position.

When the physician selects operative treatment for these injuries, he should understand that an optimal end result is not assured, particularly when the tendon is avulsed from its attachment. It is difficult to reattach the insertion of the extensor tendon so that the patient eventually has full extensor power of the distal phalanx. When a fracture is present, the same difficulties may be encountered, but ordinarily the combination of a small pin holding the fragment in place and a suture passing from the tendon through the tissues of the distal phalanx to a button over the end of the finger to protect fixation of the fracture will lead to an acceptable result. Ingenious methods in which an intramedullary pin is passed from the end of the finger across the hyperextended distal joint and even passed proximally until it perforates the proximal phalanx have been used to hold flexion of the middle joint and hyperextension of the distal joint. While good results with this method have been reported, certainly this method of stabilizing the fracture internally may lead to restriction of motion in both the distal and middle joints. Therefore, it is recommended only for surgeons with extensive experience in the method.

Chip Fractures: Chip fractures within or adjacent to one of the joints of the finger are not uncommon. Some are avulsed by ligaments placed under excessive strain. Others occur when one phalanx impacts against another as a result of excessive lateral angulating stress. With the exception of the baseball or mallet fracture, most chip fractures may be ignored.

Recovery of full motion in the finger is likely to take place sooner and the result is likely to be better if all splinting is omitted in favor of early active exercise and use of the digit. Unnecessary or particularly prolonged splinting of fingers for chip fractures predisposes to permanent limitation of motion in the joint near the chip fracture.

If the injury results in instability of the adjacent joint, splinting or perhaps even operative repair of the damage is necessary (see Chapter 20).

FRACTURES AND DISLOCATIONS OF THE LOWER EXTREMITY

Fractures and dislocations about the hip
    Fractures of the proximal portion of the femur (hip)
        Fractures of the neck of the femur (intracapsular fractures)
            Impacted fractures of the neck of the femur
            Unimpacted fractures of the neck of the femur
        Trochanteric fractures of the femur
    Dislocations of the hip
        Posterior dislocations of the hip without fractures
        Posterior dislocations of the hip with fractures of the acetabulum
        Posterior dislocation of the hip with chip fracture of the femoral
           head
        Anterior dislocation of the hip

Fractures of the shaft of the femur

Fractures of the distal end of the femur
    Supracondylar fractures of the femur
    T-fractures of the condyles
    Fractures of the medial or lateral condyle

Dislocations of the knee

Internal derangements of the knee
    Tears of semilunar cartilages
    Torn collateral ligaments
    Torn cruciate ligaments
    Loose osteocartilaginous bodies

Fractures of the patella

Fractures of the proximal end of the tibia (plateau)
    Fractures of the tibial spine
    Fractures of the lateral plateau of the tibia
    Fractures of the medial plateau of the tibia
    Fractures of lateral and medial plateaus (T-fractures)

Fractures of the shafts of the bones of the leg
    Fractures of the shafts of the tibia and fibula
    Fractures of the shaft of the tibia with an intact fibula
    Fractures of the shaft of the fibula with an intact tibia

Fractures and dislocations of the ankle
    Fractures of the ankle without displacement
    Fractures of the ankle with displacement
        Fractures of the lateral malleolus with lateral dislocation of the
           foot
        Fractures of the medial malleolus with displacement

Fractures of the bones of the foot
    Fractures of the calcaneus
    Fractures of the talus
    Fractures of the midtarsal bones (navicular, cuboid, and cuneiform)
    Fractures of the metatarsals
    Fractures of the toes
    Peritalar dislocation
    Tarsometatarsal dislocation
    Dislocation of the toes

Treatment of fractures of the lower extremity is designed to obtain (1) strong bony union with full length, (2) normal alignment and no abnormal rotation, (3) full muscle power and joint motion, and (4) stability even at the expense of mobility.

Painless weight-bearing is an important criterion of the end result. With fractures involving the hip, knee, and ankle joints, a perfect or near-perfect reduction is essential to minimize pain and restriction of motion.. Less than excellent reduction of these fractures predisposes to traumatic arthritis.

Swelling (edema) of the lower leg, ankle, and foot is likely to develop during and after immobilization for all fractures of the lower extremities. Every effort must be made to control or prevent it. Provided the arterial supply to the part is sufficient, elevation or at least the avoidance of dependency should be provided from the beginning of treatment. Regular exercise of all joints which do not cause movement of the fragments, such as the joints of the toes, helps to minimize edema. Following the removal of plaster casts or the discontinuation of traction, elastic bandages or elastic stockings should be worn to support the venous circulation. Intermittent elevation will minimize edema when the patient becomes ambulatory.

FRACTURES AND DISLOCATIONS ABOUT THE HIP

FRACTURES OF THE PROXIMAL PORTION OF THE FEMUR (HIP)

Fractures of the femoral neck and of the trochanteric region of the femur (Table 16–1) have much in common. Both are principally fractures of the elderly. The average age of the patient is between 70 and 80; almost a third occur in patients over 80. Women with this injury outnumber men

TABLE 16–1   DISTINGUISHING FEATURES OF FRACTURES OF THE HIP

Location	Intracapsular (Neck)	Extracapsular (Trochanteric)
Age	Usually 60–75 years	Usually 70–85 years
Operative treatment	Internal Fixation (Smith-Petersen nail, multiple pins or telescoping nail-plates)	Internal Fixation (Nail-plate such as Jewett, McLaughlin, Neufeld)
Nonoperative treatment	Ineffective	Continuous traction effective but hazardous because of complications; end results inferior to operative treatment
Nonunion	Common	Rare
Avascular necrosis of head	Common	Rare
Mortality before weight-bearing is resumed	15–20%	30–35%
Anticipated period for union	4–12 months	3–4 months

about four to one, probably because of a natural tendency toward coxa vara deformity, osteoporosis, and longer life expectancy.

Mortality rates are high because these patients are elderly, and because the curtailment of activity as a result of the fracture and treatment is not well tolerated. Deaths, however, do not occur from the fractures themselves, but from their complications, such as progression of cardiovascular-renal disease, pneumonia, and pulmonary embolism. Mortality in trochanteric fractures is higher than with intracapsular fractures, even though fractures of the trochanteric region almost always unite, while fractures of the neck commonly result in nonunion. Trochanteric fractures probably carry the higher mortality rate because they usually occur in older, more debilitated patients.

MECHANISM OF INJURY: Most fractures of the hip occur from a fall, as a rule, onto the injured side. Not infrequently, however, a patient will have the sensation that the hip breaks because of a misstep or stumble before the fall occurs.

DIAGNOSIS: The dominant complaint is severe pain in the hip, referred, in some instances, to the knee. The injured lower extremity appears shortened and falls into external rotation, the position of "helpless eversion," although these signs are not present if the fracture is impacted.

Roentgenograms in two planes are necessary to confirm and identify the type of the fracture. A satisfactory lateral roentgenogram is not obtained easily, but it is essential.

Fractures of the Neck of the Femur (Intracapsular Fractures of the Hip):   A fracture of the femoral neck has been called the "unsolved fracture" because it ends so often in nonunion or unites only to have the femoral head develop avascular necrosis several months or years later, and because union of the fracture always requires a long period of time.

The femoral head and even the neck have only a meager blood supply, which is a basic reason for nonunion. The head and neck receive their blood supply from intramedullary and reflected capsular arteries and the small artery of the ligamentum teres. Torn capsular vessels complicate many intracapsular fractures, often leading to nonunion or avascular necrosis (Fig. 16–40).

Fractures of the neck of the femur may be impacted or, more commonly, unimpacted. The clinical findings and choice of treatment may vary accordingly.

Impacted Fractures of the Neck of the Femur: When the fragments are well impacted, the patient has much less pain and the extremity does not fall into helpless eversion. The patient may even walk unaided although usually there is a limp. The hip may show a near normal range of

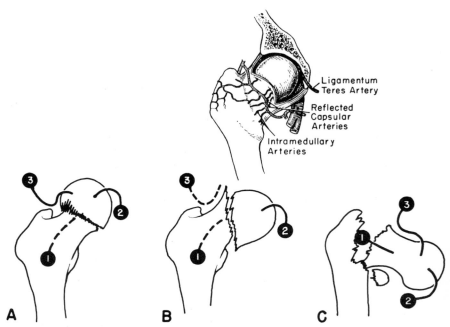

Figure 16–40   Blood supply to the head of the femur: (1) intramedullary arteries, (2) ligamentum teres artery, (3) reflected capsular arteries.

A, Avascular necrosis of the femoral head is an infrequent complication of an impacted lesion of the femoral neck. *B*, It frequently occurs after a displaced intracapsular fracture. *C*, Avascular necrosis is never seen after a trochanteric fracture. (From McLaughlin.)

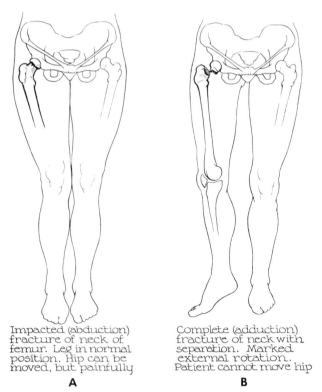

Impacted (abduction)
fracture of neck of
femur. Leg in normal
position. Hip can be
moved, but painfully

A

Complete (adduction)
fracture of neck with
separation. Marked
external rotation.
Patient cannot move hip

B

Figure 16–41 Position of the lower extremity following intracapsular fractures of the hip. *A*, Impacted (abduction) fracture of the neck of the right femur. Lower extremity in normal position. Hip can be moved actively and passively with minimal pain. *B*, Displaced fracture of the neck of the femur. Lower extremity appears shortened and is in marked external rotation. Patient cannot move the hip because of severe pain. (From Banks and Compere.)

motion in all directions. The degree and position of impaction are determined on two-plane roentgenograms. Impaction may have occurred in abduction (valgus) or in adduction (varus).

In an abduction impacted fracture, the line of fracture is near horizontal and the head is in a slight upward or valgus position (Fig. 16–41). The fragments usually are in excellent position as seen in the lateral roentgenogram. With firm impaction, the fracture is likely to unite solidly with no treatment other than a few weeks of bed rest, followed by the use of a wheel chair or crutches with minimal weight-bearing for 3 months. Some authorities advise routine internal fixation as a safeguard against disimpaction which does occur occasionally. If there is any doubt that the fracture is firmly impacted, internal fixation certainly is indicated. Moreover, even with firm impaction, it is reasonable that internal fixation will permit the patient to be out of bed and assume crutch-walking rather promptly without risk to the position of the fragments.

In an adduction impacted fracture, disimpaction is most likely to occur. These fractures, therefore, usually should be managed as unimpacted fractures.

Unimpacted Fractures of the Neck of the Femur: The majority of fractures of the neck of the femur are unimpacted and require operative treatment. Following reduction of the fragments, internal fixation is achieved, usually with multiple pins, a telescoping or nontelescoping nail-plate, or a Smith-Petersen three-flanged nail. The so-called "blind nailing" without exposing the fracture site is the procedure of choice. After accurate closed reduction and guide pin placement are confirmed by anteroposterior and lateral roentgenograms, the internal fixation device is inserted through a lateral incision below the greater trochanter. Serial roentgenograms are necessary to confirm the direction of the nail or multiple pins (Fig. 16–42). Occasionally, satisfactory closed reduction of the

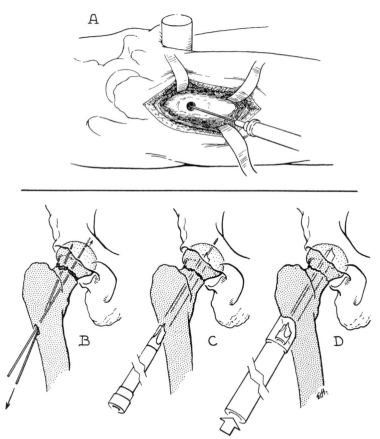

Figure 16–42 Stages of operation for internal fixation using a triflanged nail for fracture of the neck of the femur following accurate closed reduction. Note in *D* that, following removal of the guide pin, the fragments are impacted firmly over the triflanged nail. (From Hampton and Fitts.)

fragments cannot be obtained and open reduction is required to insure that the fragments are adequately reduced. Unless a good reduction is obtained, nonunion can be anticipated regardless of the internal fixation. **No patient should be removed from the operating table before final satisfactory placement of the internal fixation has been confirmed by anteroposterior and lateral roentgenograms.**

Although patients with fractures of the femoral neck are usually relatively poor surgical risks, if the operation is conducted under skillful anesthesia within 4 to 24 hours after admission, with adequate blood replacement and antibiotics, the hospital motality rate should be low. Following operation, the patient may be turned and placed in a chair several times a day without endangering the position of the fragments. The majority of these patients do not possess the necessary strength in the arms to avoid weight-bearing while using crutches. Yet, weight-bearing should be avoided until there is roentgenographic evidence of union of the fracture, which may require many months.

Operative treatment is preferable by far for patients with these fractures, not only because it gives the highest percentage of union, but because it is best for the patient's general condition. If, however, operative treatment is refused or cannot be carried out for other reasons, the Whitman abduction plaster hip spica probably offers the best chance for union of the fracture (Fig. 16–43). However, it carries a high incidence of life-endangering complications.

Because of the rather high incidence of nonunion and avascular necrosis of the head with fractures of the neck of the femur and the long period of time required to determine the end-result, some surgeons have abandoned internal fixation of these fractures in favor of primary insertion of a femoral head endoprosthesis if the patient is over 70 or 75 years of age and particularly if the line of fracture is subcapital (Fig. 16–44).

Following insertion of a prosthesis, the postoperative management is essentially the same as if the fracture had been reduced and fixed internally, except that weight-bearing may be permitted within a few days or at the most 2 weeks. This compromise treatment of fractures of the femoral neck accepts a hip somewhat inferior to one with a united fracture and a viable head, but does offer early ambulation and avoids the complications of nonunion and avascular necrosis. The patient should be told that in the future a cane may be needed as an aid to walking and that mild discomfort in the hip is to be anticipated, particularly during the first few steps after the sitting position.

Trochanteric Fractures of the Femur: These are located between the neck and about 1 inch below the lesser trochanter. The fragments have an excellent blood supply and, therefore, almost always unite, provided the patient survives and the fragments are held in a reasonably good reduction. A high mortality rate comes from the usual age (70 to 85 years) and the relatively poor general condition of people who tolerate inactivity poorly. A considerable amount of blood, estimated at about a liter, is lost

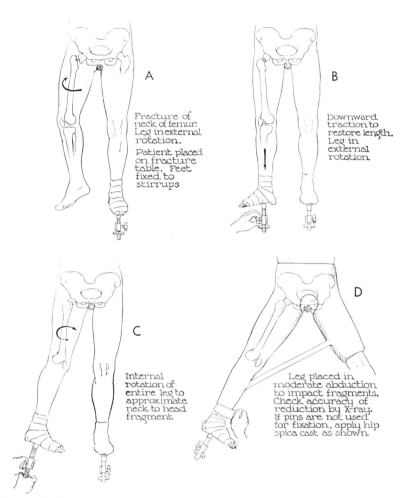

A

Fracture of neck of femur. Leg in external rotation.

Patient placed on fracture table. Feet fixed to stirrups

B

Downward traction to restore length. Leg in external rotation.

C

Internal rotation of entire leg to approximate neck to head fragment

D

Leg placed in moderate abduction to impact fragments. Check accuracy of reduction by X-ray. If pins are not used for fixation, apply hip spica cast as shown.

Figure 16–43 Whitman method of treatment for fractures of the neck of the femur. *A*, Patient is placed on a fracture table with each foot fixed in stirrups. *B*, Strong traction is applied to the injured extremity in order to restore length while it remains in external rotation. *C*, Maximum internal rotation of the extremity is provided. *D*, With the extremity in moderate abduction which tends to impact the fragments, a hip spica plaster cast is applied. The cast must include the thigh on the uninjured side. (From Banks and Compere.)

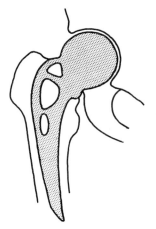

Figure 16–44 Replacement of femoral head by an intramedullary hip-joint endoprosthesis for treatment of a fracture of the femoral neck. (From McLaughlin.)

into the tissues with most trochanteric fractures, and more blood is lost during operation than occurs with operation for fractures of the femoral neck.

Trochanteric fractures should be treated by internal fixation with a nail-plate and screws. The configuration of the fracture determines whether or not a stable anatomic reduction can be achieved (Fig. 16–45). If the inferior cortex of the neck fragment and the medial cortex of the shaft fragment are intact, a stable reduction is possible in the anatomic position. However, if the inferior cortex of neck and medial cortex of shaft are comminuted, a stable reduction in the anatomic position may not be attainable. The neck and shaft fragments eventually assume a varus relationship because of the lack of a strong medial buttress. When this occurs, the nail usually cuts out of the neck fragment or the nail and plate bend or break. (See standard texts and literature for operative treatment of unstable intertrochanteric fractures.)

Subtrochanteric fractures singly or in combination with intertrochanteric fractures pose the most difficult problem in achieving a stable internally fixed reduction. Whereas internal fixation of trochanteric fractures is the method of choice to make possible early mobilization of the patient, certain precautions in mobilizing the patient with a subtrochanteric fracture may be necessary. Only the operating surgeon can judge the stability of reduction and fixation of these fractures for the individual patient and can plan the convalescence accordingly.

Union can be obtained with balanced suspension traction, but the incidence of complications and the mortality rate are much higher with traction. When treated with traction, the patient must be kept in bed constantly on the back, which predisposes to bed sores, thromboembolism pneumonia, senile dementia, and residual loss of knee motion.

The operative method permits the patients to be turned in bed promply and frequently and to be out of bed in a chair. The patient has less general discomfort and a much better mental attitude toward restriction of

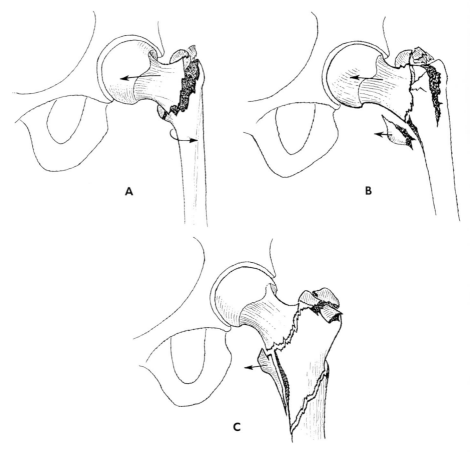

Figure 16–45   Various lines of fracture which may be present in trochanteric fractures. Internal fixation of a stable fracture as in *A* is relatively simple. However, if there is comminution of the femoral calcar as in *B* or if in addition there is a subtrochanteric fracture as in *C*, internal fixation presents a technically difficult operative problem. (From DePalma.)

activities during convalescence. The operative method is indicated because it is the best for the patient.

Weight-bearing usually must be avoided until the fracture has united as shown by roentgenograms. Union is more rapid in trochanteric fractures than in fractures of the femoral neck and usually occurs within 3 to 4 months.

DISLOCATIONS OF THE HIP

Dislocations of the hip occur only with severe trauma. In the majority, the head comes to rest behind the acetabulum and, therefore, are called posterior dislocations (Fig. 16–46*A*). Posterior dislocations often have an associated fracture of the posterior acetabular wall or of a small portion of the femoral head. Anterior dislocations (Fig. 16–46*B* and *C*) in which

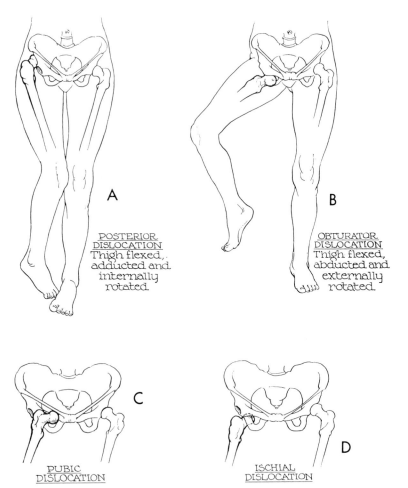

Figure 16–46 Types of dislocations of the hip. *A*, Posterior dislocation in which the thigh is flexed, adducted, and rotated internally. *B*, Anterior dislocation in which the head engages in the obturator foramen. *C*, Anterior dislocation in which the head rests on the pubis. In *B* and *C* the thigh is flexed, abducted, and externally rotated. *D*, Posterior dislocation in which the head comes to rest behind the ischium. (From Banks and Compere.)

the femoral head comes to rest in front of the acetabulum are rather rare and are seldom associated with fractures. Avascular necrosis of the femoral head may be a late complication of posterior dislocation. Central dislocations of the femoral head through a fracture of the floor of the acetabulum are discussed under Fractures of the Pelvis (see page 326).

Posterior Dislocations of the Hip Without Fractures: Posterior dislocation of the hip usually is sustained while the thigh is flexed and adducted. The injury may occur in an automobile collision from the strong force applied when the knee strikes the dashboard. A heavy weight dropped onto the low back of a person in a stooped position likewise may produce a hip dislocation.

The dislocated hip remains flexed and adducted and assumes an internally rotated position. The extremity appears shortened. These findings, except for shortening, are the exact opposite of those which occur with a fracture of the neck of the femur. The type of trauma sustained and the position of the extremity establish the clinical diagnosis, which nonetheless must be confirmed by x-ray examination of the pelvis and both hip joints in the anteroposterior view.

The sciatic nerve may be injured by the femoral head or a fragment of acetabulum in posterior dislocations of the hip. Therefore, careful motor and sensory examination of the extremity should be made and the findings recorded before reduction is attempted. Otherwise, if signs of nerve damage are found after reduction, the trauma of reduction may be blamed incorrectly.

TREATMENT: Three recognized methods are available for reduction of a posterior dislocation of the hip. One method may fail to give reduction and then another may succeed. Sufficient general anesthesia to give real muscular relaxation or spinal anesthesia usually is essential, although, in some instances soon after injury, reduction may be achieved without anesthesia.

1. Strong traction in the axis of the flexed and slightly adducted thigh is probably the most effective and safest method of reduction. Gentle maneuvering of the thigh toward external rotation and mild abduction may be advantageous. An assistant provides counter-traction by strong downward pressure against the pelvis. Traction, in effect, pulls the head back through the rent in the capsule produced by the injury. Reduction takes place with a satisfying snap or thump. These maneuvers may be carried out with the patient on a pad on the floor or on an x-ray table with the surgeon in his stocking feet standing on the table. The latter position is ideal as it positions the patient for radiological confirmation of the reduction.

2. The time-honored Bigelow method may be used (Fig. 16–47). The adducted thigh and the leg each are fully flexed over the abdomen. As traction is applied to the thigh, lateralward circumduction followed by external rotation and abduction may effect reduction. Excessive force can lead to a fracture of the neck or shaft of the femur. Sometimes a posterior dislocation is merely converted into an anterior dislocation so a roentgenogram should be obtained immediately.

3. The Stimson method, seldom used in recent years, remains a most atraumatic and effective method. The patient is anesthetized face down with the thighs flexed at the hip over the end of the table and the leg supported with the knee at a right angle. A heavy weight, up to 20 or 25 pounds, is placed on the upper leg thereby providing traction on the thigh. Traction is allowed to remain for several minutes until muscle spasm has

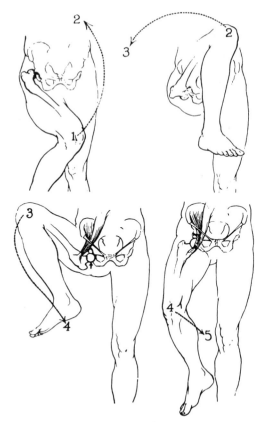

Figure 16–47 Bigelow maneuvers for reduction of a posterior dislocation of the hip. (1) The thigh is flexed, (2) over the abdomen, (3) circumducted laterally, (4) externally rotated, and (5) extended. (From Davis.)

been overcome, following which the operator merely rotates the extremity inward and outward. Reduction may be obtained with this method when other more popular methods have failed.

While reduction usually can be achieved with any of the methods, it does not always come easily. Considerable traction with only gentle rotation is often necessary. Open reduction may be required as a last resort.

POSTREDUCTION MANAGEMENT: Immobilization of the hip in a cast or prolonged traction on the extremity is not necessary. A few pounds of simple Buck's traction for a few days may help overcome spasm of the muscles and contribute to comfort of the patient. Redislocation is unlikely to occur. A safeguard against it is to keep the patient at bed rest without flexion of the hip for 3 to 4 weeks. The position of extension prevents pressure of the femoral head against the posterior rent in the capsule.

Although opinions vary as to the length of time weight-bearing should be avoided, it is recommended that weight-bearing and full function be permitted approximately 6 weeks after dislocation.

Posterior Dislocations of the Hip With Fractures of the Acetabulum: Fracture of the posterior portion of the acetabulum frequently complicates a posterior dislocation of the hip. The femoral head as it leaves the joint drives a fragment or fragments ahead of it. This combined injury is not uncommon in automobile collisions in which the knee of a front seat occupant strikes the dashboard — hence, it often is called a "dashboard dislocation." The diagnosis comes from roentgenogram findings.

TREATMENT: Reduction usually may be achieved by traction in the long axis of the thigh. As the hip is reduced, the fragment or fragments of acetabulum usually fall into position. The important consideration, however, is the size of the fragments and the defect in the acetabular wall. If the fragments are small, they may be ignored regardless of their final position and the hip may be managed as a dislocation without fracture.

On the other hand, even though large fragments go into reduction, subsequent displacement and spontaneous redislocation of the hip can occur easily through the weakened posterior acetabular wall. Therefore, open reduction and internal fixation of large reduced or unreduced acetabular fragments is indicated to provide a stable posterior acetabulum.

After either closed or operative reduction, external immobilization is not necessary. Flexion of the thigh at the hip is avoided as this position would cause the femoral head to press against the weakened portion of the acetabulum. With the thigh in extension, normal muscle tone holds the femoral head against the intact superior portion of the acetabulum. All that is necessary, therefore, is to keep the patient at bed rest with the thigh in extension for a period of 4 to 6 weeks. The patient may be turned onto either side or face down as long as the injured hip remains in extension. With very stable fixations, even these precautions may be unnecessary.

Posterior Dislocation of the Hip with Chip Fracture of the Femoral Head: As the hip is displaced, a piece of the head of the femur may be sheared off as it leaves the acetabulum. This fragment may fall into the acetabulum and prevent proper seating of the femoral head in the socket. If so, operation for excision of the fragment is necessary. If, however, reduction of the dislocation is achieved without interference by the fragment, the latter usually may be ignored as it is unlikely to interfere with subsequent hip function. Early surgical excision is to be avoided for two reasons: (1) the operation itself may further damage arterial flow to the femoral head from capsular arteries, thereby increasing the chances of avascular necrosis and (2) operative trauma may increase the chances of myositis ossificans about the joint. Late operative removal of the fragment may be necessary in some cases.

Anterior Dislocation of the Hip: Anterior dislocation, a rather rare condition, may occur when the thigh is forced into extreme abduction and external rotation. The head usually comes to rest in the obturator foramen. The extremity goes into abduction, external rotation, and some flexion, and appears longer than the uninjured limb. While the position of the extremity resembles that assumed with a fracture of the hip, it may be distinguished clinically because of the increased rather than decreased length and the mild flexion.

TREATMENT: Reduction usually may be achieved easily, often without anesthesia, by traction in the axis of the thigh, followed by internal rotation and adduction. The Bigelow method for anterior dislocations of the hip also may be used. The maneuvers are the reverse of those for posterior dislocation of the hip. The thigh and leg are flexed; then, as traction is made, the extremity is circumducted toward adduction and brought into internal rotation and extension.

POSTREDUCTION MANAGEMENT: Only a few days of bed rest and avoidance of abduction, external rotation, and hyperextension strain, and about 4 weeks on crutches are necessary. Avascular necrosis of the femoral head is unlikely to develop following anterior dislocation of the hip, particularly if reduction is performed within a few hours of injury.

FRACTURES OF THE SHAFT OF THE FEMUR

The shaft of the femur extends distally from about 1 inch below the lesser trochanter to the largely cancellous bone of the supracondylar area. Its blood supply is good, and for that reason nonunion is rare unless the fracture is not adequately reduced or immobilized. Malunion, however, occurs frequently. Powerful muscles of the body attach to the femur and tend to cause angulation and over-riding.

The femur is encircled by tight muscular and fascial compartments. Collections of fluid within them are difficult to detect by physical examination. A huge volume of blood or pus, therefore, may go unrecognized. A large unrecognized hemorrhage from fractures of the femoral shaft may be contained within these tight compartments.

Fractures in the proximal and distal portions of the shaft show the greatest displacement and are rather difficult to reduce. In proximal fractures, the upper fragment is usually flexed by the iliopsoas and abducted and externally rotated by the muscles attached to the greater trochanter. In distal-third fractures, the proximal end of the distal fragment is pulled posteriorly by the attachments of the gastrocnemius, causing posterior angulation. The sharp end of this fragment may easily injure the large nerves and blood vessels in the popliteal space (Fig. 16–48). In fractures of the middle of the shaft, the strong adductor muscles tend to angulate the fragments apex lateral.

MECHANISM OF INJURY

Because considerable violence is required to break the femoral shaft, severe displacement of fragments, extensive soft tissue damage, and considerable blood loss usually accompany the injury. The fracture may be

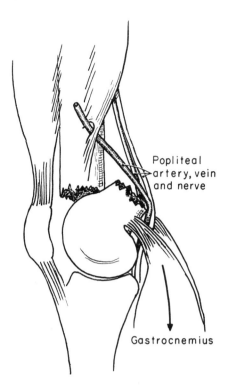

Popliteal
artery, vein
and nerve

Gastrocnemius

Figure 16–48 The proximal end of a short distal fragment of a supracondylar fracture has been pulled posteriorly by the gastrocnemius so that it encroaches on the popliteal nerves and vessels. (From McLaughlin.)

caused by a fall or by direct violence, as in an automobile crash. Gunshot fractures of the femoral shaft also occur and are seen in civilian life as well as during warfare. In contrast to fractures of the hip, which occur principally in the aged, fractures of the shaft are seen more commonly in young and middle-aged adults and children.

DIAGNOSIS

Complete fractures of the femoral shaft are easily diagnosed because contracture of the powerful thigh muscles results in severe angulation and over-riding, producing an obvious deformity. Pain is usually severe, and traumatic shock may result from the severe soft tissue and bone damage and the resulting loss of blood and extracellular fluid into the tissues.

A clinical diagnosis must be confirmed by adequate roentgenograms, only after adequate emergency splinting (see page 187), so that the exact location, type, and contour of the fracture may be determined. The entire shaft of the bone should be visualized so that double fractures will not go unrecognized. A fracture of the femoral neck or dislocation of the hip may accompany a shaft fracture.

TREATMENT

General Treatment: All methods of treatment of fractures of the femoral shaft are designed to prevent shortening, angulation, and rotational deformity, and to maintain apposition of the bone ends long enough to permit union. Satisfactory union will usually occur with less than full apposition; therefore, anatomic reduction is not required.

Limitation of knee motion and atrophy of quadriceps musculature are common complications following femoral shaft fractures and may occur following each form of treatment. Every effort must be made to minimize these complications from the time of injury. Quadriceps setting exercises must be started early, and active and passive knee exercises should be instituted when healing of the fracture permits. Foot and ankle exercises also should be initiated as early as possible.

Definitive Treatment: Fractures of the femoral shaft may be treated by one of two methods: (1) balanced traction; or (2) operative fixation. External skeletal fixation has been used by some surgeons but it has resulted in a high incidence of complications—nonunion, knee stiffness, infection along the pin tracts—and therefore is not recommended. Because of the powerful muscle pull in adults, closed reduction and immobilization in plaster are unsatisfactory, especially in comminuted, oblique, or spiral fractures. Displacement and angulation tend to occur within the cast, even though a perfect reduction may have been obtained and even though the fracture is transverse.

CONTINUOUS BALANCED TRACTION: Before the introduction of intramedullary nailing for fractures of the femoral shaft, the most generally used method was continuous balanced skeletal traction. Even now, it is an excellent method of treating femoral shaft fractures and is regaining popularity. The wire or pin for traction is drilled through the broad portion of the distal femur just proximal to the adductor tubercle or through the upper tibia about an inch posterior to the tibial tubercle. Infection along the wire or pin track is rare.

Figure 16–49 illustrates the use of balanced skeletal traction. The half-ring leg splint with a Pearson attachment in balanced suspension from an overhead frame is the most generally employed system. The splint must be long and wide enough for the extremity to rest confortably on the slings. The Pearson attachment is attached at the level of the upper border of the patella. The knee should be maintained in 170 to 175 degrees extension. The angle of the attachment to the splint should conform to the normal valgus at the knee. The foot is supported at 90 degrees by a foot rest or suspended at 90 degrees by a stockinet attached over the foot and secured to the skin by tincture of benzoin.

The distal fragment (and accordingly the leg and foot) must be allowed to remain in sufficient external rotation to conform to the uncontrolled rotation of the proximal fragment. Overpull with distraction of the fragments must be avoided. Roentgenograms must be made frequently in the early stages of treatment to detect overpull and other deformities and to allow prompt reduction of traction and other indicated adjustments of the traction apparatus.

Fractures of the upper half of the femoral shaft are best treated with a

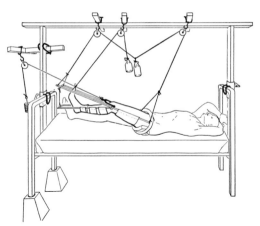

Figure 16–49 Balanced suspension skeletal traction utilizing a Thomas full-ring splint with a Pearson attachment. In this instance the pin has been inserted through the lower femur. The Pearson attachment is attached at the level of the upper border of the patella at an angle which maintains the normal valgus at the knee. The slings on both the splint and the attachment should abut each other but not overlap. They support the thigh from the ring of the splint to just proximal to the bulge of the femoral condyles. Slings on the Pearson attachment should support the leg from a point just distal to the posterior bulge of the upper tibia to the tendo Achilles for which adequate padding must be provided. The foot is supported at 90 degrees by suspension, using stockinet attached over the foot by tincture of benzoin. The ring is placed firmly against the ischial tuberosity. The weights for suspension not only support the entire splint arrangement but also aid in maintaining the ring in proper position. Elevation of the foot of the bed to increase the counter traction of the weight of the body is usually essential. (From Rhodes, Allen, Harkins, and Moyer.)

wire through the distal femur which will permit knee motion to be instituted early. In fractures of the upper third, the proximal fragment is usually sharply flexed, abducted, and externally rotated (Fig. 16–50). In such instances traction must be made with the thigh flexed, abducted, and externally rotated so as to bring the distal fragment into proper rotation and alignment with the proximal fragment.

Fractures of the lower half of the femoral shaft are usually best controlled with the wire or pin inserted through the proximal tibia posterior to the tubercle. Control of the distal fragment is difficult if the wire or pin is through the femur.

Posterior displacement or angulation of fractures of the distal end of the femoral shaft, caused by the pull of the gastrocnemius, is difficult to correct. A satisfactory method employs two wires: one at the level of the tibial tubercle for longitudinal traction and one just above the femoral condyles for anterior or vertical lift to correct the posterior angulation of the distal fragment (Fig. 16–51). Another way is as follows: the wire is placed at the level of the tibial tubercle and the hinge of the Pearson attachment at the fracture site instead of at the knee. Traction is made parallel with the leg, which is kept horizontal with the floor, rather than in the line of the proximal fragment. If a satisfactory position is not accomplished within 24

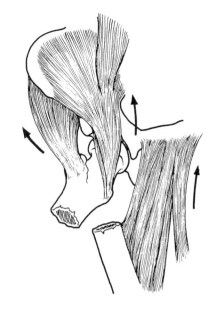

Figure 16–50 Subtrochanteric fracture. The proximal fragment is flexed by the iliopsoas, abducted by the lesser glutei, and externally rotated. The distal fragment is adducted and pulled proximally. (From McLaughlin.)

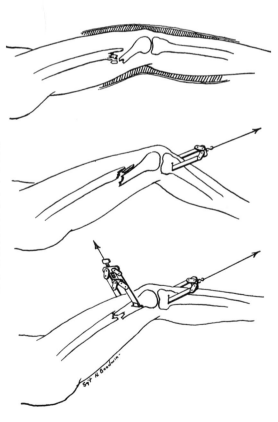

Figure 16–51 Diagrammatic representation of two-wire skeletal traction for fractures of the femur in the distal third. *Top,* Usual deformity which is difficult to correct. *Center,* Skeletal traction using a pin through the proximal tibia does not provide adequate reduction. *Bottom,* Adequate reduction is achieved when an additional wire is inserted in the lower femoral fragment and vertical lift is provided. (From Rhodes, Allen, Harkins, and Moyer.)

to 48 hours, manipulation of the fragments in the traction apparatus may be done under anesthesia.

Traction should be maintained until bony union has occurred, as shown by clinical and roentgenologic evidence which may require three to four months. Weight-bearing should not be allowed until union is solid. Patients with only precarious union should be kept in traction for an added length of time, during which active and passive knee exercises may be instituted. Further immobilization, however, may be provided by a walking hip spica cast which permits partial weight-bearing with crutches. Ischial weight-bearing leg braces may be valuable later, but they may not prevent refractures in event of falls.

OPEN REDUCTION AND INTERNAL FIXATION: Another common method of treating femoral shaft fractures is open reduction and internal fixation. Until the introduction of intramedullary nailing for these fractures about two decades ago, the operative method usually was employed only when a satisfactory reduction could not be accomplished with balanced traction. Then, internal fixation was obtained with a metal plate and screws (stainless steel or vitallium) which necessitated supplementary immobilization in a plaster hip spica. The incidence of nonunion was rather high and plaster immobilization for several months contributed to knee stiffness and muscle atrophy. Plates often broke even in a hip spica cast. For these reasons, internal fixation with a plate and screws is not ideal and intramedullary nailing has largely replaced it.

Intramedullary nailing has been used widely during the last two decades when the contour of the fracture is such as to permit stabilization by the nail (Fig. 16–52). The technique is particularly applicable for transverse or near transverse fractures of the middle two-fourths of the femur. Intramedullary nailing leads to a high rate of union and has the great advantages of allowing early weight-bearing, better preservation of joint motion, and less muscle atrophy. After a definitely stable intramedullary nailing, a patient may be up on crutches with guarded weight-bearing within a few days and may resume a sedentary occupation within a few weeks, both of which are totally impracticable with other methods. Intramedullary nailing permits ready treatment of concurrent injuries.

Intramedullary nailing usually should be done at open operation although "blind nailing" using an image intensifier is gaining popularity. A single Küntscher nail of adequate diameter is preferred.

The hazards of intramedullary nailing include infection, which may be catastrophic, and technical difficulties in the insertion of the nail. The nail may split, bend, or break. If the nail is driven too far distally, the knee joint may be injured. Fat embolism may occur, but serious effects from it are rare. In the German medical literature of World War II, many deaths attributed to fat embolism were probably the result of shock from lack of adequate blood replacement or inadequate anesthetic management.

The nail should be left in place until bony union has occurred and fully matured; it is then best removed. If infection occurs, it is probably

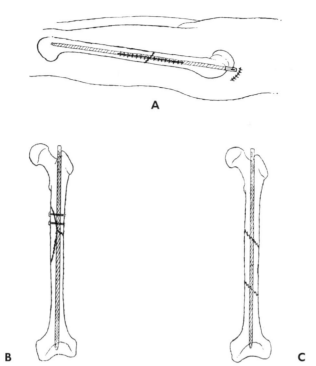

Figure 16–52 *A*, Near transverse fracture. *B*, Comminuted fracture, and *C*, segmental fracture in the middle third of the femoral shaft stabilized by an intramedullary nail. (From DePalma.)

best to leave the nail in place to stabilize the fragments, but wide dependent drainage should be maintained.

FRACTURES OF THE DISTAL END OF THE FEMUR

SUPRACONDYLAR FRACTURES OF THE FEMUR

Supracondylar fractures with severe posterior displacement may be difficult to reduce by closed methods. Occasionally manipulative reduction can be achieved and maintained by a plaster hip spica. In some instances, balanced suspension skeletal traction using a pin or wire through the proximal tibia will achieve reduction. In others, two-wire skeletal traction, using a second wire to lift the distal fragment of femur (see p. 280) may be employed advantageously.

If reduction cannot be obtained by closed methods, internal fixation may be indicated, using a blade-plate and screws somewhat comparable to those used for trochanteric fractures. Several designs of blade-plates, specifically for stabilization of supracondylar fractures of the femur, are available from producers of internal fixation devices.

T-FRACTURES OF THE CONDYLES

T-fractures of the femoral condyles are transverse supracondylar fractures with an added vertical line of fracture extending through the articular surface between the condyles. The shaft of the femur is often
wedged between the condyles. Anatomic reduction must be accomplished
if pain, disability, and traumatic arthritis are to be prevented. In most instances in which fragments are displaced, the preferred method of treatment may be open reduction and internal fixation, particularly in strong
young or middle-aged adults (Fig. 16–53). First the condyles are approximated and fixed in proper relation to each other. Then the shaft is fixed to

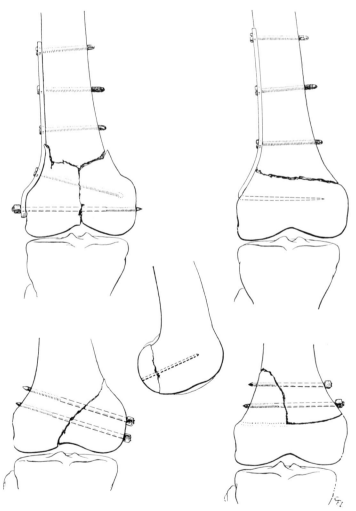

Figure 16–53 Methods of stabilization and reduction of various fractures of the distal
end of the femur. (From Crenshaw.)

the condyles using a blade-plate and screws. Following internal fixation, it might be advisable to use a plaster spica until union is solid, which usually requires 2 to 3 months. By means of modern internal fixation devices, the fragments often can be stabilized so effectively that immobilization by a supplemental plaster cast is unnecessary.

Balanced skeletal traction with a Kirschner wire inserted at the level of the tibial tubercle has been used successfully for these injuries in elderly patients with fractures so comminuted as to preclude stable internal fixation and particularly in patients for whom anesthesia and a major operative procedure are contraindicated.

FRACTURES OF THE MEDIAL OR LATERAL CONDYLE

Fractures of the medial or the lateral femoral condyle with displacement should be treated by open reduction and internal fixation. After an anatomic reduction, the condylar fragment is fixed by nails, pins, or screws (Fig. 16–53). A snug long-leg cast or hip spica may be applied for 3 or 4 weeks, after which union is usually sufficient to begin active and passive motion of the knee without weight-bearing. After operation, instead of being immobilized in plaster, the extremity may be placed in balanced suspension without traction in a Thomas or half-ring leg splint for 3 or 4 weeks. During the last 2 weeks, active knee exercises are permissible.

Undisplaced fractures usually require a hip spica for 4 to 6 weeks, although occasionally, in thin individuals, a snug long-leg cast will suffice.

DISLOCATIONS OF THE KNEE

In complete dislocation of the knee, the tibia is displaced so that it no longer articulates with the femur in any way. This relatively rare injury may occur through direct violence on the upper leg just below an extended knee or by forced hyperextension of the leg at the knee. For it to occur, both collateral ligaments and both cruciate ligaments must be torn at least partially. Probably momentary partial dislocation with spontaneous reduction occurs occasionally. If so, although a dislocation of the knee is not present when the patient is examined, marked instability in all directions is found.

A complete dislocation of the knee usually can be reduced easily by traction and manipulation. Immobilization with the knee flexed some 10 degrees in a single hip spica for 4 weeks and then a snug long-leg cast for 8 more weeks may be used, but this method may not result in an excellent and stable knee. If reduction and plaster immobilization are used, a hip spica is preferable even if the patient is thin since it serves as a safeguard against abnormal abduction or adduction movement at the knee which can occur in a long-leg cast and lead to persisting instability.

Early operative repair of torn collateral and cruciate ligaments, following reduction of a dislocation of the knee, is the method most likely to give good results. While many good results have been obtained by closed reduction and immobilization for 2 to 3 months, operative repair of the knee ligaments is recommended, unless there are contraindications.

Complications of complete dislocation of the knee include damage to the popliteal artery and to a major peripheral nerve trunk, usually the peroneal, behind the knee. The artery may be torn or pressure may obstruct the blood flow. This emphasizes the importance of rapid appraisal of the circulatory status of the leg and foot when the patient is first seen. Signs of vascular insufficiency demand immediate reduction of the dislocation which, at times, can be done without anesthesia. If after reduction of the dislocation, normal pulsations at the foot do not return, surgical exploration of the popliteal fossa is indicated to relieve obstruction or to repair a torn popliteal artery. A diagnosis of mere arterial spasm is unjustified.

The peroneal nerve is injured in dislocation of the knee more often than the posterior tibial nerve. The patient should be instructed to carry out movements of the toes just as soon as he is seen. This prereduction observation may prove advantageous in evaluating damage to the nerve trunk when paralysis of the nerve supply to the foot is found after reduction of the dislocation. While the prognosis for eventual recovery is favorable, it is by no means certain. As a rule, however, early exploration for a damaged peripheral nerve trunk is not indicated.

INTERNAL DERANGEMENTS OF THE KNEE

The knee, which is a hinge joint, depends on strong ligaments plus the strength of the musculature of the thigh for its integrity and stability. As the knee is flexed and extended, those structures hold the condyles of the femur and plateaus of the tibia snugly in contact at all points.

Internal derangements of the knee are mechanical derangements in the function of the joint caused by some lesion which eliminates the supporting strength of the major ligaments of the knee or which mechanically prevents the constant snug contact and smooth gliding of the tibial plateaus over the condyles of the femur as the leg is flexed or extended.

All acute injuries of the knee without fracture, when viewed on x-ray examination, are either contusions, sprains (a tear of the capsule of some degree or possibly a tear or contusion of the infrapatella fat pad), or true internal derangements. The physician must differentiate between these conditions, using the history of injury, the symptoms of the patient, and the findings on physical examination. Unless a definite diagnosis of an internal derangement can be established when the patient is first seen, the injury must be treated as a sprain by resting the joint, applying compression dressings (Fig. 16–54), and possibly aspirating the accumulated fluid. On the other hand, every acute injury of the knee must not be treated as a simple sprain, as many require specific treatment for one or a combination of the several internal derangements.

TEARS OF SEMILUNAR CARTILAGES

Tears of the semilunar cartilages result from twisting knee injuries. Normally, the semilunar cartilages buffer rotary grinding actions of the condyles of the femur on the tibia. At times, a cartilage becomes impinged between the bones and is torn. The medial cartilage may be torn by an abduction-external rotation strain and the lateral cartilage by an adduction-internal rotation strain. The tear may be a longitudinal split down the long axis of the cartilage (a bucket-handle tear) or it may be a flap at any point along the inner margin (Fig. 16–55). Occasionally, the entire cartilage is avulsed from its attachment to the tibia. With each type, the torn portion of the cartilage may be caught between the femur and tibia and cause symptoms of mechanical derangement. Tears of medial cartilages outnumber those of lateral cartilages about nine to one.

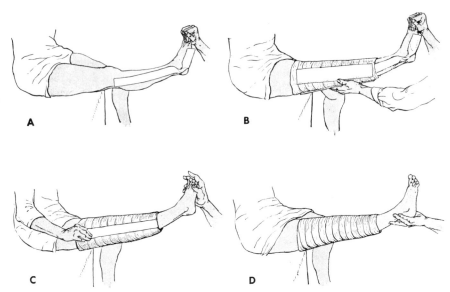

Figure 16–54 Application of the O'Donoghue cotton cast as a compression dressing. *A,* A strip of 2-inch adhesive tape about 3 feet long is applied to each side of the leg. *B,* Six to eight rolls of sheet wadding are applied from the midthigh to the midcalf over which wet yucca board splints are applied posteriorly and on each side. Yucca boards are wrapped with gauze to apply firm even pressure to the leg. *C,* Adhesive strips are turned back over the gauze and additional gauze and adhesive tape are applied. The adhesive strips support the compression dressing so it will not slip downward on the leg. (From O'Donoghue: *Treatment of Injuries to Athletes.* 2nd Edition. Philadelphia, W. B. Saunders, 1970.)

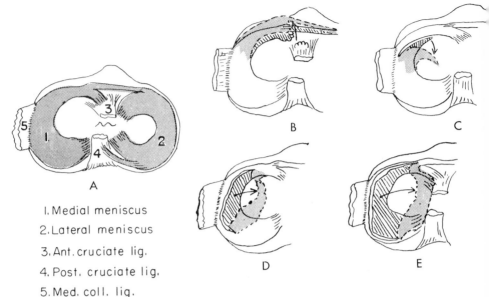

1. Medial meniscus
2. Lateral meniscus
3. Ant. cruciate lig.
4. Post. cruciate lig.
5. Med. coll. lig.

Figure 16–55   Types of tears of semilunar cartilages. *A*, Normal structure. *B*, Avulsion of anterior tibial attachment of the medial meniscus—the loose anterior horn (stippled) swings in and out of the joint interval. *C*, Single pedicle tear—the hypermobile fragment swings in and out of the joint. *D*, A splitting tear—the torn fragment swings in and out of the joint on a double pedicle. *E*, A locked bucket handle tear—a major portion of the meniscus becomes trapped in the femoral notch. (From McLaughlin.)

Diagnosis: Classically, a patient with a torn medial semilunar cartilage gives a history of a twisting injury accompanied by a painful snapping sensation on the inner side of the knee. Immediately the knee joint is locked in slight flexion. In a truly locked knee, the leg cannot be extended completely because of a mechanical block. It can be flexed fairly well although not necessarily through the full range of motion. This history indicates a bucket-handle tear with the torn portion of the cartilage displaced into the intercondylar notch of the femur. Pain persists and considerable effusion develops. Tenderness, which is fairly well localized, is found over the medial joint line. Standard roentgenograms are negative because the semilunar cartilage is not visualized by x-ray examination. This clinical syndrome establishes the diagnosis. It occurs, however, in only a small number of patients with torn semilunar cartilages.

In the majority of instances, the diagnosis of a torn semilunar cartilage is made on the history of a twisting injury to the knee, perhaps accompanied by a snap, and subsequent repeated episodes of painful, slipping, catching, near-locking sensations on the inner side of the joint. Tenderness over the cartilage usually persists after the first injury. Recurring effusions may take place. The history also is likely to reveal asymptomatic intervals between symptomatic episodes with recurrences brought on by additional twisting injuries of varying severity. Some atrophy of the quadriceps musculature may be discernible. Repeated x-ray examinations are negative. The history of repeated actual or impending mechanical derangements well localized to the inner side of the joint is more important than any other symptom or the findings on examination in arriving at the diagnosis. In an occasional patient, the diagnosis may be justified on only a history of a twisting injury, persisting pain and tenderness on the inner side of the knee, and a feeling of weakness in the joint, but the diagnosis rests on much sounder grounds if the symptoms of a true mechanical derangement are present.

The diagnosis of a torn lateral semilunar cartilage is made on comparable history, symptoms, and signs on the lateral side of the joint.

Treatment: Once a semilunar cartilage is torn, it probably never heals. The cartilages have such poor blood supply that any healing efforts are usually ineffective. On the other hand, if, instead of an actual tear of a cartilage, the coronary ligament which attaches it to the tibia is torn so that the entire cartilage is displaced, healing of the torn ligamentous attachment may readily occur if the cartilage is returned to its normal position and held there for a few weeks. With this exception, the guiding rule is once a torn cartilage, always a torn cartilage.

Surgical excision of the torn cartilage or, in selected bucket-handle tears, of the torn portion of the cartilage is the best definitive therapy once the diagnosis has been established. Surgery may be postponed, however, until a time convenient to the patient, unless the knee is locked and cannot be unlocked.

Nonoperative treatment includes aspiration of the joint, compression bandages about the knee, and protection from weight-bearing with crutches until most of the joint reaction has subsided. Nonoperative therapy is likely to be used one or more times in those instances in which the joint is not locked as the diagnosis cannot be established so as to justify surgery without a history of recurring episodes. Occasionally, in first episodes without true locking, a plaster cylinder cast may be used for 3 or 4 weeks. The rationale of the plaster cylinder cast in first episodes is based upon the possibility that the entire cartilage has been displaced and, if so, that healing of the coronary ligament as previously described may permanently relieve the patient. **With either operative or nonoperative treatment, strenuous quadriceps setting exercises throughout convalescence are highly important in rehabilitation of the patient.**

TORN COLLATERAL LIGAMENTS

Tears of the collateral ligaments result from the same type of abduction or adduction forces on the extended knee as those which may cause fractures of the tibial plateaus (see page 298). A tear of a collateral ligament of the knee on one side and a fracture of the tibial plateau on the other may

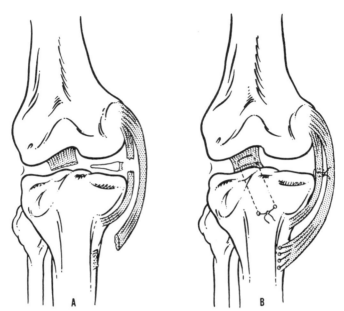

Figure 16–56   *A*, Diagrammatic representation of ruptures of both layers of the medial collateral ligament, the anterior cruciate ligament, and the medial semilunar cartilage. *B*, Torn cartilage has been removed, the anterior cruciate ligament has been reattached to the tibial spine, and each layer of the medial collateral ligament has been repaired. (From O'Donoghue, D. H.: J. Bone & Joint Surg., *32-A*:721, 1950.)

result from the same trauma. Tears of the medial collateral ligament are much more common than those of the lateral collateral ligament (Fig. 16–56*A*).

Diagnosis: Tears of the collateral ligaments are acutely painful and cause immediate disability. In all but minor injuries, the patient cannot tolerate weight-bearing. Pain and tenderness are localized over the torn collateral ligament. Hemarthrosis develops rapidly. Within 12 to 24 hours, the skin overlying the torn ligament is likely to become discolored from subcutaneous hemorrhage seeping toward the surface.

The diagnosis is confirmed on physical examination. Normally with the knee extended to about 170 degrees, abduction and adduction strains elicit little or no lateral movement. With a tear of a collateral ligament, this stabilizing function is impaired or lost so that the extended leg may be abducted (torn medial collateral) or adducted (torn lateral collateral) definitely more than the normal leg—the cardinal sign of a torn collateral ligament of the knee. The degree of abnormal mobility varies with the extent to which the ligament is torn.

Treatment: Treatment varies with the extent of the tear. Muscle guard by the quadriceps as a result of pain produced by the injury and the examination itself tends to mask the instability. Examination under anesthesia, therefore, may be necessary to demonstrate the full extent of the ligamentous tear.

When the extended leg can be abnormally abducted (or adducted) only 10 degrees or less, the injury is probably a stretching tear rather than a true rupture of the ligament. Under these circumstances, immobilization in a plaster cylinder is indicated. The cast should be applied with the knee flexed 15 to 20 degrees. The leg must be held during casting so as not to place any stretch on the torn ligament. The cast should remain in place for 4 to 6 weeks. During this time in most instances, weight-bearing is avoided by the use of crutches. When the degree of tear is minimal and when the plaster cylinder remains snug and well fitting, weight-bearing without the use of crutches may be permitted in selected instances.

When the degree of lateral instability on testing exceeds 10 degrees (Fig. 16–57), primary operative repair is usually the treatment of choice (Fig. 16–56B). This permits a thorough intra-articular inspection, so that if the adjacent semilunar cartilage is torn, it can be removed. Accurate surgical repair of the torn collateral ligament predisposes to the optimal functional result in a minimum period of time. If for any reason, operative treatment is not provided, immobilization in a plaster cylinder with the knee flexed 15 to 20 degrees should be provided for 8 weeks.

TORN CRUCIATE LIGAMENTS

The cruciate ligaments are stretched or torn in injuries which cause excessive movement of the tibia on the femur in the anteroposterior direction. The anterior cruciate ligament, which becomes taut with the leg in extension and then limits hyperextension, is often torn in twisting-hyperextension injuries. The posterior cruciate ligament, which is taut in flexion and prevents backward displacement of the tibia on the femur, is often torn when the upper portion of the flexed tibia strikes a dashboard and as a result is driven backward on the femur.

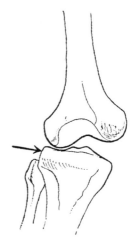

Figure 16–57 Wide gaping of the medial side of the knee joint indicative of a rupture of the medial collateral ligament. (From DePalma.)

Diagnosis: The diagnosis of a torn cruciate ligament is made on the basis of physical findings in a patient having all the symptoms of a severe sprain of the knee. Normally, when the knee is flexed to about 90 degrees, little or no passive movement of the proximal end of the tibia on the femur can be elicited. When the anterior cruciate ligament is torn, the proximal end of the tibia can be pulled forward excessively (the anterior drawer sign) (Fig. 16–58*A*). In addition, excessive hyperextension of the leg may be found. With a torn posterior cruciate ligament, the proximal end of the tibia can be pushed backward on the femur excessively (the posterior drawer sign) (Fig. 16–58*B*). Actually, with a torn posterior cruciate ligament, the proximal tibia may remain displaced backward from where it can be pulled forward passively to the normal position. When both cruciate ligaments are torn, the upper tibia can be pushed backward and pulled forward far in excess of the normal. Comparison with the range of passive anteroposterior movement on the opposite knee is always important in evaluating the findings in a suspected tear of a cruciate ligament.

Treatment: Whether a torn cruciate ligament ever heals spontaneously is subject to question. Many injuries of this structure are stretching elongations, so that after healing, the ligament remains lax. Complete tears apparently seldom, if ever, heal so as to restore continuity without operative repair. When the anterior attachment of the anterior cruciate ligament has been avulsed from the anterior tibial spine, it can be held in place by a mattress suture of silk or wire passing through two parallel drill holes in the upper tibia (Fig. 16–56*B*) (see Fractures of the Tibial Spine, page 297). Such a repair is frequently a supplemental procedure to operative repair of

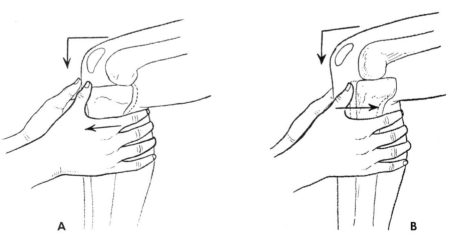

Figure 16–58   *A*, Anterior drawer sign indicative of torn anterior cruciate ligament. *B*, Posterior drawer sign indicative of a torn posterior cruciate ligament. In many such injuries, the tibia remains displaced posteriorly but can be pulled forward into normal relationship with the femur. Such a finding of a torn posterior cruciate ligament should not be interpreted as a torn anterior cruciate ligament. (From DePalma.)

a torn medial collateral ligament. A tear of the anterior cruciate ligament often is associated with a torn medial collateral ligament.

If the physician suspects a complete tear or an avulsion of a cruciate ligament in an acute knee injury, he is justified in examining the knee with the patient under anesthesia. If the diagnosis is confirmed, the torn ligament should be surgically repaired. After repair, the knee is immobilized in a plaster cylinder cast for about 6 weeks.

In an acute injury, without evidence of a tear sufficient to justify operation, therapy is the same as for a sprain of the knee. If the joint is distended, the fluid is aspirated. If a cruciate ligament has been torn, the fluid usually contains blood. A compression dressing is applied and weight-bearing is restricted or avoided by the use of crutches. The regimen is usually followed until the reaction to injury about the joint has subsided. Occasionally plaster cylinder immobilization for 4 to 6 weeks is justified. With anterior cruciate lesions, the cast should be applied with the knee in 15 to 20 degrees of flexion. With posterior cruciate tears, the tibia should be held forward and in near complete extension during application of the cast. Strenuous quadriceps and hamstring-setting exercises during convalescence are exceedingly important in minimizing residual disability.

When a torn cruciate ligament is diagnosed as part of a chronic instability of the knee due to other than a most recent (up to 7 to 14 days) injury, about all that can be accomplished without operative reconstruction is strengthening of the quadriceps and hamstring muscles by an intensive course of exercises. Strong quadriceps and hamstring musculature may compensate in a large measure for loss of the stabilizing effect of a cruciate ligament.

LOOSE OSTEOCARTILAGINOUS BODIES

The exact cause of these is not known. They are considered to be secondary to injuries which cause necrosis of a portion of articular cartilage and its subchondral bone. This piece of bone and cartilage is gradually separated from its bed until it falls free into the joint cavity. The most common site of origin of a loose body is the inner or anterolateral surface of the medial condyle of the femur.

Diagnosis: The symptoms of a loose body in the knee joint are pain in the knee and recurring slipping, snapping, catching episodes usually without true locking of the joint. The patient may experience frequent "giving-way" sensations. Recurring effusions are common. The patient actually may feel a movable particle on either side or on the front of the knee.

On examination the surgeon may feel the movable particle. Some atrophy of the quadriceps musculature may be found. Otherwise, the physical findings are usually not remarkable.

The diagnosis often is made (or confirmed if a loose body has been palpable) by x-ray examination which discloses a loose radiopaque particle varying in size from that of a pea to a large bean. It may lie in the inter-condylar notch of the femur or in the knee joint bursa. Occasionally, a loose body may be palpable and not shown on x-ray examination. This in-dicates that the loose body is cartilaginous rather than osteocartilaginous.

Treatment: The indicated therapy is arthrotomy and removal of the loose body or bodies. If this is not done, nonoperative therapy is the same as for a sprain of the knee.

FRACTURES OF THE PATELLA

The patella is a large sesamoid bone in the extensor mechanism of the thigh at the knee. Although practically full function of the extremity may be maintained if removal of the patella becomes necessary, the bone serves several useful purposes. It provides some protection for the joint cavity and its contents; it serves as a fulcrum as the flexed leg is extended, thereby per-mitting better and smoother extensor action; and, cosmetically, it improves the contour of the knee.

Fractures of the patella, frequently open fractures, result from direct trauma to the front of the knee such as a fall on the knee or impact against a dashboard. Fractures with the fragments separated are easily identified by palpation but unseparated fractures can be determined only by x-ray examination.

Fractures of the patella are of real clinical significance only to the ex-tent that the extensor mechanism is divided. An undisplaced or un-separated fracture of the patella, as seen on x-ray examination, indicates that the surrounding tendon and the retinaculum patellae have remained intact. While these injuries are painful and cause some temporary loss of function, the intact extensor mechanism preserves some power of exten-sion of the leg. On the other hand, separation or displacement of the frag-ments means that the soft tissue structures about the patella have been severed to some extent. In these instances, the extensor mechanism has been interrupted and power to extend the leg at the knee is lost.

TREATMENT

Treatment of fractures of the patella is designed to achieve a smooth articular surface of the patella, strong musculature of the thigh, particu-larly of the quadriceps muscle group, and the maximum range and power of extension and flexion of the leg at the knee.

Fractures Without Separation: These frequently are accompanied by considerable hemarthrosis, for which aspiration followed by some form of compression dressing is all that is needed. Immobilization is not neces-sary if the patient will avoid a sudden uncontrolled flexion of the leg at the knee which could result in a tear of the soft tissues about the patella and separation of the fragments. Usually, the use of crutches or perhaps only a cane for several weeks will serve as an adequate safeguard against such a complication. Since early mobility of the knee joint is permitted, this application of the no-immobilization method of management predisposes to the maximum return of motion in the knee and minimizes temporary disability.

When a patient cannot be trusted to protect the knee against additional injury or if he prefers to avoid the use of crutches, an undisplaced fracture of the patella may be protected for 4 to 6 weeks by a plaster cylinder cast extending from the upper thigh to a short distance above the ankle with the knee extended to about 175 degrees. The plaster cylinder should be applied over a stockinet which is secured to the skin by tincture of benzoin or some comparable preparation. With the distal end of the stockinet turned back and incorporated in the cast, the cast itself is supported in place and does not tend to drift downward when the patient is ambulatory.

Fractures With Separation: These present classic indications for primary operative management. Closed methods are inadequate. The operation is expected to include accurate approximation of the patellar fragments and repair of the defects in the soft tissue portion of the extensor mechanism.

Separated fractures of the patella are of three types; (1) two major fragments and practically no comminution, (2) one major fragment with comminution of the other, usually the distal but occasionally the proximal fragment, and (3) comminuted fractures of the entire bone (Fig. 16–59).

The operative technique for each type varies. In fractures with two major fragments, a circumferential loop of strong stainless steel wire, properly inserted, will permit accurate approximation of the raw surfaces of bone. In fractures with comminution of the distal or proximal fragment, removal of the comminuted pieces is indicated, followed by approximation of the patella tendon to the raw distal surface of a proximal fragment or of the quadriceps tendon to the raw proximal surface of a remaining distal fragment. In severely comminuted fractures of the entire patella, patellectomy is usually the procedure of choice.

In each of these operative techniques, the tears in the extensor mechanism, that is, the expansions of the quadriceps tendon and capsule, are accurately repaired with interrupted sutures. When the patella has been removed for a comminuted fracture, imbrication of the torn tissues is mandatory. An accurate repair of torn tendon and capsule is an integral part of the operative treatment of fractures of the patella.

Postoperative immobilization may or may not be used. If the operative repair has been entirely satisfactory, immobilization is not really necessary and, after soft tissue healing, quadriceps exercises and early motion may be instituted. If there is some doubt about the operative repair, a plaster cylinder as previously described may be employed for 6 weeks.

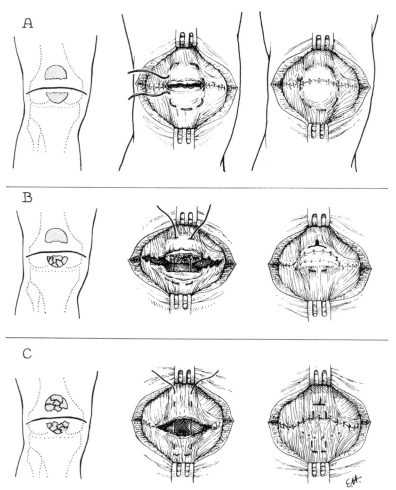

Figure 16–59 Several varieties of separated fractures of the patella and the surgery indicated to restore both a smooth articular surface and the extensor mechanism. In *A* the two fragments of the patella are approximated with a circumferential wire. In *B* comminuted lower portion of the patella is excised and the patella ligament approximated to the raw surface of the upper fragment. In *C* the entire patella is removed because the entire patella was comminuted. Note that the torn tendinous expansions on each side of the patella are repaired in each instance. (From Hampton and Fitts.)

FRACTURES OF THE PROXIMAL END OF THE TIBIA
(PLATEAU)

In all fractures of the proximal end of the tibia, a line or lines of fracture extend into the knee joint through articular cartilage. Objectives of management are to restore a smooth articular surface of the tibia and establish stability of the joint.

These fractures may be diagnosed only by adequate x-ray studies. Oblique views supplementing the routine anteroposterior and lateral views will be valuable in many instances.

FRACTURES OF THE TIBIAL SPINE

The tibial spine is avulsed by the anterior cruciate ligament which is attached to it. The fracture may be an isolated injury; it may be part of a comminuted fracture involving one or both plateaus, or it may complicate a tear of a collateral ligament, usually the medial.

Treatment: An undisplaced fragment or one which drops into perfect position with moderate extension of the knee requires merely aspiration of blood from the joint and a long-leg plaster cast for 4 weeks.

Displaced fragments usually require open operation to fix the fragment in perfect position (Fig. 16–60). A mattress suture of catgut, silk, or fine wire is made to pass through two parallel drill holes beginning over the anterior medial surface of the tibia and emerging through the defect in the articular surface of the tibia. It then passes through two comparable drill holes in the small bony fragment. As the loop of suture material is tightened, it becomes buried in the substance of the anterior cruciate ligament. A long-leg cast then is applied for 4 to 6 weeks with the knee at an angle of about 165 degrees.

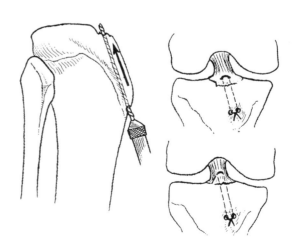

Figure 16–60   Procedure by which a displaced fracture of the tibial spine may be fixed in excellent reduction. (From De-Palma.)

FRACTURES OF THE LATERAL PLATEAU OF THE TIBIA

These result from a force applied from the lateral side to an extended knee (Fig. 16–61*A*) such as that produced by the bumper of a moving automobile (the common bumper fracture). They may also occur from a fall which produces a strong abduction strain on the knee. Either mechanism forces the leg into forced abduction at the knee. The same mechanisms place a great strain on the medial collateral ligament (see page 289). A

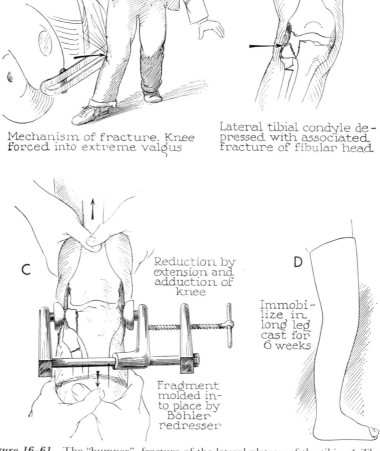

Mechanism of fracture. Knee forced into extreme valgus

Lateral tibial condyle depressed with associated fracture of fibular head

Reduction by extension and adduction of knee

Immobilize in long leg cast for 6 weeks

Fragment molded into place by Böhler redresser

Figure 16–61   The "bumper" fracture of the lateral plateau of the tibia. *A*, The mechanism which forces the extended knee into extreme valgus. *B*, The separated and depressed fracture of the lateral plateau with an associated fracture of the neck of the fibula. *C*, A technique of closed reduction. With the knee extended and adducted a redresser or C-clamp is used to force the fragment into good apposition. *D*, Immobilization is provided in a long-leg plaster cast. (From Banks and Compere.)

fracture of the lateral plateau of the tibia or a tear of the medial collateral ligament or both may result. The lateral semilunar cartilage may be torn to complicate a fracture of the lateral plateau.

A fracture of the lateral plateau may consist of one large fragment or it may be severely comminuted. The fracture may remain undisplaced or may be widely displaced. Several fragments, including portions of the articular cartilage of the lateral plateau, may be driven downward into the adjacent cancellous bone.

Treatment: In some undisplaced fractures, the fragments are so well impacted that immobilization may be omitted and only a compression dressing used for 10 to 14 days. Active motion of the joint and quadriceps exercises are immediately instituted. Weight-bearing is avoided, but the patient may be up on crutches. When the fragments are in good position but unimpacted, a long-leg plaster cast is usually provided for 5 to 6 weeks. Blood in the joint is removed before any form of immobilization is applied.

A large fragment displaced laterally or downward must be reduced accurately and maintained until it is united. At times, closed reduction can be achieved by using lateral compression, perhaps with a carpenter's C-clamp (Fig. 16–61C). After x-rays have verified reduction, a long-leg plaster cast extending to the groin is applied.

Open reduction and internal fixation of a large displaced fragment in good position, however, may be preferable. While the knee joint is open, any small chips of bone or cartilage or torn lateral semilunar cartilage may be removed. If firm fixation in good position is achieved, plaster immobilization may be omitted or removed after only a few weeks so that early active exercises are possible. In comminuted fractures of the lateral plateau, several fragments are usually depressed downward and spread laterally, defying adequate closed reduction (Fig. 16–62). For these, operative treatment is likely to give the best obtainable result. Reference is made to standard text books for the various techniques which are applicable for various kinds of fractures. Following operation for comminuted fractures, immobilization in a long-leg plaster cast for 6 to 8 weeks is advisable.

In all fractures of the lateral plateau, whether managed by closed reduction or open reduction and internal fixation, prolonged protection from weight-bearing is necessary. Ambulation with crutches is permissible but weight-bearing must be avoided until there is mature bony union of the fragments. This may require from 3 to 6 months, depending upon the severity of the fracture. Too early weight-bearing while bony union is immature may cause some depression of the lateral plateau with resulting knock-knee, instability, and subsequent traumatic arthritis.

FRACTURES OF THE MEDIAL PLATEAU OF THE TIBIA

These fractures may result from forces applied from the medial side to an extended knee, the reverse direction of forces which cause a lateral plateau fracture. A fall from a height is unlikely to produce a fracture of the

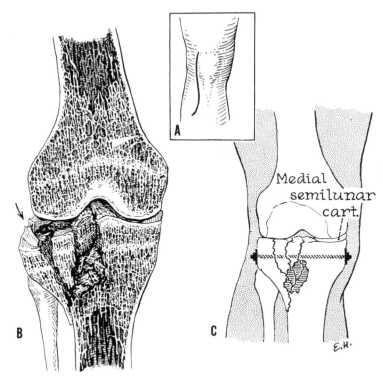

Figure 16–62   Comminuted depressed fracture of the lateral plateau of the tibia as seen in coronal section before and after open reduction and internal fixation. (From Hampton and Fitts.)

medial condyle as the extremity is seldom adducted at the hip when the feet strike the ground. Also, the slight normal valgus of the leg at the knee minimizes the chances of an impact causing a varus strain. A force producing a fracture of the medial plateau may simultaneously cause tears of the lateral collateral ligament.

Treatment: Treatment for fractures of the medial plateau of the tibia is entirely analogous to that of fractures of the lateral plateau. The same principles are applicable for obtaining reduction of the fracture, for providing immobilization when necessary, and for early mobilization and exercise. Prolonged protection from weight-bearing is also advisable.

FRACTURES OF LATERAL AND MEDIAL PLATEAUS (T-FRACTURES)

These may occur as a result of a compression force applied to an extended knee which impacts the upper tibia against the femur. They result from falls from a height onto a foot or in vehicle accidents from the force of an uprising floor board which jams an extended knee. Each plateau may be essentially a large single fragment or both may be severely comminuted.

Treatment: The choice of treatment depends largely on the degree of comminution of the fragments. Occasionally displacement of the fragments will be so minimal that reduction is not necessary. After aspiration of the knee, mildly displaced fragments can be reduced in some instances by closed manipulation using manual traction applied at the ankle and side-to-side compression at the proximal end of the tibia. In either instance, immobilization is provided by a long-leg cast. A knock-knee or a bow-leg deformity during application of the cast must be avoided assiduously.

When the fragments are significantly displaced, open reduction and internal fixation or continuous skeletal traction is usually indicated. At times, a combination of these will give the best result. Separated large condylar fragments often can be approximated with a tibial bolt so as to restore the articular surface of the tibia. The fixation of the condyles may provide sufficient stability at the fracture site to permit the use of a long-leg plaster cast for immobilization.

In other instances, continuous skeletal traction on the shaft of the tibia will be necessary to avoid some telescoping of the shaft between the condyles and resulting displacement and shortening. Continuous traction requires a Steinmann pin or Kirschner wire inserted through the lower end of the tibia. The extremity may be placed in a Thomas splint or on a Bohler-Braun splint for traction or in a long-leg plaster cast incorporating the Steinmann pin to which traction is applied with the extremity resting on a pillow (see pages 304 and 305).

Traction may be used similarly when the plateau fragments are severely comminuted and displaced. Traction must be continued until sufficient healing has occurred to prevent the fragments from again telescoping. Usually 6 to 8 weeks in traction are required. Further immobilization in a cast is usually necessary. As with fractures of single plateaus, weight-bearing must be avoided until bony union is solid and mature.

FRACTURE OF THE SHAFTS OF THE BONES OF THE LEG

Fractures of the shafts of the bones of the leg result from direct trauma, such as the impact of an automobile bumper, and from indirect trauma, such as the rotation or leverage strain caused by a person stepping into a deep hole while running. Either one or both bones may sustain fractures which may be transverse, oblique, spiral, double or even triple, or minimally or severely comminuted (Fig. 16–63). Because the tibia is entirely subcutaneous on its anterior and medial surfaces, open fractures of this bone are common.

Diagnosis of fractures of both bones or of the tibia alone usually is established easily by the clinical symptoms and signs. Adequate roentgenograms, however, identify the extent and contour of the fractures as a preliminary to the selection of a method of management.

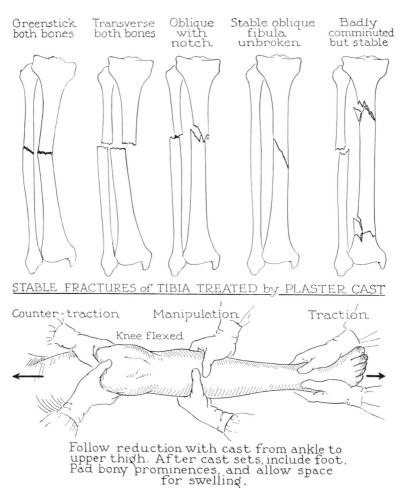

Greenstick both bones   Transverse both bones   Oblique with notch   Stable oblique fibula unbroken   Badly comminuted but stable

STABLE FRACTURES of TIBIA TREATED by PLASTER CAST

Counter-traction   Manipulation   Traction

Knee flexed

Follow reduction with cast from ankle to upper thigh. After cast sets, include foot. Pad bony prominences, and allow space for swelling.

Figure 16–63 Diagrams of fractures of the tibia with varying contours which permit a stable reduction and immobilization in a long-leg plaster cast. (Banks and Compere.)

A possible pitfall is to conclude erroneously that only a fracture of the tibia is present when actually both bones are broken. It is important to know if the fibula is also broken, not because the fragments of the fibula must be reduced, but because when the fibula is broken, its splinting effect on the tibia is lost, a factor which may influence the choice of method in managing the tibia. Failure to recognize a fracture of the fibula is most likely to occur when films of the lower half of the leg show a spiral or oblique fracture of the lower third of the tibia in fairly good position with minimal displacement and over-riding. Since a fracture of the fibula is not visualized, it may be wrongly concluded that the fibula is intact and that further displacement of the fracture of the tibia will not occur. Actually, the fibula may be broken in the unvisualized proximal third, a not uncommon location for such a fracture in association with spiral or oblique fractures of the tibia in the lower third. It is important, therefore, that the entire shafts of both the tibia and fibula be well visualized on roentgenograms before the diagnosis of a fracture of the tibia alone or even of the fibula alone is made.

FRACTURES OF THE SHAFTS OF THE TIBIA AND FIBULA

Fractures of the shafts of both bones of the leg present problems for several reasons. Many are open fractures, so that the hazard of wound infection and prolonged drainage is introduced. Reduction is often not only difficult to obtain but even more difficult to maintain. Circulation to the soft tissues of the leg on the anteromedial surface in the lower third is at times so precarious as to preclude operative intervention. Nonunion of a fracture of the tibia occurs not infrequently, not only because of the reasons just cited, but also because this bone, particularly in the lower half, has meager muscle attachments and blood supply.

Treatment: There are four methods of management—(1) closed reduction and immobilization, (2) balanced skeletal traction, (3) open reduction, and (4) external skeletal fixation (usually by transfixion pins incorporated in plaster)—which may be selected depending upon the characteristics of the fracture. The fact that one of four different methods may be chosen is further evidence of the complexity of these injuries. Precise surgical judgment is required for the selection of the best method.

The choice of a method should be based upon several factors. The contour of the fracture as revealed by the roentgenograms is probably the most important. Other factors include the general condition and age of the patient, the quality of the circulation to the foot and leg, the character of the skin overlying the fracture site, the presence of other injuries, the equipment at hand, and the experience and ability of the surgeon.

CLOSED REDUCTION AND IMMOBILIZATION: When a stable reduction of the tibia is possible (or is already present in undisplaced fractures), a long-leg plaster cast is usually selected for fractures of the shaft of both bones of the leg. A reduction is considered stable when significant displacement of the fragments is unlikely, provided they are kept in good alignment by the cast.

Reduction is achieved under general or spinal anesthesia by means of strong traction on the foot and ankle against equally strong counter-traction usually applied at the knee, together with direct manipulation of the fragments at the fracture site, bringing the distal fragment first into apposition in proper rotation and then into alignment with the proximal fragment. The stability of reduction may be tested by gently compressing the distal fragment against the proximal fragment while good alignment is maintained. If the reduction is not sufficiently stable to withstand this compression force, it may not be maintained in a plaster cast.

When a satisfactory stable reduction has been achieved (check-roentgenograms at this stage are quite valuable), a lightly padded long-leg cast is applied. It extends from the upper thigh to the toes and holds the foot at a right angle and in neutral version and, conventionally, the knee in 10 to 15 degrees of flexion. The cast should be well molded, especially about the knee and the foot and ankle.

Excellent results in the Army Medical Service produced by using routinely closed reduction and an almost unpadded long-leg walking plaster cast with the knee in full extension for all fractures of both bones of the leg has led many surgeons to use this method. Usually the first cast is split and the extremity is kept elevated as precautions against excessive swelling. A second cast often is applied a few days later, perhaps again with the patient under anesthesia. Early weight-bearing with or without crutches is encouraged. The method accepts slight shortening, incomplete apposition and at times a few degrees of angulation, but avoids complications which may occur with other methods. Those who use this method report an exceedingly low incidence of nonunion and strongly recommend it.

Closed reduction and immobilization in a plaster cast can be applied for a large percentage of the fractures of the shaft of both leg bones in adults. It offers many advantages: it is a conservative method with few pitfalls and complications; it entails no added risk to life or limb; it makes the patient immediately ambulatory on crutches; and it gives a very high percentage of good results. However, other methods may be preferable even though they are more confining and may entail some risk.

When an inadequate reduction is to be anticipated from the contour of the fracture or when efforts to achieve a good reduction have failed, one of the other methods may be selected. The choice of method will rest a great deal on the contour of the fracture, although the other factors mentioned must also be carefully evaluated.

CONTINUOUS TRACTION: This method may be elected for varying reasons. In comminuted fractures precluding a satisfactory reduction, traction will serve to maintain length and usually adequate apposition and alignment. If open reduction appears preferable but is contraindicated because of bad skin, the general condition of the patient, inadequate equipment or facilities, or inexperience on the part of the surgeon in the open treatment of fractures, continuous traction, using a pin or Kirschner wire through the os calcis or lower tibia, affords an acceptable method of management.

Skeletal traction may be provided with the extremity suspended in a Thomas splint or on a Bohler-Braun frame (Fig. 16–64). More effective and comfortable splinting, however, may be provided by the use of a plaster cast combined with traction.

Skeletal traction combined with a cast is provided as follows: A pin or wire is inserted and attached to a traction bow; strong manual traction is

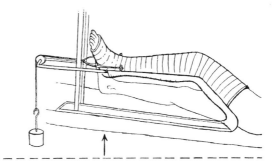

Figure 16–64 Skeletal traction in a plaster cast using a pin through the distal tibia and a Böhler-Braun frame for treatment of fractures of both bones of the leg. The pin and traction bow are incorporated in the cast. Traction may be provided also with the leg resting on a pillow. (From DePalma.)

provided, and the fragments are manipulated toward apposition and then held in good alignment. With traction maintained, a long-leg padded plaster cast is applied. The padding is usually made rather heavy at the knee in order that the fixation there will not be absolute. The plaster incorporates the traction bow and pin or wire. The foot is immobilized at a right angle, with the knee preferably in slight flexion. As the plaster is hardening, every effort is made to maintain perfect alignment of the fragments, although the cast may be wedged later to correct malalignment.

Postoperatively, 10 to 12 pounds of traction are provided with the extremity elevated on pillows or a Bohler-Braun frame. The patient may be turned to either side as long as the indicated direction of the traction is maintained. Traction is continued until sufficient healing has occurred to hold apposition and length, usually 5 to 6 weeks. Then, the wire or pin may be removed and perhaps a new cast applied for further immobilization. Throughout the period of traction, check-roentgenograms in two views are made to ensure that the amount of traction is adequate but not excessive and that good alignment is being maintained. Overpull is to be avoided.

OPEN REDUCTION AND INTERNAL FIXATION: This method may be selected for fractures having a contour which permits a stable internal fixation, provided the equipment, facilities, and experience of the surgeon are adequate. Oblique or spiral fractures of the tibia may be selected for operative fixation with screws alone, a plate and screws, or an intramedullary nail. The operative treatment for fractures of both bones of the leg carries with it dangers of infection, poor wound healing, and other complications. **The method is being used less and less because of its inherent hazards and because of the success of those methods which use routinely closed reduction and an early walking cast as previously described.**

Supplemental immobilization in a plaster cast is essential following all forms of internal fixation, including intramedullary nailing. With the latter, early weight-bearing in a walking cast is feasible. This often can be initiated a few weeks after operation.

EXTERNAL SKELETAL FIXATION: This method has been used to some extent for fractures of both bones of the leg when a stable reduction cannot be achieved. Its application with standard external skeletal fixation apparatus (that is, transfixion or half pins clamped to longitudinal metal bars) is not recommended. (See page 201.) Certainly such apparatus should be used only by surgeons with extensive experience in the method.

An acceptable substitute is provided by a long-leg plaster cast incorporating transfixion pins through the upper and lower major tibial fragments. The pins are inserted, the fracture is held reduced, and the cast is applied (Fig. 16–65). The pins are removed and a new cast substituted after enough healing of the fracture has occurred to prevent displacement and over-riding of the fragments. This modification of external skeletal fixation also has many pitfalls such as distraction of fragments, infection about pins, and broken pins. The method requires adequate previous experience for good results.

Period of Immobilization: The period of time required for solid healing of fractures of both bones of the leg will vary with the age of the patient, the contour and location of the fracture of the tibia, and the quality of the reduction and immobilization of the fragments. With each method, healing is slow and requires many months. While in general, union is secured faster in closed than in open fractures and when apposition of the fragments is adequate and is maintained, even under these favorable circumstances, a long time may be required for solid union of the fracture of the tibia.

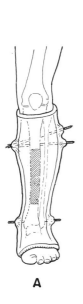
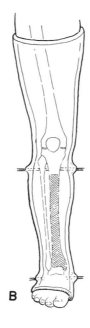

Figure 16–65   Treatment of comminuted tibial fractures by "pins and plaster." *A*, Fixation of shattered fracture (shaded segment) of tibia by transfixion pins and plaster boot. Two proximal pins are required, otherwise the proximal fragment would pivot upon a single pin. The two proximal pins should not be parallel. Knee motion can be maintained while the fracture heals.

B, If only a single proximal pin is used, the plaster dressing should be extended to the upper thigh. (From McLaughlin.)

A   **B**

The average period for adequate union is at least 4 or 5 months and this may be extended to 8 or 10 months. Immobilization must be continued until the fracture of the tibia is solidly united, clinically and roentgenographically. The immobilization may be discontinued before union of the fracture is complete only in those fractures adequately stabilized by intramedullary nailing, and even with these a walking plaster cast for several months is less hazardous than early removal of the immobilization.

FRACTURES OF THE SHAFT OF THE TIBIA WITH AN INTACT FIBULA

Fractures of the shaft of the tibia alone usually are not significantly displaced and require only immobilization in a long-leg plaster cast with the knee in 10 to 15 degrees of flexion and the foot at 90 degrees and in neutral version. The early walking cast with the knee extended also may be used. The splinting effect of the intact fibula tends to effect a stable reduction of a tibial fracture with a contour which otherwise would indicate an unstable situation (Fig. 16–63). Occasionally, however, significant displacement of a fracture of the tibia will occur even with an intact fibula. Usually this can be overcome and reduction obtained by closed manipulation, following which the cast is applied.

The period of time required for solid healing of a fracture of the tibia alone, just as with fractures of both bones of the leg, will vary with its contour and location and the age of the patient. Certainly, 8 to 10 weeks of immobilization is the minimum, 12 to 14 the average, and 16 to 18 not uncommon. The prognosis for union of a fracture of the tibia alone is excellent but it is not certain especially in transverse fractures of the shaft of the tibia in the middle third. In this region, absorption about the fracture may lead to poor contact of fragments because they are strutted apart by the intact fibula.

FRACTURE OF THE SHAFT OF THE FIBULA WITH AN INTACT TIBIA

Fractures of the shaft of the fibula are not important skeletal injuries. In fractures of the shafts of both bones of the leg, all efforts are directed toward obtaining and maintaining adequate reduction of the tibia, and the fracture of the fibula for practical purposes is ignored. When the shaft of the fibula alone is broken, the intact tibia splints the fragments and they practically always remain in adequate reduction.

Fractures of the shaft of the fibula alone are usually immobilized in a walking plaster cast in order to minimize pain and maintain the foot in a good functioning position, although healing would undoubtedly occur without immobilization. Definitely, a plaster cast applied for a fracture of the shaft of the fibula need extend only to the knee. Three to four weeks of immobilization usually suffices, although six to eight weeks may be necessary for solid union of the fracture.

FRACTURES AND DISLOCATIONS OF THE ANKLE

Ligaments as well as bony structures provide integrity for the ankle joint. The inferior tibiofibular ligaments contribute materially to the stability of the ankle by helping to maintain the ankle mortise, the bony framework formed by the malleoli about the talus. The large deltoid ligament on the medial side and the calcaneofibular and the talofibular ligaments on the lateral side of the joint tend to retain the talus in the mortise and prevent abnormal lateral movement.

In treating injuries about the ankle, the status of the ligaments must be considered. A torn deltoid ligament, for example, is probably as significant as a fracture of the medial malleolus. Figure 16–66*B* shows a bimalleolar fracture with lateral displacement of the fragments and the foot. Figure 16–66*C* shows a fracture of only the lateral malleolus, yet the foot is displaced. For this to occur without fracture of the medial malleolus, the deltoid ligament must be torn. The injuries shown in Figures 16–66*B* and *C*, then, are entirely comparable insofar as the integrity of the articulation at the ankle is concerned. Similarly, Figure 16–66*D* shows a laterally

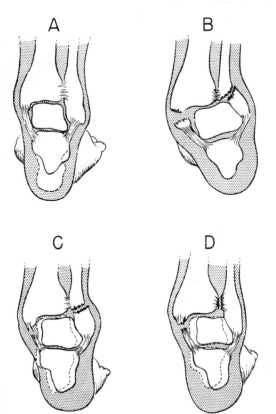

Figure 16–66 The major ligamentous support of the ankle mortise. *B*, Bimalleolar fracture with lateral displacement of the foot. The ligaments are intact. *C*, Fracture of the lateral malleolus with a torn deltoid ligament permitting lateral displacement of the foot. The injuries depicted in *B* and *C* are quite comparable. *D*, Torn deltoid ligament and the disruption of the ligament supporting the inferior tibiofibular synchondrosis with lateral displacement of the foot. (From Hampton and Fitts.)

displaced fracture of the medial malleolus and an intact fibula with a lateral dislocation of the foot. For this to occur, a disruption of the inferior tibiofibular ligaments must have occurred. A clear appreciation of the foregoing is essential to the proper treatment of fractures about the ankle joint.

FRACTURES OF THE ANKLE WITHOUT DISPLACEMENT

These injuries require only plaster cast immobilization. Sometimes the cast may extend only to the knee, although it should extend to the upper thigh if there is any danger of subsequent displacement of the fragments in the cast as exists with many trimalleolar and bimalleolar fractures. The foot should be held at 90 degrees and in neutral version. Immobilization in plantar flexion and inversion is to be avoided as this pernicious position predisposes to prolonged disability after the cast is removed. Usually a walking-type cast is advantageous.

Healing of an undisplaced fracture of the lateral malleolus alone is not rapid and fracture lines may be visible on x-ray films for several months. Usually, however, 6 weeks of immobilization in a cast will permit sufficient union to make further immobilization unnecessary. A well-reduced fracture of the medial malleolus unites more rapidly, so that 4 weeks of immobilization usually suffices. The most rapidly healing fractures about the ankle are those of the undisplaced posterior malleolus. These fracture lines have been observed to disappear on roentgenogram in 2½ to 3 weeks. Undisplaced bimalleolar and trimalleolar fractures should be immobilized for 8 weeks, largely because the combination of bony injuries includes a fracture of the lateral malleolus.

FRACTURES OF THE ANKLE WITH DISPLACEMENT

These require precise reduction and immobilization in a plaster cast. While closed reduction will suffice in many instances, open reduction and internal fixation often are necessary.

Fractures of the Lateral Malleolus with Lateral Dislocation of the Foot: Precise reduction of the dislocation and the fracture is required for an optimal result. General anesthesia is advisable. Reduction is achieved by a combination of direct pressure on the lateral malleolus and internal rotation of the foot on the vertical axis of the tibia. This does not imply inversion of the foot which contributes nothing to the reduction and is a poor position for immobilization of the foot in plaster. Internal rotation of the foot closes the space between the talus and the medial malleolus, provided the deltoid ligament is not interposed between them. These maneuvers should be carried out with the knee flexed from 45 to 90 degrees to avoid tension of the gastrocnemius muscle. Flexion of the knee over the side or end of a table will secure the desired flexion.

If precise reduction of the dislocation cannot be obtained by manipulation, probably torn fibers of the deltoid ligament have become engaged between the talus and the medial malleolus. If so, operative intervention is mandatory. Some surgeons stabilize the lateral malleolus in reduction with an intramedullary pin introduced retrograde from the tip of the malleolus. All agree that the torn deltoid ligament should be repaired.

In these injuries treated by closed reduction or open reduction without internal fixation of the lateral malleolus, the plaster cast should extend well above the knee. This immobilizes the ankle and avoids rotation strains which might cause recurrence of the dislocation. With internal fixation of the lateral malleolus and good operative repair of the torn deltoid ligament, the danger of redisplacement is practically nonexistent and a short plaster leg cast will suffice.

Fractures of the Medial Malleolus with Displacement:

WITH DISPLACEMENT BUT WITHOUT DISLOCATION OF THE ANKLE: The medial malleolus frequently is displaced downward, Usually under anesthesia, an effort may be made to replace it by dorsal flexion and perhaps slight inversion of the foot and upward pressure on the fragment. If the raw edges can be well approximated, immobilization of the leg and foot in a below-the-knee walking plaster cast for 4 weeks will permit union of the fragment.

Frequently the separated medial malleolus cannot be approximated to the body of tibia because tags of periosteum and deltoid ligament have dropped into the fracture site. If so, operation is advisable to permit removal of the soft tissues from between the fragments, especially if the fracture line of the malleolus is at or above the level of the ankle joint. Fixation of the medial malleolus is provided with a screw or a threaded pin (Fig. 16–67). The internal fixation must be supported by a below-the-knee plaster of Paris cast for at least 4 weeks.

WITH DISPLACEMENT AND LATERAL DISLOCATION OF THE FOOT: As

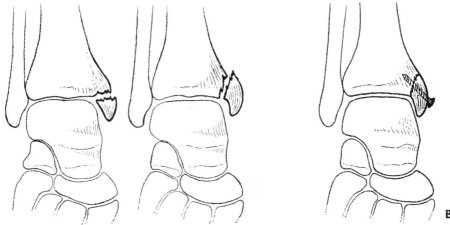

Figure 16–67   *A,* Contour of common fractures of the medial malleolus, *B,* Precise reduction and internal fixation of a fracture of the medial malleolus. The same technique is applicable to a fracture with the other contour shown on the left. (From DePalma.)

outlined previously, for this injury some disruption of the inferior tibiofibular syndesmosis has occurred. Under these circumstances, manipulative
reduction may reduce the fracture of the medial malleolus and restore the
fibula to its proper place against the tibia. Operative fixation, however,
often is preferable. With the medial malleolus fixed in accurate reduction,
the fibula is pulled back against the tibia and the ankle mortise is restored.
Surgery on the medial side of the ankle may suffice in some instances, but
bolt or screw fixation of the fibula to the tibia a short distance above the
ankle is advisable to insure that the mortise will be maintained. The fixation of the fibula to the tibia and of the medial malleolus permits use of a
below-knee walking cast after the wounds have healed. The cast may be
eliminated after 6 weeks.

With nonoperative treatment of this combined injury, at least 6 weeks
in a long-leg plaster cast followed by a snug below-the-knee cast for an additional 2 or 3 weeks is indicated. The use of a walking heel is hazardous as
the force of weight-bearing may lead to some spread of the mortise.

BIMALLEOLAR FRACTURE-DISLOCATION: These injuries present a combination of the problems previously mentioned for displaced fractures of
either malleolus. Frequently, closed manipulation will provide adequate
reduction of both malleoli. Immobilization in a long-leg nonwalking cast
for at least 8 to 10 weeks is indicated.

If manipulation provides a stable reduction of the lateral malleolus,
but fails to achieve reduction of the medial malleolus, then internal fixation
of the medial malleolus is indicated. On the other hand, if neither the
medial nor the lateral malleolus can be reduced by manipulation, then both
should be internally fixed in precise reduction; the medial malleolus is
fixed with a screw or pin and the lateral malleolus with a retrograde intramedullary pin (Fig. 16–68).

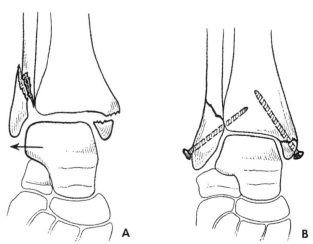

Figure 16–68 A, Bimalleolar fracture of the ankle with lateral displacement of the
foot. B, Perfect reduction of each fracture following internal fixation. The crucial element
of the procedure is the stabilization of the medial malleolus in perfect position. Stabilization
of the lateral malleolus is optional. (From DePalma.)

TRIMALLEOLAR FRACTURE-DISLOCATION OF THE ANKLE: The addition of a fracture of the posterior malleolus (the posterior lip of the distal tibia is called the "posterior malleolus" clinically) to those of the medial and lateral malleoli with dislocation of the foot creates a more complex problem (Fig. 16–69). If the posterior malleolar fragment is of significant size, maintenance of accurate reduction is essential to provide for a smooth articular surface of the tibia. In spite of a perfect initial closed reduction, displacement of a large fragment and posterior subluxation of the foot may occur in a cast.

Actually the size of the posterior malleolar fragment may determine the preferable method of management. When it includes one-third or

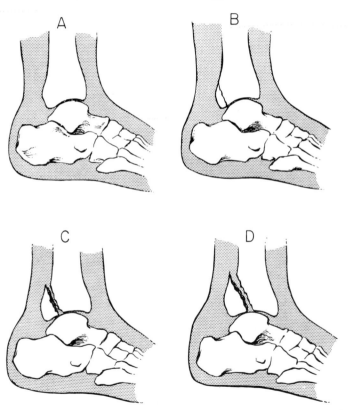

Figure 16–69   Fractures of the posterior malleolus of the tibia. *A*, The uninjured ankle. *B*, Fragment involves only 10 per cent of the articular surface and may be ignored even if it is not reduced. *C*, If fragment makes up about 25 per cent of the articular surface and the foot is displaced posteriorly, perfect reduction is crucial. At times it may be maintained following closed reduction, but internal fixation in perfect position may be necessary. *D*, If the fragment makes up about 35 per cent of the articular surface, efforts to maintain closed reduction in a plaster cast are unlikely to be successful. Primary open reduction and internal fixation of the fragment in perfect position is justified. (From Hampton and Fitts.)

more of the articular surface of the tibia, closed reduction usually will not be maintained in the cast and, therefore, operative fixation of this fragment in reduction is indicated (Fig. 16–70). When it includes less than one-third of the articular surface of the tibia, reduction by manipulation may be attempted and if precise replacement is obtained, a long-leg plaster cast may maintain the reduction. Check x-ray films every 4 or 5 days for 2½ to 3 weeks are essential to make certain that displacement has not recurred. Delayed open reduction may be indicated. If the posterior malleolar fragment includes only a small portion of the articular surface — 10 per cent or less — it requires no special attention. Incomplete reduction of this small fragment is not likely to have any effect on future function of the ankle and, therefore, operation to replace it is not justified.

Management of the fractures of the medial and lateral malleoli as part of a trimalleolar fracture conforms to that recommended for single malleolar or bimalleolar fractures.

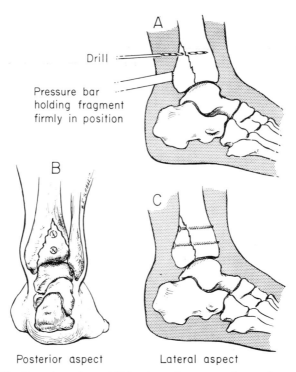

Figure 16–70 Procedure for stabilizing large fragment of posterior malleolus in perfect position. *A*, Following reduction, a pressure bar and a drill hold the fragment in perfect position. *B* and *C*, Reduction is stabilized with two parallel screws which extend just through the anterior tibial cortex. Note that the screws are placed parallel to the articular surface. (From Hampton and Fitts.)

FRACTURES OF THE BONES OF THE FOOT

FRACTURES OF THE CALCANEUS

These exceedingly painful injuries are the most significant fractures of the bones of the foot. Except in the case of minor chip fractures, temporary disability is likely to be prolonged and considerable permanent disability is to be expected far beyond that indicated by the findings on roentgenograms. Disability comes from pain on weight-bearing, loss of inversion and eversion of the foot, and restricted motion in the ankle joint.

Falls onto the heels are the most common cause of fractures of the calcaneus, but explosions of land mines, or the upsurge of the deck of a torpedoed ship or comparable trauma in civilian life may also cause them. Compression fractures of the spine are often associated with fractures of the calcaneus. The presence of either indicates a thorough examination and perhaps x-ray visualization to see if the other fracture is also present (Fig. 16–71).

Fractures of the calcaneus are crush fractures (Fig. 16–72*B*). At impact, the calcaneus is crushed between the object onto which the patient falls and the talus. Lines of fracture may occur in many directions. A downward crushing of the central portion including the posterior articular facet into the substance of the bone, lateral and medial spread of cortical fragments, or upward displacement of a large posterior fragment to which the tendoachilles is attached may be present.

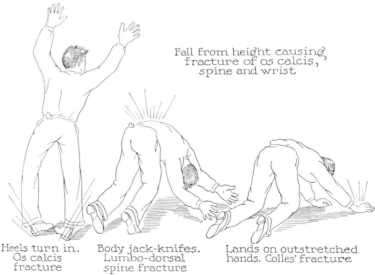

Fall from height causing fracture of os calcis, spine and wrist

Heels turn in. Os calcis fracture

Body jack-knifes. Lumbo-dorsal spine fracture

Lands on outstretched hands. Colles' fracture

Figure 16–71 Mechanism by which a fall from a height on to the heels followed by jack-knifing of the trunk may cause fractures of both the os calcis and a vertebral body. As the body falls forward, efforts to protect it with the outstretched arms may lead to a Colles' fracture. (From Banks and Compere.)

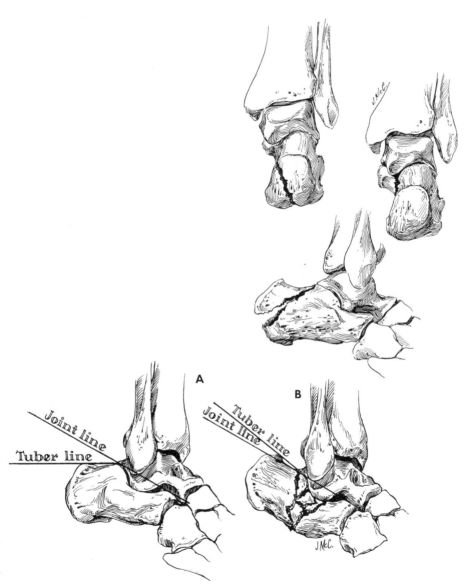

Figure 16–72   *Upper,* Several varieties of fractures of the os calcis. *A,* Uninjured foot showing the normal tuber angle. *B,* Fracture of the body of the os calcis with marked reduction in the tuber angle. (From Davis.)

Fractures of the calcaneus often result in marked swelling and discoloration as a result of hemorrhage. Massive bleb formation and even spotty necrosis of the skin on the sides of the heel may result from the intense swelling.

Special x-ray views are indicated to confirm the presence of a fracture and to determine its type and extent. In addition to a standard lateral view, a special anteroposterior view of the calcaneus must be made according to techniques known to all qualified x-ray technicians. At times only the anteroposterior view will demonstrate the fracture. It should be routine, therefore, in all suspected fractures of the calcaneus. Comparable views of the uninjured heel at times will be helpful.

Treatment: The principles to be considered in treatment of fractures of the calcaneus include reduction of swelling prior to efforts at reducing the fracture (a definite exception to the rule of prompt reduction of fractures); restoration of the contour of the bone as best possible, particularly its articular surface and Böhler's angle (the tuber angle) (Fig. 16–72A); immobilization of the foot and ankle only as long as a useful purpose is being served; early mobilization of the foot and ankle in order to minimize any permanent restriction of motion; avoidance of weight-bearing until mature bony healing has taken place; and minimizing of postimmobilization edema by adequate elastic support. The means of applying these principles varies according to the type, severity, and displacement of the fragments.

Usually before an effort is made to reduce a displaced fracture, the severe swelling about the heel and ankle must be allowed to subside so that the swollen, edematous soft tissues overlying the calcaneus will not be irreparably damaged during the reduction. When the patient is first seen, a large compression dressing is applied immediately to the foot and ankle and the foot is elevated markedly (Fig. 16–73). Depending upon the severity of the fracture, 5 to 10 days is usually required for the swelling to decrease sufficiently to permit reduction.

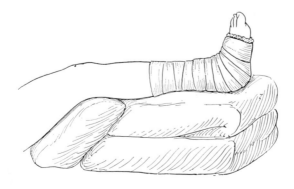

Figure   16–73 Compression dressing to the foot and ankle with marked elevation of the extremity for reduction of swelling that follows a fracture of the os calcis. (From Banks and Compere.)

From the standpoint of treatment, fractures of the calcaneus may be grouped as (1) those requiring no reduction, (2) those which can be reasonably well reduced by closed methods, (3) those which are likely to be helped by open reduction, and (4) those in which reduction is impossible.

1. **No reduction:** Undisplaced and many minimally displaced fractures need no reduction. Compression dressings and elevation for a few days may suffice. A cast may minimize discomfort but it should be removed after 1 to 2 weeks. Early mobilization is highly desirable but weight-bearing should not be permitted until x-ray examination shows a disappearance of the lines of fracture.

2. **Closed reduction:** Several steps are involved in the closed reduction of fractures of the calcaneus. Firm impaction of displaced fragments must be broken up as a first step. Strong manipulation of the heel with the hands or forcibly striking each side of the padded heel with a large wooden or rubber mallet may be used. Upward displacement of the posterior fragment must be overcome by downward traction on it. During this maneuver, the knee should be fully flexed to relax the calf muscles as much as possible. Traction on the heel may be made manually or on a Steinmann pin inserted through or just above the posterior fragment. Traction is made in a posterior direction in an effort to restore the length of the bone after the fragment has been pulled downward. Downward and backward traction tends to restore the tuber angle. Bulging of comminuted fragments is overcome by side-to-side compresssion, preferably with a padded large C-clamp or a special calcaneus redressor made for this purpose. A pin, if used, is removed after reduction of the fracture.

Immobilization is provided with a padded plaster cast under which additional heavy felt pads are placed on each side of the heel. As the plaster is setting, firm pressure is made over the felt pads in an effort to minimize exuberant callus formation beneath the malleoli. The foot is immobilized in about 15 degrees of plantar flexion and in slight inversion, rather than the usual 90 degrees and neutral version for casts over the ankle and foot. If a posterior fragment has been pulled downward, the cast must be extended to the midthigh with the knee immobilized in some 30 degrees of flexion for several weeks.

The duration of immobilization varies with the type of fracture, the degree of displacement, and what has been achieved by efforts at reduction. If a good reduction has been obtained, the cast should remain in place for 4 to 6 weeks.

If efforts at reduction are not successful and fragments remain out of position, prolonged immobilization is inadvisable. The cast should be removed within a few weeks and active exercises initiated. In this way, even though the fracture has not been accurately reduced, permanent restriction of motion, especially in the ankle, will be minimized.

When the patient is allowed up on crutches without a cast, elastic bandage support from the base of the toes to just below the knee is advisable in an effort to minimize edema. Persisting edema itself tends to cause restriction of foot and ankle motion. If it can be prevented by the constant use of elastic support until the tendency toward edema has disappeared, a better end-result will be obtained. Weight-bearing must be avoided until the fracture is soundly healed.

3. **Open Reduction:** In those fractures consisting principally of a downward impaction of the posterior articular facet into the substance of the bone, efforts at closed reduction are unlikely to be worthwhile. In these instances, open reduction is often advantageous. The fragment containing the articular facet is elevated into normal position which restores the contour of the articular surface. A small block of bone from the ilium or upper tibia is used to fill the defect and maintain elevation of the fragment. In these cases, plaster immobilization should be maintained for about 6 weeks, but an additional period of 4 to 6 weeks without weight-bearing is advisable.

4. **Reduction Impossible:** In severely comminuted fractures, particularly those involving the articular surface, efforts to reduce them are probably not worthwhile. The best result may be obtained by omitting immobilization altogether and starting exercise immediately. In these severe fractures, primary subtalar arthrodesis may give the best end-result. In late cases with persisting pain and disability, this procedure is often used to alleviate these symptoms.

FRACTURES OF THE TALUS

These fractures result from trauma which produces excessive dorsal flexion of the foot. A fracture across the neck of the talus occurs as it is forced against the lower tibia.

Treatment: The fracture may remain undisplaced but some upward displacement of the distal fragment is common. For a good end-result, accurate reduction is essential. Often closed reduction can be accomplished under anesthesia by strong plantar flexion of the foot (Fig. 16–74). Open reduction is indicated if the fragments cannot be reduced accurately by closed methods. Following closed or open reduction, a boot cast with the foot in some plantar flexion is applied for 5 or 6 weeks. Weight-bearing must be avoided by using crutches until solid union of the fracture occurs.

A partial or complete dislocation of the body of the talus may complicate a displaced fracture of the neck. Incomplete dislocations or subluxations are easily overlooked. Closed manipulation for the fracture may reduce the dislocated body but, if not, open reduction is essential.

Avascular necrosis of the body of the talus is the outstanding complication of fracture of the neck. The nutrient arteries for the talus enter through the distal portion of the bone. A fracture through the neck destroys the major blood supply to the body. Avascular necrosis is uncommon in undisplaced fractures but rather common when the fracture has been displaced. Complete or near complete dislocations of the body, in which ligamentous attachments to the bone are torn, make avascular

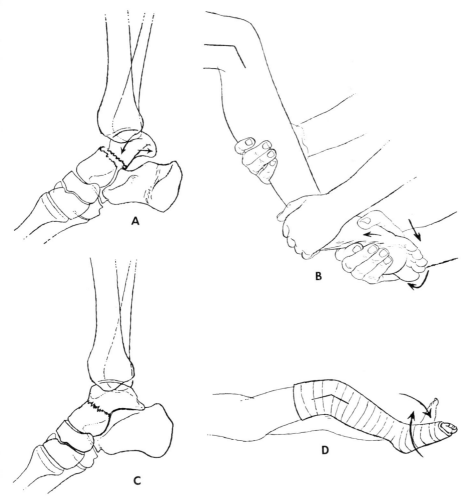

Figure 16–74   *A*, Displaced fracture through the neck of the talus. *B*, Manipulation to achieve closed reduction. Strong plantar flexion is essential. *C*, The reduced fracture. *D*, Reduction is maintained in a long-leg plaster cast which holds the foot in plantar flexion and mild eversion. (From DePalma.)

necrosis a probability. This complication requires prolonged protection from weight-bearing until new blood vessels grow into the body and the dead bone is replaced with living bone, a process which may require many months. Too early weight-bearing will cause an irreparable collapse of the talus and will lead to severe traumatic arthritis of the ankle.

FRACTURES OF THE MIDTARSAL BONES (NAVICULAR, CUBOID, AND CUNEIFORM)

These result from side-to-side crushes or from a heavy weight falling on the foot. The skin and other soft tissues of the foot are often badly bruised or torn. After these fractures have healed, there is often considerable disability from pain and soreness on twisting strains of the foot and loss of motion in the midtarsal joints. Prolonged walking is usually painful.

Displacement of fragments usually may be reduced by manual manipulation. Open reduction and some form of internal fixation is advantageous in many cases. In other instances the midtarsal bones are so crushed that they can only be molded so as to restore the general contour of the foot.

A boot cast is used for immobilization. It should be well molded about the foot so as to conform to and support the arches. A walking heel may be advantageous as weight-bearing in the cast during the healing period tends to minimize demineralization of the bones of the foot. Immobilization is discontinued after 4 to 8 weeks, depending upon the severity of the fractures.

FRACTURES OF THE METATARSALS

These may be grouped into (1) fractures of the shafts or necks of the metatarsals, (2) fractures of the base of the fifth metatarsal, and (3) "march" fractures.

Fractures of the Shafts or Necks of the Metatarsals: These fractures result from compression injuries of the foot: front-to-back, side-to-side, or top-to-bottom. The latter type of trauma would result from a heavy object dropping on the foot. These injuries also result from falls onto the balls of the feet — a front-to-back compression.

TREATMENT: Undisplaced fractures require only a compression dressing and crutches for 4 to 6 weeks. A walking boot cast may be preferable as it makes the patient ambulatory without crutches. A long plantar slab to protect the toes is advisable, since a subsequent blow on the toes might displace the metatarsal fracture(s).

Displaced fractures should be reduced. Those of the first and fifth metatarsals require excellent reduction so that the weight-bearing heads of these bones are in their normal position. Alignment of a fracture of each metatarsal must be restored so that after the fracture is united, the head or heads will not project into the sole or dorsum of the foot and lead to painful callus formation.

In many transverse or near transverse fractures reduction can be achieved by closed manipulation. In oblique or comminuted fractures, continuous traction is often advisable to hold reduction (Fig. 16–75). Skeletal traction may be provided by a small Kirschner wire through the bone or the tough tissue of the distal phalanx of the toe of the broken metatarsal. Traction is provided on the wire by use of a rubber band connected to a loop of heavy wire incorporated into a boot cast. Skeletal traction may be applied simultaneously for fractures of several metatarsals. Traction is advisable for about 4 weeks. Open reduction may be required for some displaced metatarsal fractures (Fig. 16–76).

Fractures of the Base of the Fifth Metatarsal: These fractures, which are relatively unimportant injuries, may result when the foot gives way into inversion as the patient is running or walking rapidly. The major-

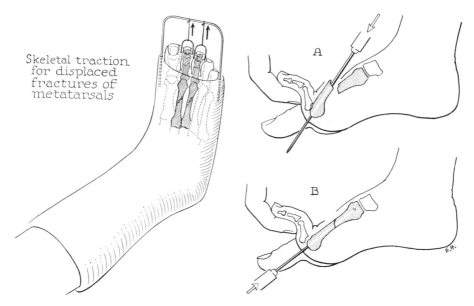

Skeletal traction for displaced fractures of metatarsals

A

B

Figure 16–75 Skeletal traction in a banjo-cast for over-riding fractures of the second and third metatarsal. (From Banks and Compere.)

Figure 16–76 Procedure for stabilizing reduction of a fracture of a metatarsal which cannot be held reduced following efforts at closed reduction. (From Hampton and Fitts.)

ity remain undisplaced, although occasionally the small proximal fragment is separated by the pull of the peroneus brevis muscle attached to it.

TREATMENT: Undisplaced fractures require little active treatment. An elastic bandage may suffice and even weight-bearing, perhaps with the aid of a cane, may be permitted. Crutches for 10 to 14 days may be necessary. A walking-boot cast rarely is justified. Significant displacement of the proximal fragment may indicate a boot cast. The degree of displacement is seldom enough to predispose to nonunion.

"**March**" **Fracture:** A "march" (fatigue) fracture of the second, third, or fourth metatarsal results from prolonged strain rather than from any known trauma. Unconditioned military personnel who have been subjected to a long fatiguing hike are prone to this injury. Pain in the metatarsal region develops and persists. X-ray films may not be obtained because the pain is relatively mild and no injury has occurred. If made, the films may show a faint line of fracture. Later, a palpable lump develops in the metatarsal region, leading to roentgenographic examination which shows a healing fracture with some exuberant callus formation. Recognition that a march fracture and not a bone tumor is present is crucial.

TREATMENT: A march fracture may be treated with a walking-boot cast for several weeks or, in many instances, merely by a metatarsal pad in the shoe or a metatarsal bar on the shoe combined with restricted activity.

FRACTURES OF THE TOES

These result from a falling object or when a toe is struck forcibly against an object. Fractures of the fifth toe occur frequently when a barefoot person catches it on a piece of furniture. Only fractures of the great toe are of real consequence.

Treatment: Only protection from additional injury is necessary in undisplaced fractures, including those of the great toe. Strapping of the injured toe to the adjacent toe or toes with small strips of adhesive tape affords some protection and tends to minimize discomfort. Crutches may be used for comfort during the first week or 10 days. A metatarsal bar applied to the shoe may permit patients to resume activity rather promptly.

In displaced fractures of the great toe, particularly in the proximal phalanx, reduction is necessary. This may be achieved by manipulation. Some may require continuous skeletal traction in a banjo cast as described for fractures of the metatarsals. Open reduction is seldom necessary. These fractures usually have sufficient union in 3 or 4 weeks to permit weight-bearing.

In displaced fractures of the small toes, efforts at reduction usually are not indicated. The bones are so small that even with perfect reduction redisplacement is likely. Reasonably good alignment usually can be maintained by strapping the broken toe to the adjacent toe or toes.

PERITALAR DISLOCATION

The injury may be closed or open. The talus remains seated in the ankle joint, the articulations between the talus and the calcaneus and between the talus and the navicular are disrupted, and the foot is dislocated medially.

Prompt closed reduction as an emergency is indicated using traction and manipulation. General anesthesia is usually necessary. A plaster cast should be applied to the foot and leg, so that the ankle is held at 90 degrees and the foot in neutral version for a period of about 4 weeks. With good reduction, the prognosis is good, especially for so severe an injury.

TARSOMETATARSAL DISLOCATION

This rather severe foot injury is produced by some levering force at the midfoot, such as when the forefoot is caught and the body is forced medially or laterally. The metatarsals are torn loose from their articulations with the tarsus. Multiple chip fractures usually occur along these joints.

Closed reduction in many instances may be obtained by traction and manipulation and maintained by a plaster cast which includes the foot and leg. In other instances, usually those markedly displaced, operative reduction and usually some form of internal fixation are necessary.

DISLOCATION OF THE TOES

Dislocation of a toe without fracture is an unusual injury but occasionally one of the toes, particularly the great toe, is dislocated at the metatarsophalangeal joint. Reduction is usually easy by traction and manipulation. Reduction often may be achieved without anesthesia, or a local anesthesia may be used.

FRACTURES OF THE PELVIS

Fractures of the pelvis are produced by falls from a height, automobile crashes, and crushing trauma. One or both rami of the pubis or the ischium, the wing of either ilium or all of these bones may be broken. Because of the design of the pelvis, significant displacement of a fracture often does not occur. However, with fractures involving both rami and the wing of the ilium on one side, upward and inward displacement of the outer fragment of that innominate bone may occur. With fractures through both rami on each side, as may occur in side-to-side crush injuries, the pelvis may collapse so that the fragments override; or with such fractures following front-to-back crush injuries, separation of the fragments and spread of the pelvis may occur.

Prime consideration with fractures of the pelvis, particularly when the fragments are displaced, concerns not the fractures themselves but the close-by soft tissues which may have been injured: the bladder, urethra, intestine, or the iliac vessels. Unless the patient can void clear urine immediately, catheterization is indicated to determine whether the bladder has been damaged. Such an investigation is necessary even though the fragments are undisplaced, because a full bladder may have been ruptured by the force of the impact. Absence of urine or the presence of bloody urine indicates injury to the lower urinary tract. (See Chapter 14.).

Repeated examination of the abdomen is indicated to search for signs of injury to an intra-abdominal viscus. The absence of normal peripheral arterial pulsations in either lower extremity would indicate the probability of a torn iliac artery. The management of these life-endangering complications takes precedence over management of the fractures of the pelvis.

Even without complicating injuries to soft tissue structures, multiple fractures of the pelvis may be life-endangering because of massive shock-producing hemorrhage from the fractures into the spaces and tissues surrounding them. Before treatment of fractures is initiated, blood volume replacement (see Chapter 3) must be provided concurrently with examinations to determine whether essential soft tissues have been damaged.

TREATMENT

Most fractures of the pelvis have little or no displacement and require nothing more than bed rest on a hard bed for a few weeks, followed perhaps by the support of a canvas corset for a few days. With fractures of a single ramus or even two rami on the same side, the patient may easily become ambulatory on crutches in 2 to 3 weeks, but full weight-bearing should be postponed until about 6 weeks after injury.

In undisplaced fractures involving rami on both sides (Fig. 16–77*A*), the period of bed rest should be 4 or 5 weeks, and crutch-walking postponed for several more weeks. The prognosis in undisplaced fractures of the pelvis is excellent for practically full function. Elderly individuals, for whom bed rest may be inadvisable, often can be safely lifted into a chair after a few days.

In fractures through both rami and the wing of the ilium on the same side with upward and perhaps inward displacement of the lateral fragment of the innominate bone (Fig. 16–77B, C, D), closed reduction may be achieved by manipulation with the patient on the uninjured side and maintained in a hip spica cast which extends to the knee on the injured side. In some instances, however strong skeletal traction must be applied to the extremity early in the management of the fracture in an effort to pull the displaced fragment back into position; efforts at reduction will be more successful if the patient is anesthetized for relaxation. While strong manual traction is being made on the involved extremity, a strong downward and rotary manual thrust is made against the upward displaced wing of the ilium by an assistant. After reduction, traction must be maintained for 5 to 6 weeks to avoid recurrence of the upward displacement.

Those fractures with separation of the fragments and spreading of the lower pelvis require some compressing force. This may be easily accomplished using a pelvic sling which serves barely to lift the weight of the pelvis from the mattress and to supply a binding force which tends to mold the fragments back into proper position (Fig. 16–78). Some caution is necessary to avoid converting a spreading type of fracture into a collapsing type as a result of excessive compression. Bilateral skin traction on the extremities may aid in obtaining reduction of the fragments and, in the early stages, contributes to patient comfort.

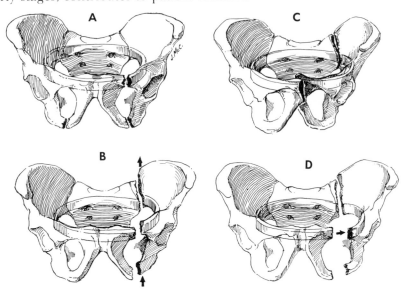

Figure 16–77   *A*, Fractures of one ramus of pubis and rami of the ischium, undisplaced and stable.

B, Displaced unstable segment of left innominate bone as a result of fractures of rami of both pubis and ischium and of the wing of the ilium near the sacroiliac joint.

C, Fractures of rami of pubis and ischium and a separation of the sacroiliac joint on the left with fragments of the rami over-riding.

D, Separated fractures of same portions of pelvis as in *C* but with spread of the segment of the innominate bone. (From Davis.)

In bilateral fractures of both rami with overriding and collapse of the pelvis, a pelvic sling with a wide spreader may be used. Strong bilateral traction with the lower extremities in abduction may effect some improvement in the position of the fragments.

In displaced fractures of the pelvis, treated in a pelvic sling, or when some displacement is accepted without attempts to improve the position of the fragments, bed rest is indicated for 6 to 8 weeks, following which the support of a canvas corset should be provided. Other than following manipulative reduction of displaced fractures of an innominate bone as described above, immobilization in a plaster cast is seldom worthwhile. If used, it must incorporate the trunk and one or both thighs.

FRACTURE OF THE ACETABULUM WITH CENTRAL DISLOCATION OF THE FEMORAL HEAD

A blow or fall onto the greater trochanter may drive the head of the femur through the floor of the acetabulum and into the pelvis, with fragments pushed ahead of it. The dislocated femoral head usually can be reduced by skeletal traction by means of a pin or wire through the lower femur. In some instances, supplemental lateral traction in which a wire is passed in the anterior posterior direction through the greater trochanter is helpful (Fig. 16–79). Skeletal traction should be continued for a minimum of 8 weeks.

At times, the acetabular fragments fall into good position, but frequently they are not pulled back into place by traction and the acetabulum remains distorted. Fortunately sufficient scarring of the acetabular floor often occurs to prevent or minimize redisplacement of the femoral head.

When traction is discontinued after 8 weeks, the head may return to a somewhat centrally displaced position. Even so, open reduction of the ace-

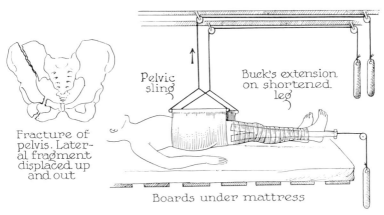

Pelvic sling

Buck's extension on shortened leg

Fracture of pelvis. Lateral fragment displaced up and out

Boards under mattress

Figure 16–78 Separated and upward displaced fracture of right innominate bone treated in a pelvic sling with traction to the leg. (From Banks and Compere.)

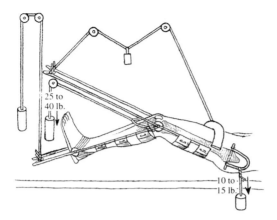

25 to
40 lb.

10 to
15 lb.

Figure 16–79 Two-direction skeletal traction for central fracture-dislocation of the hip. Longitudinal traction is provided with the extremity suspended in a Thomas or half-ring leg splint. A wire in an anteroposterior direction through the greater trochanter is utilized for lateral traction. (From DePalma.)

tabular floor is an extensive and dangerous procedure and should seldom be attempted in these circumstances, especially since a satisfactory functional result is often obtained by closed reduction even though the acetabular fragments are not reduced accurately. The explanation probably is that the weight-bearing part of the acetabulum is chiefly the superior undisplaced aspect rather than the central, displaced portion. If traumatic arthritis develops later, arthrodesis or arthroplasty may be performed.

Chapter 17

Fractures and Epiphyseal Injuries in Children

CARDINAL PRINCIPLES OF DIAGNOSIS AND MANAGEMENT

Fractures in children are different.   Unlike in adults whose bones break with increasing ease in advancing age, producing complex fracture patterns, bone injuries in children are usually simple with characteristic bone changes and a predictable outcome. Younger bones are very apt to break incompletely in a greenstick fashion without significant displacement of the fragments. The tough periosteum of children's bones often remains intact following fracture, thus helping to prevent displacement and to maintain reduction. The abundant blood supply of the periosteum and bone make nonunion an almost unknown complication. However, in certain fractures, such as fracture of the neck of the femur in the child, the prognosis is no better than in the adult.

Due to growth in the epiphyses at the ends of the long bones, children's bones continue to grow after the fracture heals. This growth provides spontaneous correction of shortening, lateral displacement and angulation by remodeling of the deformed bone within the limits of the child's age and remaining bone growth, and the nature and degree of deformity.

CORRECTABILITY OF ANGULATION

The degree of spontaneous correctability of angular deformities in long bone fractures of children is dependent upon several factors: (1) the age of the child, (2) the distance of the fracture from the end of the bone, and (3) the amount of angulation.

The younger the child and the nearer the fracture to the end of the bone, the more angulation one may accept. The older the child and the nearer the fracture is to the middle of the bone, the more accurate the reduction must be. The most complete spontaneous correction of angular deformity occurs when moderate angulation is in the plane of motion of a neighboring joint. Just proximal to the wrist joint, angulation of the radius with the apex toward the flexor surface produces surprisingly little immediate disability. Alignment and function are eventually normal unless the fracture occurs near the end of the growth period (Fig. 17–34).

CORRECTABILITY OF SHORTENING

Apposition (the amount of end-to-end contact of the fragments) and moderate shortening are of little significance in children. Long bones may be allowed to unite with bayonet (side-to-side) apposition in girls as old as 10 years and in boys as old as 12 years, with assurance that modeling will produce a nearly normal bone before growth is complete. Although the bayonet position is usually not acceptable in adults it is desirable in *displaced* fractures of the long bones of younger children. The stimulus that follows a displaced fracture results in accelerated longitudinal growth of the bone involved and sometimes of another distal to it. The average overgrowth of the individual bones following displaced fractures may be used as an index of the desirable overlap during healing: 2 cm. for the femur, and 1 cm. for the tibia and humerus. Undisplaced fractures do not result in permanent overgrowth.

ROTATIONAL DEFORMITY

Rotational deformity *must* be corrected at an early stage of treatment. It does not correct spontaneously. Failure to heed this fact results in deformity, which could have been avoided.

EPIPHYSEAL INJURIES

Special problems arise in the diagnosis and treatment of epiphyseal injuries. The dread complication is growth disturbance. Knowing what the prognosis is for a specific injury to an epiphyseal plate in a particular child is of paramount importance to the surgeon, who has both the responsibility of treating the child and advising the parents.

TYPES OF EPIPHYSES

There are two types of epiphyses in the extremities; pressure epiphyses and traction epiphyses.

Pressure Epiphyses: The epiphyses at the ends of the long bones are subjected to pressure, may be considered as articular epiphyses, and through their epiphyseal plates contribute to longitudinal growth of the long bones.

Traction Epiphyses (Apophyses): The traction epiphyses (apophyses) are the sites of origin or insertion of major muscles and are subjected to traction rather than pressure. They are nonarticular and do not contribute to the longitudinal growth of bone, for example, the greater and lesser trochanters of the femur.

THE EPIPHYSEAL LESION

When an epiphysis is separated by injury, the plane of separation occurs consistently through the zone of calcifying cartilage, structurally the weakest area of the epiphyseal plate. The constant location of this

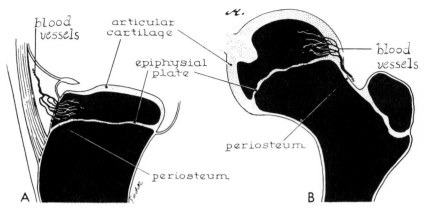

Figure 17–1   The two methods by which blood vessels enter epiphyses. *A*, Blood vessels entering side of epiphysis remote from the epiphyseal plate. *B*, Blood vessels traversing the rim of the epiphyseal plate. Rupture of these vessels may lead to avascular necrosis of the epiphysis. (From Salter, R. B., and Harris, W. R., J. Bone Jt. Surg., *45A*:590, 1963.)

plane of cleavage is of great significance because the growing cells remain attached to the epiphysis. Thus, if the nutrition of these cells is not damaged by the separation, there is no reason why normal growth should not continue.

The crux of the problem is not the mechanical damage to the plate, but whether the separation interferes with the blood supply of the epiphysis. In long-bone epiphyses the blood vessels penetrate the side of the epiphysis at a point remote from the epiphyseal plate. These vessels usually are not injured by epiphyseal separation and the nutrition of the epiphysis is preserved. A notable exception is the proximal femoral epiphysis where the blood vessels enter the epiphysis by traversing the rim of the plate. These vessels may be ruptured at the time of epiphyseal separation with subsequent avascular necrosis of the epiphysis (Fig. 17–1).

Fractures that cross the epiphyseal plate and injuries that crush the epiphyseal plate present additional problems that are discussed later. (See pages 334 and 335.)

INJURIES INVOLVING PRESSURE EPIPHYSES

Of all injuries to the long bones during childhood approximately 15 per cent involve an epiphyseal plate.

AGE AND SEX INCIDENCE

Although injuries to the epiphyseal plates may occur at any age during childhood, they are more common in periods of rapid skeletal growth—in the first year and during the prepubertal growth spurt, 9 to 12 years for girls and 12 to 14 years for boys. The growth spurt for the distal humerus, however, is 4 to 5 years for girls and 5 to 8 years for boys. Epiphyseal injuries are more frequent in boys than in girls.

SITE

The lower radial epiphyseal plate is by far the most frequently separated by injury. In order of decreasing frequency, epiphyseal injuries are found in the distal humerus (including injuries of the epicondyles), distal tibia, phalanges (fingers), distal fibula, distal ulna, proximal radius, proximal humerus, distal femur, proximal ulna, proximal tibia, metacarpals, proximal femur (head), and proximal fibula.

ETIOLOGY OF INJURIES TO THE EPIPHYSEAL PLATE

Trauma to an epiphyseal plate is usually one of four main types: shearing, avulsing, splitting, or crushing. Each mechanism tends to produce a characteristic type of lesion. The injury may be closed or open. Open injury, although rare, is more likely to be associated with disturbance of growth.

Iatrogenic damage to epiphyseal plates is preventable. Such damage may occur by forceful or multiple closed manipulations, by instrumentation at open reduction, and by injudicious use of metal fixation across epiphyseal plates.

DIAGNOSIS OF EPIPHYSEAL PLATE INJURIES

CLINICAL DIAGNOSIS

While an accurate diagnosis depends upon roentgenographic examination epiphyseal injury should be suspected clinically in any child who shows evidence of pain, swelling, tenderness, and spasm at a joint. Sprains in children are uncommon and the burden of proof rests with the surgeon to exclude epiphyseal injury or fracture. A positive x-ray confirms the diagnosis but a negative x-ray does not exclude the possibility of an epiphyseal injury.

The diagnosis may be established on clinical grounds alone by demonstrating focal tenderness exactly at the epiphyseal plate. This can be done by running an object such as the blunt end of a ballpoint pen along the bone and watching the child's face. Nothing happens with metaphyseal pressure. However, as the pen exerts pressure at the epiphysis, the child will wince. As the pen pressure travels beyond the epiphysis over the adjacent ligament, there is no facial reaction. Tenderness exactly at the epiphysis indicates a separation of the epiphysis without displacement. The roentgenogram is negative.

Such an epiphyseal injury is less likely to cause growth disturbance than one with displacement, unless the history suggests a crushing injury. Treatment is the same as for a displaced epiphyseal injury and the parents should be informed of the character of the lesion, the possibility of growth disturbance, and the need for follow-up examination.

ROENTGENOGRAPHIC DIAGNOSIS

Accurate interpretation of the roentgenograms of bones and joints in children necessitates a knowledge of the normal appearance of epiphyses and epiphyseal plates at various ages. Two views at right angles to each other are essential, and comparable views of the opposite uninjured extremity should always be taken. These are invaluable in interpreting what the appearance of the normal epiphysis should be for the injured child at his age. Similarly, right and left comparable views should be taken after healing when follow-up examinations are conducted.

POSSIBLE EFFECT ON GROWTH AFTER INJURY INVOLVING THE EPIPHYSEAL PLATE

Fortunately, most epiphyseal plate injuries are not associated with disturbance of growth. The clinical problem associated with premature cessation of growth depends on the bone involved, the extent of involvement of the epiphyseal plate, and the amount of remaining growth normally expected in the involved epiphyseal plate.

If the entire epiphyseal plate ceases to grow, the result is progressive shortening without angulation. However, if the involved bone is one of a parallel pair (such as tibia and fibula or radius and ulna), progressive shortening of one bone will produce progressive deformity in the neighboring joint. If growth in one part of the epiphyseal plate ceases but continues in the rest of the plate, progressive angular deformity occurs.

CLASSIFICATION OF EPIPHYSEAL PLATE INJURIES

The Salter classification is used in this text. It is based on the mechanism of injury and the relationship of the fracture line to the growing cells of the epiphyseal plate. The classification is also correlated with the prognosis concerning disturbance of growth.

TYPE I (Fig. 17–2)

There is complete separation of the epiphysis from the metaphysis without any bone fragment. The growing cells of the epiphyseal plate remain with the epiphysis.

This type, the result of a shearing or avulsive force, is more common in birth injuries and in early childhood when the epiphyseal plate is relatively thick. Wide displacement is uncommon because the periosteal attachment is usually intact.

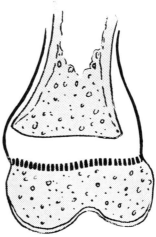

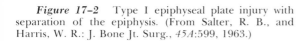

Figure 17-2   Type I epiphyseal plate injury with separation of the epiphysis. (From Salter, R. B., and Harris, W. R.: J. Bone Jt. Surg., *45A*:599, 1963.)

Reduction is not difficult, and the prognosis for future growth is excellent unless the epiphysis involved is entirely covered by cartilage (for example, at the upper end of the femur). In this case, the blood supply frequently is damaged with consequent premature closure of the epiphyseal plate.

TYPE II (Fig. 17–3)

There is epiphyseal separation along the epiphyseal plate and out through the metaphysis, leaving a characteristic triangular fragment of metaphysis attached to the epiphysis. It results from a shearing or avulsive force and is the most common type of epiphyseal injury. It generally occurs in children 10 years or older. The growing cartilage cells remain with the epiphysis, the circulation remains intact, and the prognosis is good.

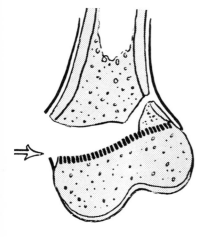

Figure 17–3   Type II epiphyseal plate injury: fracture-separation of the epiphysis. (From Salter, R. B., and Harris, W. R.: J. Bone Jt. Surg., *45A*:604, 1963.)

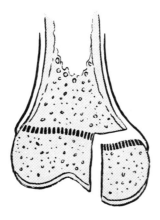

Figure 17-4   Type III epiphyseal plate injury: fracture of part of the epiphysis. (From Salter, R. B., and Harris, W. R.: J. Bone Jt. Surg., *45A*:606, 1963.)

TYPE III (Fig. 17–4)

There is an intra-articular fracture through the epiphysis, extending from the articular surface to the weak zone of the epiphyseal plate and then along the plate to its periphery. It results from an intra-articular shearing force and occurs usually at the upper or lower tibial epiphysis. Accurate reduction is essential and open reduction and pin fixation may be necessary.

TYPE IV (Fig. 17–5)

There is an intra-articular fracture across the epiphysis extending from the joint surface across the full thickness of the epiphyseal plate and through a portion of the metaphysis to produce a complete split. It most commonly occurs at the lateral condyle of the humerus. Perfect reduction is essential both to prevent growth disturbance and to provide a smooth

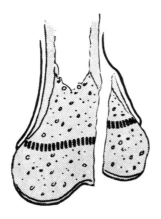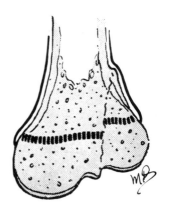

Figure 17–5   Type IV epiphyseal plate injury: *A*, fracture of the epiphysis and epiphyseal plate; *B*, bone union and premature closure. (From Salter, R. B., and Harris, W. R.: J. Bone Jt. Surg., *45A*:608, 1963.)

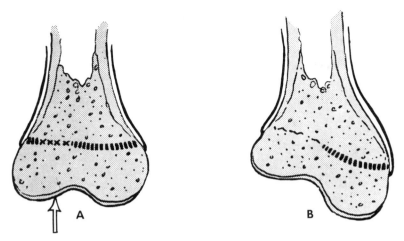

Figure 17–6   Type V epiphyseal plate injury: *A*, crushing of the epiphyseal plate; *B*, premature closure. (From Salter, R. B., and Harris, W. R.: J. Bone Jt. Surg., *45A*:609, 1963.)

joint surface. If the fracture is not reduced, cross union can occur between the displaced epiphyseal fragment and the metaphysis of the main fragment. This produces growth retardation or premature epiphyseal closure with deformity. Nonunion of the displaced fragment may also occur and produce a severe deformity. Unless the fragment is undisplaced, open reduction is almost always necessary. A fixation pin or screw across the metaphyseal fragment, securing it to the main fragment, is preferable to metal traversing the epiphyseal plate, although a small pin across the plate may be used for a few weeks if necessary.

TYPE V (Fig. 17–6)

A severe crushing force applied through the epiphysis at one area of the epiphyseal plate may result in growth retardation or premature epiphyseal closure by mechanical derangement of the epiphyseal plate. Fortunately, it is an uncommon injury. Initial diagnosis is based on clinical suspicion from a knowledge of the force applied and the clinical findings of epiphyseal tenderness with joint motion restricted by pain, swelling, and muscle spasm. Treatment consists of splinting and no weight bearing for 3 weeks or until the epiphyseal tenderness disappears.

OPEN REDUCTION AND INTERNAL FIXATION

In children the treatment of fractures is usually nonoperative. The long bones of children do not react kindly to open reduction and internal fixation. In fact, a generalization may be stated that, *a no more deliberate way exists to produce unnecessary complications in shaft fractures of the long bones in a child than open reduction and internal metal fixation.* Many reasons support this statement:

1. The introduction of infection with osteomyelitis, nonunion, permanent loss of length, prolonged disability, and numerous subsequent operations to correct the damage. Meanwhile, bony union would have occurred and a normal extremity have resulted by nonoperative treatment.

2. Loss of fixation as a result of the metals loosening or breaking, producing nonunion or malunion and requiring additional operative procedures.

3. Distraction of the fragments by improperly applied metal plates, resulting in delayed union or nonunion.

4. Metal plates, left in situ, become permanently imbedded in young bone. Refracture at the junction of the rigid section of plated bone and the resilient normal bone occurs frequently enough to make it mandatory that metal plates, if used, be removed when healing occurs to prevent the dilemma of repeated refracture and an imbedded, unremovable plate.

5. Displaced fractures of the shaft of the femur in a young child, if operated upon, with normal length restored, will result in permanent overgrowth and inequality of leg length. *Never open a shaft fracture of the femur in a child under 12.*

Open reduction may be necessary in certain epiphyseal injuries to restore a smooth joint surface or lessen the possibility of growth disturbance. The joint most commonly involved, which may require open reduction, is the elbow joint, with injuries to the lateral humeral condyle, the medial humeral epicondyle, or the proximal radial epiphysis with displacement. Other joint injuries which involve an epiphysis and which may require open reduction are Types III and IV epiphyseal fractures, separation of a proximal femoral epiphysis, and rare intra-articular fractures.

In older children, who may be approaching epiphyseal closure and bone maturity, the indications for open reduction of long-bone fractures more nearly approximate those outlined for the treatment of adult fractures in Chapter 16.

GENERAL CONSIDERATIONS IN THE TREATMENT OF CHILDREN'S FRACTURES AND EPIPHYSEAL INJURIES

1. **The principles of treatment are simple.** Alignment is the chief requirement. The fracture should not be rotated or grossly angulated. Rotational deformities are avoidable.

2. **Angulated greenstick fractures** near the center of the long bones, particularly the forearm bones of older children, must be completely broken through and accurately aligned to prevent recurrence of angulation in plaster and permanent deformity and disability.

3. **Method and technique of reduction:** In most cases, excellent results are obtained either by continuous traction or by manipulative reduction and plaster. When overlapping is desirable, traction is the method of choice.

4. **Epiphyseal fractures** in general are best treated by closed methods. Exceptions are fractures at the proximal end of the femur and certain joint fractures, particularly at the elbow. This subject is further discussed in the section dealing with specific fractures.

It is important to bear in mind that the initial injury may cause damage to the epiphyseal plate. So may the first reduction, with increasing likelihood of further damage with each successive manipulation. An effort should be made to achieve an anatomic or satisfactory reduction with the first attempt.

In open reduction of epiphyseal injuries avoid instrumental prying and levering which can damage the epiphyseal plate.

It is not only the responsibility of the surgeon but a measure of his competence to inform the parents of the possibility of growth disturbance and subsequent deformity due to epiphyseal damage at the time of injury. The need for periodic follow-up examinations should be explained to the parents, not to alarm them, but to reassure them that such visits permit early recognition of growth disturbance and an opportunity to elect timely remedial measures if necessary.

5. **Immobilization** should be efficient in order to prevent deformity. Children are active. It is wise to immobilize one or more joints on either side of the fracture until the callus is solid. Permanent stiffness of joints due to such immobilization is unknown in children.

6. **Physical therapy** is almost never necessary in the management of children's fractures. Manipulative reduction should be gentle to avoid soft tissue damage. There must be no obstruction to circulation in the application of casts, splints, bandages, and traction. Apply ice locally and elevate the part to minimize swelling. At the proper time active motion in unlimited quantities is supplied by the healthy child. Passive joint motion or manipulation should be strictly avoided. It does more harm than good.

INJURIES OF THE SHOULDER GIRDLE

FRACTURE OF THE CLAVICLE

The clavicle is one of the most frequently fractured bones in the body, particularly during childhood. It serves as the only bony connection between the shoulder girdle and the trunk. Any medially directed blow on the shoulder is transmitted to the clavicle. This bone may break when force is applied to the outstretched hand, the elbow, or the shoulder.

FRACTURES AT BIRTH AND DURING INFANCY

Compression of the shoulder girdle during delivery will occasionally cause a fracture of the clavicle. The common symptom is pseudoparalysis of the arm with obvious pain when the arm is moved. If the fracture is complete with over-riding, the pain will be considerable. A newborn infant with a greenstick fracture can be moved quite freely. Supine rest and gentle handling is the only treatment necessary. Early abundant callus and remodeling of the clavicle can be expected.

The symptoms of a displaced fracture in the toddler may be relieved by the addition of a figure-of-eight bandage. Healing is rapid and the fracture may be ignored after 10 days. The mother should be assured that the bump caused by the callus and any deformity will disappear in a few months. Reduction is seldom necessary in a child under 6 years of age.

FRACTURES IN CHILDREN 6 TO 12 YEARS OLD

Greenstick fractures are still frequent in this age range but over-riding fractures are more common. The greenstick fracture is treated by a figure-of-eight dressing made of stockinette, padded inside with felt under the axillae, and pinned in back. The bandage may be tightened by the mother each morning (Fig. 17–7) and is worn for 3 to 4 weeks.

FRACTURES IN CHILDREN OVER 12 YEARS OF AGE

A markedly displaced and over-riding fracture in an older child should be reduced. Satisfactory anesthesia is obtained by injecting procaine into the fracture hematoma. With the child seated in a chair the shoulders

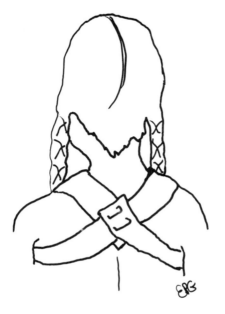

Figure 17–7   Simple figure-of-eight bandage made of stockinette with felt padding inserted into the stockinette under the axillae. The bandage may be tightened each morning by the mother.

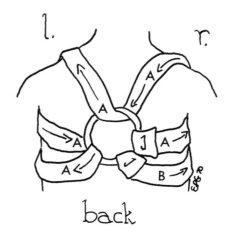

back

Figure 17–8 Figure-of-eight bandage for the older child designed with posterior ring which affords gliding for self-adjustment and constant effective tension. Felt pads are inserted into the stockinette under the axillae.

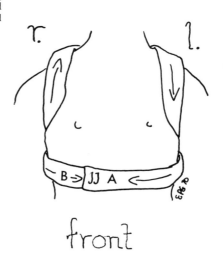

front

are pulled backward toward the spine, thus restoring the maximum length of the clavicle (see Fig. 16–3*B*). Reduction is maintained with a stockinette dressing padded inside for the axillae and constructed to act as an adjustable figure-of-eight dressing by means of a posterior centrally placed metal ring between the scapulae with the loops of the eight passed through the ring. The tension on the eight is adjusted in front by tightening and pinning the ends (Fig. 17–8). A long piece of stockinette is fastened with safety pins to a 1½ inch metal ring as at A in Figure 17–8 and the free end is passed under the right axilla and upward in front of the right shoulder and back to the ring through which it is passed. The end is then passsed over the left shoulder and circled downward in front of the left shoulder and back through the left axilla and again passed through the ring. The free end is then circled around the left chest to the front. A second short

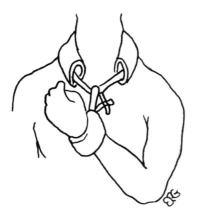

Figure 17–9   Collar and cuff to which an elastic bandage swathe encircling the arm and chest may be added for greater stability when indicated.

length of stockinette is fastened to the ring at B and passed around the right chest to the front. The two ends in front are pinned together at the desirable tension and this tension can be adjusted daily, facilitated by the stockinette gliding through the ring in back. This is the most practical and comfortable of all figure-of-eight clavicular dressings, it provides minimal axillary pressure on vessels and nerves and can be kept constantly under effective tension. With practice the technique is easily acquired.

INJURIES AT THE SHOULDER JOINT

FRACTURES IN CHILDREN 2 TO 7 YEARS OLD

Children from 2 to 7 years sustain injuries at the upper end of the humerus while at play. Dislocations and epiphyseal injuries are rare. A transverse greenstick fracture of the neck of the humerus is common in the younger child. Angulation of 10 to 15 degrees is compatible with a normal end result. A collar and cuff is the only treatment necessary (Fig. 17–9).

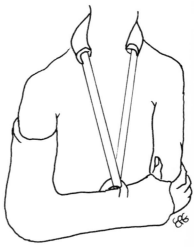

Figure 17–10   A hanging cast may be suspended from the neck with a padded muslin bandage or stockinette.

A displaced neck of humerus fracture is aligned by the application of a hanging cast (Fig. 17–10). Bayonet apposition with 1 cm. of over-riding is ideal. Ten to twenty degrees of angulation is permissible. Shortening and angulation will be outgrown.

FRACTURES IN CHILDREN 8 TO 14 YEARS OLD

In children from 8 to 14 years fractures of the neck of the humerus are less common. Epiphyseal fractures of the proximal end of the humerus can occur during games and sports. Dislocations are uncommon until adolescence.

Treatment of an epiphyseal fracture of the proximal humerus is nonoperative. Open reduction is not required and can be harmful by causing damage to the epiphyseal plate. Closed reduction by manual traction on the arm and the application of a hanging cast or sling and swathe is all that is necessary. Occasionally it will be found difficult to reduce such a fracture unless the arm is placed in the overhead position with olecranon pin traction for several weeks until firm callus is formed (Fig. 17–11).

The younger the child with an epiphyseal fracture, the greater the displacement which may be permitted. A 10-year-old boy with bayonet apposition of an epiphyseal fracture may be treated conservatively with every assurance that the result will be perfect. When a child is 12 years old, 50 per cent apposition is satisfactory but there should be less than 10 degrees of angulation (Fig. 17–12).

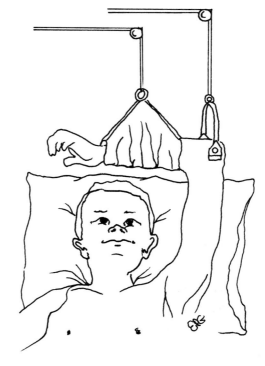

Figure 17–11 Traction on the humerus by a Kirschner wire through the olecranon with care to avoid the olecranon epiphysis and the ulna and dorsal interosseous (radial) nerves in placing the wire.

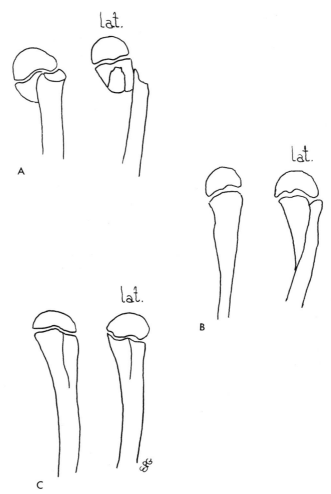

Figure 17–12   Epiphyseal fracture of the proximal end of the left humerus in an 8-year-old child. Treatment with a hanging cast and then a sling. *A*, Original position; *B*, 4 months later; *C*, 3½ years later. There is almost complete elimination of the deformity. The humeri are the same length.

FRACTURES OF THE SHAFT OF THE HUMERUS

Fracture through the middle of the humerus is rather rare in children compared to its frequency in adults. It may occur with rough handling of infants or may result from direct trauma in older children.

TREATMENT

In infancy the fracture is ideally treated by lateral traction for a week in bed with the elbow flexed and the forearm pointing straight up from the bed in neutral rotation to avoid rotary displacement (Fig. 17–13). When

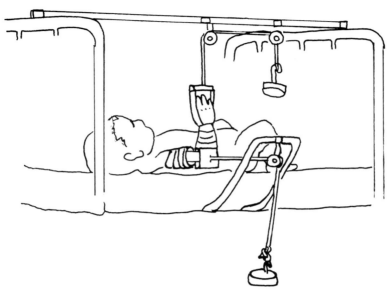

Figure 17–13   Flannelette secured with a skin adherent may be used for lateral traction. To prevent rotation of fragments, the forearm should be suspended perpendicular to the bed.

soft callus has formed, traction can be discontinued and a collar and cuff with swathe substituted. Apposition is not necessary and 15 degrees of angulation is permissible. If there is no displacement, a collar and cuff with swathe can be used primarily, but it is less comfortable than traction.

Ambulatory children are best treated with a hanging cast or collar and cuff with swathe. Bayonet apposition with 1 cm. of over-riding is acceptable and even desirable because of overgrowth as in the femoral shaft fractures. An undisplaced fracture does not overgrow. Healing is rapid and all support may be removed in 4 weeks (Fig. 17–14). A plaster spica, with the arm abducted, tends to cause angulation. Open reduction is not justified.

Complications are almost unheard of in closed fractures of the shaft of the humerus in children. Nonunion is not encountered and radial nerve palsy occurs less frequently in children.

In multiple injury cases, lateral traction in bed as described for an infant can be used. In an older child, overhead skeletal traction with a wire or pin through the olecranon is preferred.

INJURIES ABOUT THE ELBOW

SUPRACONDYLAR FRACTURES

Supracondylar fracture of the humerus is the most frequent elbow fracture sustained in children. The terms supracondylar and transcon-

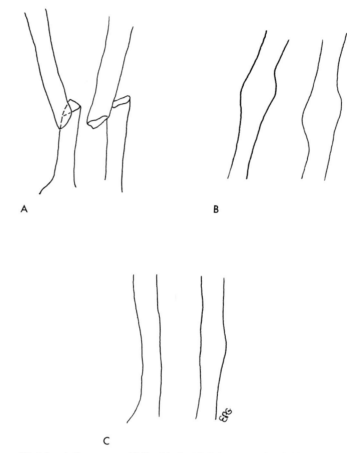

A   B

C

Figure 17–14   *A*, Fracture, middle third of left humerus in child age 12. Bayonet position is desirable. *B*, Solid union with good alignment and 2 cm. shortening 3 months after injury. *C*, Two years after original injury. There was 1 cm. of shortening.

dylar are identical for all practical purposes. The fracture is sustained by a fall on the outstretched hand with the force transmitted through the radius and ulna to the lower end of the humerus which becomes fractured through or just above the broadest portion of the condyles. The most common deformity is posterior angulation or displacement of the distal fragment of varying degree. In addition to the usual posterior displacement of the lower fragment, there is often lateral or medial displacement and there may be rotation of the distal fragment as well. The bony deformity may vary considerably, from no deformity to extreme deformity (Fig. 17–15).

DIAGNOSIS

The bony landmarks at the elbow are helpful in differentiating between a supracondylar fracture with displacement and a dislocation of

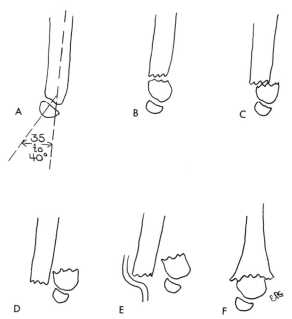

Figure 17–15   Sketch of lateral view of lower humerus to show: *A*, normal forward tilt of articular process (capitellum); *B*, loss of forward tilt; *C*, same plus partial posterior displacement; *D*, complete posterior displacement with over-riding; *E*, possible relation of brachial vessels to anterior distal end of proximal fragment; *F*, rotation deformity showing an anteroposterior view of the proximal fragment and a lateral view of the distal fragment.

the elbow. Normally, with the elbow flexed at 90 degrees the medial and lateral epicondyles and the tip of the olecranon form an isosceles triangle, and the epicondyles are in line with the shaft of the humerus. This triangle is preserved with a supracondylar fracture, but if posterior displacement of the distal fragment has occurred the epicondyles will be posterior to the axis of the humerus. With dislocation at the elbow, the isosceles triangle is disrupted by posterior displacement of the olecranon with elongation of the triangle. However, the axis of the epicondyles to the humerus is preserved.

This is one of the most potentially serious of all fractures. Hemorrhage, swelling, and displacement of the distal fragment may cause compression or actual kinking or stretching of the brachial artery, and, consequently, a serious threat to the circulation of the forearm and hand can occur. If improperly treated and unrelieved, this circulatory embarrassment may rapidly lead to Volkmann's ischemia and paralysis (see page 349).

Nerve injuries are not infrequent, with the radial nerve or its motor branch (posterior interosseous) being the most frequently, the ulnar nerve next, and the median nerve the least often injured. In most cases impairment of nerve function is the result of contusion or stretching rather than laceration.

TREATMENT

Successful reduction of a supracondylar fracture is accomplished by restoring the following anatomic features of the elbow. Viewed from the lateral side, the condylar component (capitellum) normally has a forward tilt of approximately 35 to 40 degrees to the humeral shaft (Fig. 17–15). Viewed from the front, with elbow extended, there is a normal carrying angle of 5 to 15 degrees. Persistence of posterior tilt and displacement can limit elbow flexion. Lateral or medial displacement with external or internal rotation of the distal fragment can produce an increased carrying angle or a reversed carrying angle with gun stock deformity (Fig. 17–16). The accuracy of restoration of forward tilt is easily determined by the lateral roentgenogram. Also the degree of rotary deformity is assessed by lateral roentgenogram. Rotary deformity is indicated by a flare of the distal end of the proximal fragment caused by an anterior or oblique position of the supracondylar ridges. This "fishtail" flare disappears and malrotation is corrected when the transverse diameter of the lower shaft of the humerus and the distal fragment are identical (Fig. 17–17). Persistence of medial or lateral displacement is determined by the anteroposterior roentgenogram. Residual displacement requires correction (Fig. 17–18).

Reduction is accomplished by manual traction-countertraction with correction of posterior displacement, rotation and medial or lateral shift before apposition, and correction of posterior tilt after the bone ends engage. The surgeon requires an assistant to apply traction-countertraction, permitting the surgeon to use both hands to accomplish the reduction (Figs. 17–19 and 17–20). The surgeon stands behind the elbow so he may

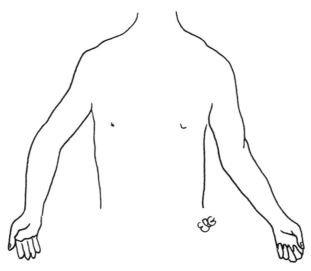

Figure 17–16   Reverse carrying angle with gun stock deformity (cubitus varus) due to persistent medial displacement and malrotation of distal fragment (right arm).

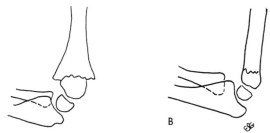

Figure 17–17   *A*, Sketch of lateral roentgenogram of elbow showing "fishtail' appearance of the distal end of the proximal fragment indicating malrotation. *B*, Shows correction of the rotary deformity. Both fragments present an identical transverse diameter in the lateral roentgenogram.

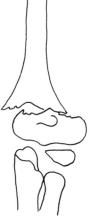

Figure 17–18   Anteroposterior view showing lateral displacement of the distal fragment.

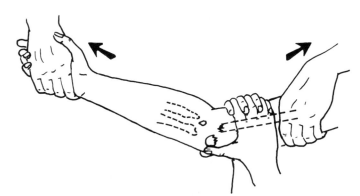

Figure 17–19   Manual reduction showing assistant exerting traction on the patient's hand and countertraction on the upper arm. Both hands of the surgeon are free to perform the reduction as shown and also illustrated in Figure 17–20.

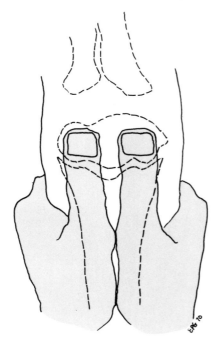

Figure 17-20   Close-up of bimanual reduction with the thumbs placed behind the medial and lateral epicondyles to control and correct medial or lateral displacement and rotation and to finally push the distal fragment forward to correct posterior displacement and angulation.

place one thumb on the back of each epicondyle and clasp his fingers in front of the arm. After adequate distraction of the fragments by the assistant, the surgeon pushes the distal fragment forward, with his thumbs controlling lateral displacement and rotation. Once the bone ends engage, further thumb pressure restores the forward tilt and the elbow is flexed beyond 90 degrees to maintain reduction without obliteration of the radial pulse.

A successful closed reduction is maintained with a posterior plaster moulded splint with the degree of flexion monitored by the radial pulse and circulation in the hand (Fig. 17–21). It is mandatory that all patients with supracondylar fractures of the elbow be admitted to the hospital for observation, regardless of the method of reduction, until the circulatory status is satisfactory and stable. Immobilization should be continued 3 to 4 weeks, followed by active use and a complete avoidance of passive stretching.

If reduction cannot be achieved or satisfactorily maintained without threat to the circulation, manual reduction is abandoned and overhead skeletal traction with an olecranon wire or pin is instituted (Fig. 17–22). The latter may not accomplish an immediate complete reduction but will provide an adequate reduction which, together with elevation of the extremity, is sufficient to prevent the serious consequences of ischemia. Several days later, when the swelling recedes, manual completion of the reduction can be accomplished in skeletal traction at the bedside with

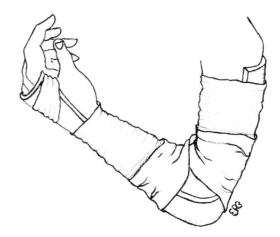

Figure 17-21 To maintain reduction of a supracondylar fracture a posterior moulded plaster splint is applied from the level of axilla to the metacarpophalangeal joints with the circular bandage applied as a figure-of-eight anterior to the elbow to avoid antecubital bandage constriction. Note supination of forearm and hand pointing toward the shoulder. This position lessens internal rotation effect on the fracture caused by usual across chest and pronated position.

appropriate anesthesia. When the callus permits, at 10 days to 2 weeks, a posterior moulded splint can be applied with the elbow flexed and the olecranon pin traction removed.

VOLKMANN'S ISCHEMIC PARALYSIS

The basic etiology of this dreaded, crippling lesion is of vascular origin, including spasm and mechanical blockage of the brachial artery at the fracture and an impeded venous return. The most significant warnings of early ischemia are: pain, swelling, coldness, cyanosis or pallor, and loss of ability to move the fingers. *Remember the four P's: pain, pallor, pulselessness,*

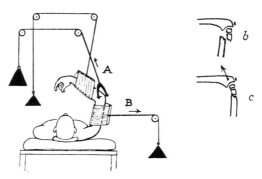

Figure 17-22 Overhead skeletal traction and suspension by means of Kirschner wire through olecranon. This method plus manipulation helps to bring about reduction of the fragments. The traction maintains the fragments in the reduced position. *A*, Traction on wire in olecranon; *B*, pull to keep shaft of humerus in a posterior position if necessary. High elevation assists gravity drainage of veins and lymphatics and gets rid of excessive swelling rapidly. Note that position of acute flexion is not necessary to maintain reduction by this method; also note absence of constricting bandage around elbow. Insets (*b* and *c*) show position of fragments before and after reduction by this method. (From Smith, F. M.: Surg. Clin. North America, *31*:554, 1951.)

and paralysis. The most important and constant of these signs is pain. A well-reduced fracture in a child should require no sedative other than aspirin. Pain severe enough to require opiates should be a warning that there is some complication. *The pain of anoxia is severe.*

The primary cause of anoxia is displacement of the fracture fragments, and the only potentially efficient single corrective measure is prompt reduction of this displacement. Until this has been accomplished, procaine block of the stellate ganglion or use of vasorelaxing drugs or local instillation of hyaluronidase or decompression of the antecubital space by incision of the deep fascia will prove of little avail. When these ancillary measures are carried out as the primary therapy, time passes, and often also the point of no return from tissue anoxia. *The urgent primary measure for relief of impending or early Volkmann's ischemia is reduction of the fracture.*

FRACTURES OF THE LATERAL CONDYLE OF THE HUMERUS

Forced abduction of the forearm may produce a shearing fracture of the lateral condyle. This is a classical Type IV epiphyseal fracture with the fracture line extending from the joint surface across the full thickness of the epiphyseal plate and through a portion of the metaphysis, producing a complete split. The extent of the injury is not fully apparent on the roentgenogram because the ossification centers of the capitellum and trochlea are not fully developed. The fracture through the bone of the lateral condyle is readily apparent. However the split in the cartilaginous epiphysis dividing the capitellum and trochlea cannot be visualized. If displacement occurs, a roentgenogram shows the fragment of lateral condyle and the capitellum ossification center to be pulled away. Part of the unvisualized trochlea is often included in the displaced fragment. The attached forearm extensor muscles rotate and further displace the fragment (Fig. 17–23).

Complete accuracy of reduction is a necessity in the management of this injury. Incomplete reduction invariably leads to growth disturbance by cross union between metaphysis and epiphysis or to a fibrous nonunion and further lateral displacement of the fragment. The eventual result in both instances is a progressive cubitus valgus deformity of the elbow which may produce a late ulnar nerve palsy (Fig. 17–24).

TREATMENT

If no displacement has occurred, immobilization of the elbow in a posterior moulded plaster splint with the elbow flexed for 3 to 4 weeks is recommended. If displacement has occurred one attempt at closed reduction is justified, and, if successful, immobilization as above is followed by healing and a relatively low incidence of growth disturbance.

Open reduction and internal fixation is mandatory if a "hair-line" closed reduction cannot be obtained. Operation is performed through a

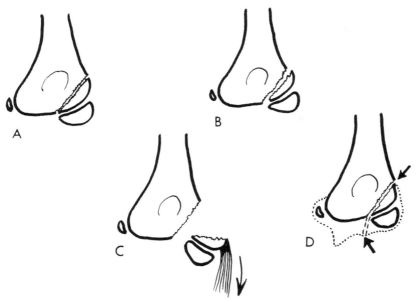

Figure 17–23   Sketch showing types of fracture of the lateral condyle of humerus. *A*, No displacement; *B*, minimal displacement; *C*, marked displacement in distal direction by pull of extensor muscles originating from the lateral condyle; and *D*, fracture line passing through cartilaginous lower end of humerus (designated by dotted line) but not visible on roentgenogram. The visible part of the displaced fragment always consists of the ossification center of the capitellum plus a variable sized portion of the diaphysis of the lower humerus. (From Smith, F. M.: Surgery of the Elbow. 1954, Courtesy of Charles C Thomas, Publisher, Springfield, Illinois.)

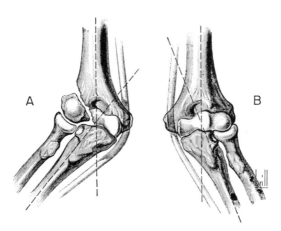

Figure 17–24   *A*, Schematic representation of nonunion of the right lateral humeral condyle with increase in the carrying angle. *B*, Prolonged trauma to the ulnar nerve results in delayed ulnar nerve palsy. (From Blount, W. P.: Fractures in Children. Williams and Wilkins Company, Baltimore, 1955.)

lateral approach to the elbow. Exposure of the fragment requires very precise dissection lest the circulation carried by its few remaining soft-part attachments be destroyed. Internal fixation can be obtained with a Kirschner wire. If the metaphyseal fragment is large enough, it is preferable to transfix this fragment. If not, the epiphysis may be transfixed with a Kirschner wire or two which must be removed when healing occurs (Fig. 17–25). A posterior moulded plaster splint with the elbow flexed is indicated for 3 to 4 weeks following operation.

FRACTURES OF THE MEDIAL EPICONDYLE OF THE HUMERUS

Medial epicondylar avulsion is the result of sudden valgus strain of the elbow with or without dislocation of the elbow joint. The fragment is a traction epiphysis and takes no part in longitudinal growth. If it is displaced no more than a few millimeters, the aponeurosis to the flexor muscles is not completely torn. Brief immobilization in flexion is all that is necessary. Bony healing will usually take place without deformity or disability. If the displacement is greater than 5 mm., one must decide between leaving the fragment displaced or opening the fracture and pinning the fragment in its normal position. Attempts at closed reduction are futile. If the displacement is allowed to persist, nonunion is the rule. Usually there is slight deformity but no disability.

There are only two urgent indications for operation. (1) If there are symptoms of ulnar nerve injury, the nerve must be explored promptly, and the fracture can be dealt with at the same time. (2) Temporary dislocation of the elbow joint not infrequently leaves the bone fragment incarcerated in the elbow joint (Fig. 17–26). It is a valuable axiom to scrutinize the anteroposterior view of a dislocated elbow to ascertain if the medial epicondyle is absent from its normal position as compared to the anteroposterior x-ray of the opposite normal elbow and, if so, to look for it in the joint.

Closed reduction of the dislocated elbow with the medial epicondyle trapped in the joint may be possible by angulating the elbow under anesthesia into a valgus position to dislodge the fragment. The possibility of overstretching the ulnar nerve by this maneuver must be kept in mind. If this closed maneuver does not extricate the fragment from the joint, open reduction is mandatory. Operation is performed through a medial approach to the elbow and the fragment is located by identifying the shiny aponeurosis of the flexor pronator group attached to the fragment. A skin hook placed in the aponeurosis and traction applied to the hook extricates the attached medial epicondylar fragment from the joint. The fragment can be reattached with a Kirschner wire to its site of origin or it can be excised and the aponeurosis sutured in place. The elbow is immobilized in a posterior plaster moulded splint with the elbow at right angles for 3 to 4 weeks and the pin can be removed at that time.

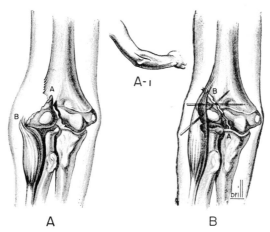

Figure 17–25   *A*, Sketch of fracture of lateral condyle. The extensor muscles of the forearm have displaced and rotated the fragment. *B*, Open reduction is performed through a lateral incision. The fragment is fixed with two small pins which are allowed to protrude slightly under the skin. (From Blount, W. P.: Fractures in Children. Williams and Wilkins Company, Baltimore, 1955.)

Figure 17–26   Sketch of anteroposterior view showing displacement of the avulsed medial epicondyle into the elbow joint. The aponeurosis of origin of the flexor-pronator muscles is attached to the fragment and is drawn into the joint with it. Extrication of the aponeurosis will eject the medial epicondylar fragment from the joint. The fragment can then be reattached to its site of origin.

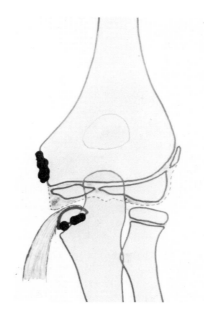

EPIPHYSEAL INJURIES OF THE RADIAL HEAD AND NECK

The longitudinal thrust that produces a compression fracture of the radial head in an adult causes a fracture of the radial neck or a separation of the proximal radial epiphysis with displacement in a child. These injuries are comprised of four main types.

TYPE I

These are injuries to the proximal radial epiphysis diagnosed on clinical grounds alone. Children who sustain a fall on the outstretched hand or forearm and complain of elbow pain and show tenderness centered at the upper radial epiphysis with painful limited elbow motion and hemarthrosis of the elbow joint, despite a negative roentgenogram, are considered to have injured the proximal radial epiphysis and not to have just a "sprained" elbow.

Treatment: Treatment consists of a protective splint or sling for 1 to 3 weeks or until epiphyseal tenderness subsides, whichever occurs first. Then full use of the elbow is permitted. Full elbow motion is quickly regained and no clinical or x-ray evidence of growth disturbance is to be anticipated.

TYPE II

These injuries are characterized by roentgenographic evidence of a fracture of the radial head and neck but with minimal or no displacement. Roentgenogram shows a tilt of the radial epiphysis of 15 degrees or less with buckling of the cortex of the neck.

Treatment: The treatment is the same as for Type I injuries. Growth disturbance is not to be anticipated. Some widening of the radial head may occur.

TYPE III

Fractures of the radial epiphysis and neck with a tilt of the proximal fragment of greater than 20 degrees, if unreduced, result in enlargement of the radial head and may lead to premature epiphyseal closure. If unreduced some limitation of elbow motion occurs (Fig. 17–27).

Treatment: Closed reduction is accomplished with the elbow extended and a varus force applied to the forearm and the displacement corrected by thumb pressure over the proximal fragment (Fig. 17–28). The varus force is thought to assist the reduction by exerting traction on the orbicular ligament which encircles the radial head and neck. If the tilt is severe and cannot be corrected by closed reduction, open reduction is warranted. However, damage to the epiphyseal plate is to be avoided.

TYPE IV

This group is comprised of fractures of the radial epiphysis associated with a dislocation at the elbow. There is complete avulsion with displace-

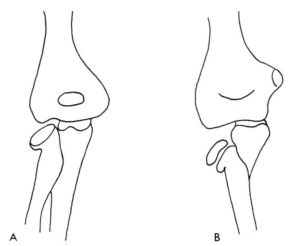

Figure 17-27   Epiphyseal fracture of the proximal radius; *A*, a 30-degree tilt of the radial epiphysis; *B*, a 70-degree tilt of the radial epiphysis.

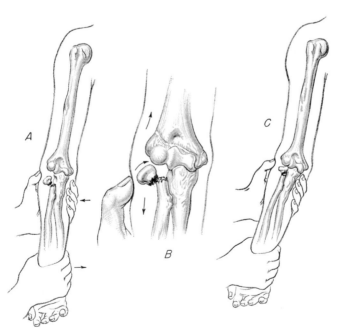

Figure 17-28   Reduction of tilt or displacement of radial neck fracture can sometimes be accomplished under general anesthesia by *A*, angulating the elbow into varus and *B* and *C*, reducing the fragment with firm thumb pressure. With gross displacement, this method is not usually successful. (From Blount, W. P.: Fractures in Children. Williams and Wilkins Company, Baltimore, 1955.)

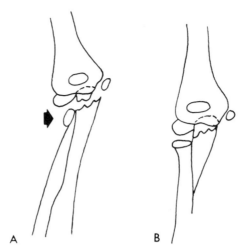

A   B

Figure 17–29   Complete avulsion of the proximal radial epiphysis is usually associated with a dislocation of the elbow. The dislocation may have been reduced when the child is first seen. *A*, Dislocation of the elbow with complete avulsion and end-to-side position of the radial epiphysis. Note fracture of olecranon, a frequently associated injury. *B*, Closed reduction using method illustrated in Figure 17–28. Open reduction is mandatory if closed reduction fails.

ment and rotation of the radial epiphysis with roentgenographic findings of an end-to-side position of the radius and epiphysis. It is unlikely that complete avulsion of the epiphysis occurs without dislocation. Fracture of the olecranon may be an associated injury. Although dislocation of the elbow may not be found when the child is first seen, it may be assumed to have occurred (Fig. 17–29).

Treatment: One attempt at closed reduction should be tried. Under general anesthesia the same maneuver is employed as described under the treatment of Type III injuries. If reduction is successful, the elbow is flexed to 90 degrees and protected by a posterior moulded splint which should not be changed or removed for a minimum of 4 weeks. Loss of reduction following successful closed reduction has occurred by premature removal of the immobilizing splint.

Open reduction is mandatory if closed reduction fails. A lateral approach to the elbow joint exposes the lesion. Damage to the dorsal interosseous nerve in the substance of the short supinator, two finger-breadths distal to the radial neck, is to be avoided in obtaining the exposure. Usually a paucity of periosteum following replacement prevents suture fixation of the epiphysis. If no fixation is used, the epiphysis can displace postoperatively unless immobilization is meticulously preserved for a minimum of 4 weeks. A recommended method of internal fixation is to introduce a Kirschner wire transfixing the capitellum from behind and drilling the wire through the center of the radial epiphysis into the intramedullary radial shaft. This is done with the elbow at 90 degrees. The pin can be removed in 3 to 4 weeks. If an accurate reduction is obtained and maintained, an excellent functional result can be anticipated. Growth disturbance is minimal unless nonunion occurs. *Never remove the radial head in a growing child.* This leads to cubitus valgus, radial shortening, and disparity of the length of the radius at the wrist with radial deviation of the hand and malfunction of the distal radio-ulnar joint.

DISLOCATIONS AT THE ELBOW JOINT

The diagnosis of the common posterior or posterolateral type of dislocation of the radius and ulna upon the humerus is usually not difficult on clinical examination. The clinical diagnosis of dislocation can be made on the basis of disturbed relationship of the three points making up the bony triangle at the elbow (see page 344).

Nerve lesions may occur from stretching or contusion or later may result from compression by scar tissue formed during the process of healing. The ulnar nerve is most commonly affected as a result of dislocation, but the radial and median nerves may also be involved. Avulsion of the medial epicondyle with the epicondyle sucked into the joint may occur (see page 352). Complete avulsion of the proximal radial epiphysis may be an associated injury (see page 354).

TREATMENT

Reduction of a dislocation can be accomplished usually by closed methods. General anesthesia is advisable if the dislocation is more than one hour old in order to alleviate pain and especially to obtain complete muscle relaxation. Without muscle relaxation it may be necessary to use considerable force in the reduction which predisposes to additional joint and soft-part injury.

Reduction is accomplished by traction on the forearm and counter-traction upon the humerus with the elbow slightly hyperextended. When the forearm bones are felt or appear to come forward, the elbow is flexed. If reduction is complete, the joint can be fully flexed with ease (see Fig. 16–19).

Following reduction of a simple dislocation, subsequent treatment should be directed toward prevention of recurrence. Therefore, the elbow should be immobilized in a posterior moulded plaster of Paris splint (extending from the axilla to the metacarpophalangeal joints) with the elbow at an angle of approximately 100 to 110 degreees of flexion. This splint should be worn for 2 weeks. Following removal of the splint, elbow motion is regained by normal active use. Passive stretching and "pump-handling" exercises are to be avoided.

MISCELLANEOUS ELBOW INJURIES

OLECRANON FRACTURES

Olecranon fractures occur rarely as isolated injuries in children. Plaster fixation in adequate extension is the treatment of choice. Immobilization for 5 weeks or longer does not cause prolonged or permanent stiffness in a child as it does in the adult. Ordinary unguided activity soon restores normal motion. Physical therapy is contraindicated.

MONTEGGIA FRACTURE

A *Monteggia fracture* is an angulated fracture of the shaft of the ulna with dislocation of the radius at the elbow. Due to the intimate parallel relationship of the radius and ulna supported by the interosseous membrane, angulation of the shaft of the ulna forces a dislocation of the radial head in the direction of the apex of ulnar angulation. Thus the radial head will dislocate anteriorly with ulnar angulation apex volar, or posteriorly with ulnar angulation apex dorsal (Fig. 17–30).

Diagnosis: Diagnosis depends chiefly on considering three factors:

1. Include the elbow joint in the roentgenogram of the forearm.

2. Study the relationship of the longitudinal axis of the radius to the capitellar epiphysis in the lateral roentgenogram. Regardless of the degree of flexion or extension of the elbow, the longitudinal axis of the radius normally passes through the center of the capitellar epiphysis (Fig. 17–31).

3. Assume that the radial head is dislocated in any angulated fracture of the shaft of the ulna until proved otherwise.

Treatment: Closed reduction is usually successful in children.

The angulation of the ulna is corrected and the radial head is reduced by manipulation. The elbow is immobilized in flexion. If the reduction of the radial dislocation is unstable or angulation of the ulna persists, open reduction is indicated.

It is recommended that the radial head be reduced through a lateral incision and the orbicular ligament dealt with as necessary. The radial head may be avulsed from and found lying upon an invaginated orbicular ligament or buttonholed through the joint capsule, either of which prevents successful closed reduction. The ulnar fracture may be treated with an intramedullary pin inserted through the olecranon apophysis. If it is necessary to open the ulnar fracture site, a separate incision over the subcutaneous ulna is recommended. The pin can be removed through a window cut in the cast at 3 weeks, and the cast left on for 2 weeks longer.

SUBLUXATION OF THE HEAD OF THE RADIUS
(THE "PULLED ELBOW")

This is a very common injury in young children and usually occurs between the ages of 2 and 6 years. The mechansim of the injury is a sudden pull, jerk, or lift on the child's wrist or hand by a playmate or by a tired and

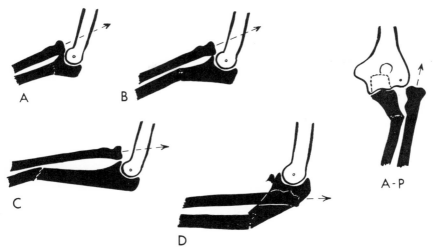

Figure 17–30   Varieties of Monteggia fractures: *A, B,* and *C* show extension types and *D,* the flexion type. Arrow shows failure of the axis of the radius to pass through the center of the capitellum when the ulnar fragments are angulated. The displacement of the upper radius is *always* in the direction pointed to by the apex of the angle formed by the ulnar fragments. (From Smith, F. M.: Surgery of the Elbow. 1954. Courtesy of Charles C Thomas, Publisher, Springfield, Illinois.)

annoyed parent (or nursemaid), who is trying to hurry the youngster across the street or up the steps. Sometimes while holding the parent's hand, the child stumbles and the parent in an attempt to protect him from the fall pulls up quickly on his hand and wrist.

The pathology is not definitely understood, but probably one of two things occurs: (1) the radial head is pulled distally and jammed into the orbicular ligament which grips it tightly or (2) the orbicular ligament is split and a portion of the ligament is interposed between the radial head and capitellum and is temporarily caught.

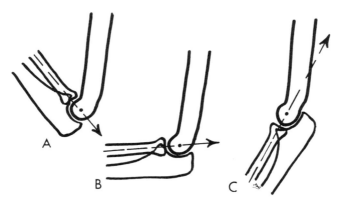

Figure 17–31   Sketches of lateral roentgenograms of the elbow in: *A,* acute flexion; *B,* at 90 degrees; and *C,* in full extension to show how the longitudinal axis of the radius normally passes through the center of the capitellum or the capitellar epiphysis. (From Smith, F. M.: Surgery of the Elbow. 1954. Courtesy of Charles C Thomas, Publisher, Springfield, Illinois.)

The main symptoms are pain and refusal to use not only the elbow but frequently the entire arm. The history of a jerk on the arm is invaluable. Flexion and extension at the elbow are usually not limited but are painful. Supination is definitely limited. There is no characteristic palpable deformity. Roentgen examination is of no value except to rule out other bony injury.

Treatment: *Anesthesia is unnecessary.* Reduction is accomplished with the elbow flexed and with the examiner's thumb placed over the radial head. The forearm is slowly supinated and thumb pressure applied to the radial head. A snap or click is usually heard. The forearm should again be tested in pronation and supination to make certain that the latter motion has been definitely regained. The elbow should then be moderately flexed and rested in a sling. The child within a few hours will usually begin to use the arm spontaneously. The prognosis is excellent.

FRACTURES OF THE FOREARM AND WRIST

Fractures of the forearm occur in order of frequency in the distal third (75 per cent), the middle third (18 per cent), and the proximal third (7 per cent). Fractures of the distal third are produced by a fall on the hyperextended, outstretched hand. Fractures of the middle third may be produced by direct or indirect trauma, and fractures of the proximal third are complex in etiology.

There are three main types of fracture.

1. The *torus fracture* usually occurs in the distal radius about 1 inch proximal to the epiphysis and consists merely of buckling of the cortex of the radius with minimal angulation and no displacement.

2. A *greenstick fracture* occurs usually in the distal third in young children and in the middle third or at the junction of middle and distal thirds in children from ages 6 to 12. The apex of angulation in a greenstick fracture is characteristically volar.

3. *Displaced fractures* of one or both bones may occur at any level. They are the most difficult to treat.

TORUS FRACTURE: TREATMENT

The torus fracture of the distal radius requires no reduction, only protection. A sugar tong splint of moulded plaster of Paris over canton flannel is applied with the wrist in neutral position and the forearm in midrotation for 2 or 3 weeks (Fig. 17–32).

GREENSTICK FRACTURE: TREATMENT

Treatment of a greenstick fracture of one or both bones is quite simple if one important principle is borne in mind. It does not suffice simply to straighten the bone and apply a plaster cast. In a greenstick fracture one

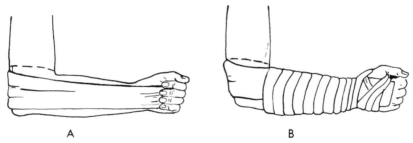

Figure 17–32   *A,* moulded "sugar-tongs" splint extending from the knuckles on the dorsum of the hand around the elbow, to end at the flexion crease in the palm: *A,* palmar view without bandages, and *B,* bandaged in place.

cortex remains unbroken, and in the characteristic deformity it is the dorsal cortex. This intact cortex acts as a spring to cause recurrence of angulation even within the plaster cast. It is essential that the fracture be completed by the surgeon thus removing the spring effect. This is accomplished by grasping the forearm with both hands with the thumbs applied over the apex of the angulation. With the thumbs used as a fulcrum, the angular deformity is over-corrected until one hears the dorsal cortex snap (Fig. 17–33). It is important to avoid displacing forces and permit the intact periosteum to protect against displacement of the fragments. Following this a long-arm circular plaster can be applied from axilla to the metacarpophalangeal joints with the elbow at right angles and the forearm in midrotation. Whereas the fracture will heal in 6 weeks, refracture is

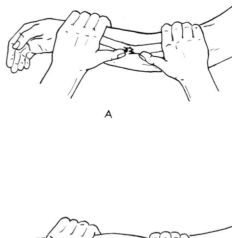

Figure 17–33 An angulated greenstick fracture of both bones of the forearm. *A,* The dorsal cortices are still intact, and to merely straighten the bones will lead to recurrence of angulation, even in plaster. *B,* It is necessary to break the dorsal cortices, by overcorrection of the angulation using the thumbs as a fulcrum. The bones are broken but the periosteum remains intact. Recurrence of deformity does not occur.

A

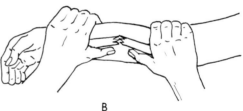

B

common and to protect the child against reinjury it is important to continue the immobilization for a minimum of 8 weeks.

FRACTURES OF BOTH BONES OF THE FOREARM WITH DISPLACEMENT: TREATMENT

Treatment in this instance can be difficult and requires considerable skill. If both bones are reduced simultaneously, one is fortunate. If one bone is reduced, it may be possible to use that bone as a fulcrum to reduce the other bone. Of the two bones, reduction of the radius is the more important. If reduction is not possible, slight over-riding can be accepted but angular deformity should be corrected. It is mandatory that rotary deformity be corrected. In assessing the accuracy of reduction it is important to include the elbow as well as the wrist in the postreduction roentgenograms taken in two planes. Beware of the film which shows a lateral view of the forearm bones at the elbow and an anteroposterior or oblique view at the wrist. Sometimes multiple views are helpful in assessing rotary deformity.

The first step in reduction is traction and countertraction to regain length. To correct over-riding and obtain end-to-end apposition, it may be necessary to angulate the bones 90 degrees to the normal axis in order to slip one end onto the other. Proper rotation and alignment are restored. Partial displacement is less important and will be corrected by remodeling in the young child. It is important to accept very little angular deformity in the midshaft fractures. The closer the fracture to the distal extremity of the bone or bones, the more angulation can be accepted when the child is under 10 (Fig. 17–34).

The importance of traction cannot be over-emphasized in correcting displaced fractures of the forearm bones in children. For the purpose of accomplishing reduction, Japanese finger trap traction may be used. Traction is maintained until the plaster hardens and is then removed (Fig. 17–35).

As long as rotation and major angulation are corrected and there is a minimal amount of over-riding an excellent result can be anticipated through remodeling of the bone (Fig. 17–36).

A knowledge of the muscle motors attached to the forearm bones is essential to proper positioning of the forearm. The short supinator and the biceps (long supinator) supinate the proximal fragment when the fracture is in the proximal third of the radius. The short and long supinators are balanced by the radial attachment of the pronator teres in fractures of the midshaft of radius. The pronator quadratus influences the position of the radius in fractures of the distal shaft of the radius (Fig. 17–37).

Therefore, fractures of the proximal third of the radius should be treated with the forearm in supination. Fractures between the pronators should be treated with the forearm in neutral rotation.

Recurrence of deformity following an apparently successful reduction occurs with sufficient frequency to make it mandatory that roentgenograms

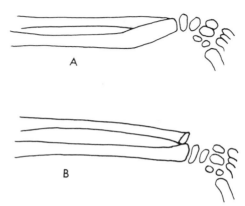

Figure 17–34   *A*, Angulation of distal radius 5 months after fracture. *B*, Sketch of follow-up roentgenogram 4 years later. Moral: Angular deformities in the plane of motion of a joint of a young child straighten out to a remarkable degree.

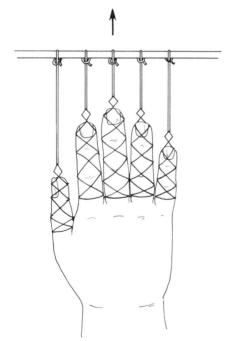

Figure 17–35   Japanese finger trap traction aids reduction of forearm fractures. Traction is maintained until the immobilizing plaster hardens.

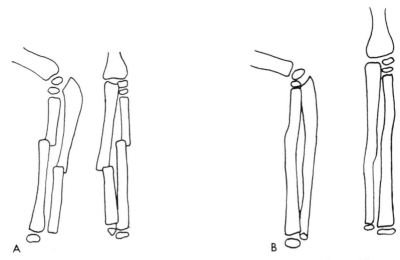

Figure 17–36   *A*, Fracture shaft of radius and ulna in a 6-year-old boy. Alignment and rotation were considered acceptable. *B*, Sketch of a roentgenogram 6 months later. Normal function. End-on apposition in a young child is not essential to a good result; strive for proper rotation and the best possible alignment.

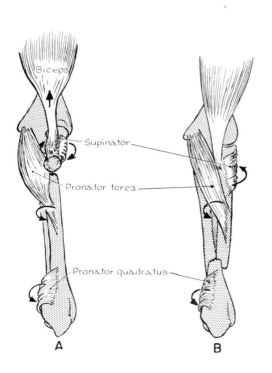

Figure 17–37   Rotary muscle forces affecting radial shaft fractures. *A*, In a fracture between the supinator and pronator teres insertions the proximal fragment is flexed and supinated by the biceps and supinator; the distal fragment is pronated by the pronator teres and quadratus. *B*, In a fracture between the pronators, the proximal fragment remains in neutral rotation; the distal fragment is pronated. (From McLaughlin, H. L.: Trauma. W. B. Saunders, Philadelphia, 1959.)

be repeated in a few days and at one week and again at two weeks post-reduction. Within this period of time, recurrence of deformity can be corrected by closed reduction.

Fracture of the distal shaft of the radius with over-riding may be irreducible by closed reduction. This is due to the fact that the proximal end of the distal fragment is buttonholed through the periosteal sleeve, and the more traction that is applied the tighter the buttonhole becomes, preventing reduction. If the child is of an age where the over-riding and tilt of the distal fragment is not acceptable, it may be necessary to open the fracture and slit the periosteal sleeve to permit a reduction. Internal fixation is not necessary.

Refracture of both bones of the forearm at the same level is more frequent than generally realized. It usually occurs within the first 6 months after the original injury but may be delayed longer.

Fracture of the Distal Radial Epiphysis

The equivalent of a Colles' fracture in the adult is a fracture of the distal radial epiphysis in the child. The mechanism of injury is the same — a fall on the outstretched hand. The force transmitted by the carpus displaces the distal radial epiphysis dorsally, usually with a small dorsal triangular metaphyseal fragment attached to the epiphysis (Fig. 17–38).

Reduction is accomplished in the same manner as with a Colles' fracture. The surgeon grasps the hand and an assistant provides countertraction on the arm. After a few minutes of traction the dorsally displaced epiphyseal fragment is pushed volarward by thumb pressure applied to the dorsum of the displaced epiphysis (see Fig. 16–24B, C, D).

If a perfect reduction is not obtained and the displacement is slight, it is better to allow it to remain. Multiple attempts at reduction can damage the growing cells on the displaced epiphysis. Residual displacement will remodel up to the age of 10, affording a normal wrist in most instances.

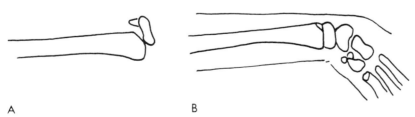

A   B

Figure 17–38   *A*, Epiphyseal fracture of the distal radial epiphysis is the most frequently encountered epiphyseal injury. Note dorsal displacement and tilt of the displaced epiphysis; Type II epiphyseal injury. *B*, Reduction is accomplished by traction-countertraction and downward thumb pressure on the epiphysis. Residual displacement of a few millimeters is preferable to repeated reductions. Reduction is maintained by a sugar-tongs splint with the wrist in flexion and ulnar deviation.

Immobilization with the wrist in volar flexion and pronation in a sugar tong moulded plaster splint is maintained for 3 weeks.

As with all epiphyseal injuries, the possibility of growth disturbance is explained to the parents, and the child should be followed for 3 years both clinically and roentgenographically.

INJURIES OF THE FEMUR

FRACTURES OF THE SHAFT OF THE FEMUR

A tranverse fracture of the middle third of a child's femur is usually produced by direct trauma. A long spiral fracture is usually produced by torsion. Birth fractures of the femur are usually transverse in the middle third.

TREATMENT

Closed fractures of the shaft may be treated by nonoperative measures with a routinely satisfactory outcome. An incomplete fracture without deformity is immobilized in a plaster of Paris spica cast for 6 to 8 weeks, depending upon the age of the child. In treating the displaced fracture, only a few principles need be observed. Rotation and angulation of the distal fragment must be avoided. Both can be eliminated by traction with the legs held in symmetrical positions. In the child 2 years of age or under, this can be accomplished by Bryant's traction.

Bryant's skin traction is in common use for the treatment of femoral shaft fractures in infants (Fig. 17–39). Both legs are suspended by adhesive skin traction from an overhead frame, so that the buttocks are just lifted from the mattress. The vascular status of both limbs must be determined frequently to avoid risk of Volkmann's ischemic paralysis (refer to page 349). This dreaded complication can result from the circular bandages supporting the adhesive skin plaster, and the results are as disastrous as those described under Volkmann's ischemia complicating supracondylar fracture of the humerus in a child. The uninjured extremity is in the greatest danger. This is because hyperextension of the knee can occur causing excessive stretch on the popliteal vessels. For this reason, it is advisable to apply a posterior moulded splint to the uninjured leg with the knee in slight flexion. Pain in the leg, swelling, cyanosis, or impaired motion of the toes require immediate removal of the bandages and inspection of the extremity. Never disregard the complaint of pain. The pain from a fracture should not be sufficient to require opiates in a child. Pain of this magnitude usually indicates ischemia.

In a very young child, the fracture will be solid in as short a time as 2 weeks, but traction should not be removed until the tenderness of the callus

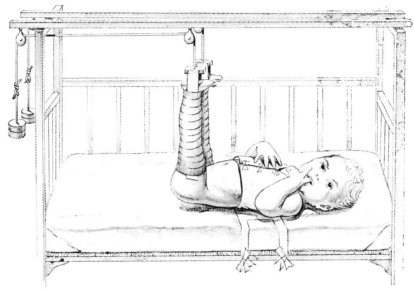

Figure 17–39   Bryant's skin traction applied to both legs. Traction may be adjusted better if separate weights and pulleys are used. Some form of restraint is imperative. (From Blount, W. P.: Fractures in Children. Williams and Wilkins Company, Baltimore, 1955.)

has disappeared. Application of a plaster spica affords protection for another 2 weeks.

Another method of treatment for femoral shaft fractures used as an alternative to Bryant's traction for infants and children up to 5 years of age is skin traction applied to the legs with the child supine on an inclined Stryker frame (Fig. 17–40). This frame provides safe traction with a flexion band behind the knees. No weights are required. The legs are fastened to the end of the frame with the pull of the body on the inclined frame furnishing the traction. The angle of inclination determines the amount of

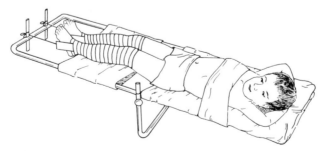

Figure 17–40   Stryker frame traction on an inclined plane. Skin traction is applied to both legs and attached to the end of the frame. No weights are required. The weight of the body on the inclined plane furnishes the traction. The angle of inclination determines the amount of pull. A flexion band is added back of the knees.

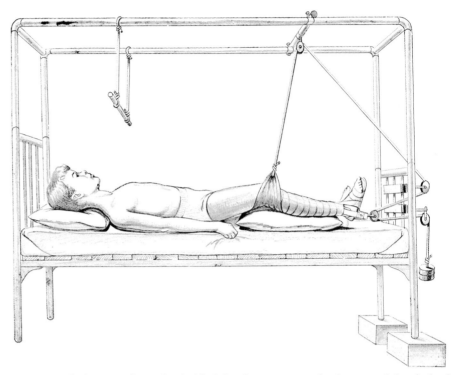

Figure 17–41   Russell traction is ideal for the treatment of a fracture of the shaft of femur in older children. If the position is difficult to maintain, the other leg should be treated similarly. If the child is cooperative, unilateral traction may be used. (From Blount, W. P.: Fractures in Children. Williams and Wilkins Company, Baltimore, 1955.)

pull. Subsequent treatment with a plaster spica follows the same guidelines as with Bryant's traction.

Russell skin traction with a weight of three to six pounds is used for children 5 years of age or older (Fig. 17–41). The knee sling must be soft and placed so as to avoid pressure on the peroneal nerve. A steady pull on the fractured leg will usually maintain correct alignment. If there is angulation it may be corrected by application of traction to the other leg.

Skeletal traction and balanced suspension may be helpful in children over 10 years of age if skin traction proves to be inadequate. The wire or pin is placed in the distal femoral fragment proximal to and avoiding the distal femoral epiphysis.

In fractures of the junction of middle and upper thirds, there is frequently adduction of the proximal fragment. This is overcome not by increasing the pull on the injured side but by diminishing it and pulling harder with traction on the opposite side. This tilts the pelvis downward on the other side, thus reducing the adductor spasm (Fig. 17–42).

There is less chance of complication and a higher percentage of good results with traction than any other form of treatment. Union is more

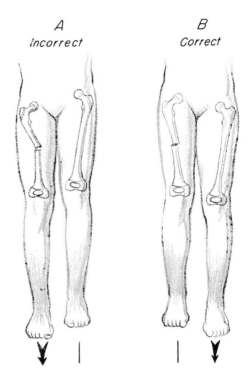

Figure 17-42 When the proximal fragment is adducted *A*, do not increase the pull; apply traction to the other leg *B*, tilt the pelvis downward on the other side, and release the adductor spasm. (From Blount, W. P.: Fractures in Children. Williams and Wilkins Company, Baltimore, 1955.)

prompt than with a cast and there is less likelihood of angulation. It usually is a mistake to discontinue traction and apply a cast while the callus is soft. The fragments are likely to angulate. When the callus is no longer tender, traction may be discontinued safely and a spica cast applied.

In the usual *displaced* fracture of the shaft of the femur in a child 12 years or younger, end-to-end apposition is not only unnecessary but is undesirable. End-to-end apposition by closed reduction or open reduction results in overgrowth in the length of the extremity. Such overgrowth averages 1.7 to 2.5 cm. and is permanent (Fig. 17-43).

An acceptable reduction consists of fragments angulated less than 15 degrees with the fragments in contact and over-riding (side-to-side or "bayonet" position) not in excess of 2 cm (see page 328). If these tenets are observed, a normal result may be anticipated (Figs. 17-44 and 17-45).

An *undisplaced* fracture of the shaft of femur should be treated with a plaster spica. Overgrowth does not occur.

As the patient approaches epiphyseal closure, the accuracy of reduction must approach that required for an adult.

FRACTURES OF THE PROXIMAL END OF THE FEMUR

Fractures of the proximal end of the femur in children are difficult to treat. Fortunately, they are rare.

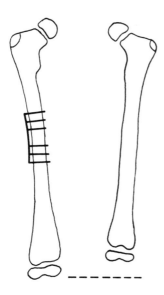

Figure 17–43   Displaced fracture shaft of right femur in a 5-year-old child. Sketch of scanogram of both femurs 5 years after open reduction, *restoration of normal length*, and internal fixation with plate and screws. Note permanent overgrowth of 2.3 cm. on the injured side.

Figure 17–44   *A*, Fracture shaft of femur in a 5-year-old child with 2 cm. over-riding in the "bayonet" position. *B*, Six weeks later. Treated with Bryant's traction. Note callus beneath stripped-up periosteum at the ends of the over-riding fragments. Over-riding favors healing. *C*, Four and one-half years later. Equal leg lengths. Shaft displacement remodeled. Over-riding of 2 cm. is desirable in a displaced fracture of the shaft of femur in a child 12 years of age or younger.

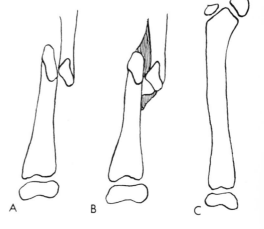

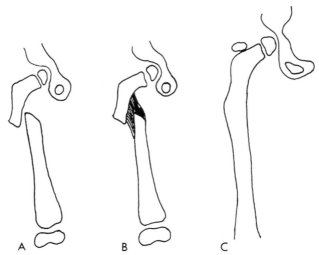

Figure 17–45   *A*, Fracture shaft of femur in a 7-year-old child with abduction of the proximal fragment and approximately 15 degrees of angulation. *B*, Three months later. Angulation persists. *C*, Seven years later. Angulation deformity has been fully corrected by bone remodeling. Leg lengths are equal.

The injury occurs in children from 3 to 16 years and is most common from 11 to 13 years. The fracture usually follows severe violence, especially falls from a height or motor accidents.

Complications are frequent and include avascular necrosis, coxa vara, delayed union or nonunion, and growth disturbance. Avascular necrosis occurs in 45 per cent of cases, is always apparent within a year, and occurs in all groups of fractures whether or not they are displaced. No treatment appears available to influence the course of avascular necrosis. Delayed union or nonunion occurs more frequently in those patients treated by closed reduction and plaster than by internal fixation. Therefore, internal fixation is recommended.

The fractures may be classified as transepiphyseal, transcervical, cervicotrochanteric, and intertrochanteric. A description of these fractures and the treatment for each follows.

TRANSEPIPHYSEAL FRACTURES

This fracture, not to be confused with slipping of the capital femoral epiphysis, is an acute traumatic separation of a previously normal epiphysis. It may occur with dislocation of the femoral head and carries a high incidence of aseptic necrosis of the proximal femoral epiphysis.

Treatment.   Treatment depends on whether the femoral head is dislocated.

Without dislocation of the femoral head treatment consists of gentle closed manipulation and insertion of two or three parallel Knowles pins.

With dislocation of the femoral head, treatment involves open reduction, internal fixation with two or three Knowles pins, and prolonged nonweight bearing.

It is recommended that the Knowles pins be inserted parallel to each other and if three are used that their bases form an equilateral triangle. The normal size Smith-Peterson nail, because of the firmness of the femoral head, can displace the femoral head or distract it during insertion. For this reason it is recommended that Knowles pins or a modified smaller size 3 flange Smith-Peterson nail be used. The nail is introduced over a guidewire with the guidewire penetrating the epiphysis and protruding a short distance into the acetabulum to stabilize the head as the nail is inserted. After the nail is inserted, the guidewire is removed.

TRANSCERVICAL FRACTURES

This fracture occurs through the neck of the femur and is the most common type of fracture involving the proximal end of the femur.

Treatment: Undisplaced fractures may be treated in a single-leg plaster spica, but displacement has been known to occur in the spica.

Displaced transcervical fractures should be treated by gentle closed manipulative reduction and insertion of three Knowles pins plus a single-leg plaster spica. This is also a more assured method of maintaining reduction with undisplaced fractures.

CERVICOTROCHANTERIC FRACTURES

This is also referred to as a basal fracture at the junction of base of neck and trochanter.

Treatment: Good results have been reported from treatment of an undisplaced cervicotrochanteric fracture by an abduction single-leg spica. However, varus deformity has also been reported to occur in the spica. The safest treatment is internal fixation with Knowles pins and a single-leg spica.

Displaced cervicotrochanteric fractures are treated by gentle manipulative reduction and internal fixation with Knowles pins, followed by a single-leg plaster spica.

INTERTROCHANTERIC FRACTURES

Intertrochanteric fractures of the hip in children are rare compared with their incidence in adults.

Treatment: Treatment consists of gentle manipulative closed reduction with immobilization in a single spica cast in wide abduction.

SUBTROCHANTERIC FRACTURES OF THE FEMUR

Subtrochanteric fractures of the femur are treated by skin or skeletal traction similar to fractures of the shaft and follow the same rules of aftercare. However, the muscle motors on the proximal fragment require a different positioning of the distal fragment to achieve proper correction of displacement, angulation, and rotation. The proximal fragment is flexed by the iliopsoas, abducted by the abductors, and externally rotated by the external rotators (see Fig. 16–50). Therefore, the extremity is placed in the degree of flexion, abduction, and external rotation required by clinical and radiologic assessment.

FRACTURES OF THE DISTAL END OF THE FEMUR

SUPRACONDYLAR FRACTURES

Supracondylar fractures of the femur just above the epiphyseal plate are rare. They may be treated with skin or skeletal traction on the leg with the extremity in balanced suspension and the knee extended with the axis of pull in the direction of the shaft of the femur. When the callus is firm enough and nontender, a single-leg spica is applied until bony union has occurred.

INJURIES TO THE DISTAL FEMORAL EPIPHYSIS

Such injuries are usually Type II, III, or IV. (See page 333).

Forced hyperextension of the knee may produce an epiphyseal separation of the distal end of the femur with gross anterior displacement (the wagonwheel injury of the horse and buggy days). If the injury is seen promptly, accurate closed reduction under general anesthesia usually offers no problem. Once the fracture is reduced there is no tendency to displacement. A single-leg plaster spica with the knee in slight flexion will immobilize the fracture until union is solid in 3 to 4 weeks (Fig. 17–46).

Manipulative reduction is performed with the patient face down and the knee flexed. Traction is applied to the leg and downward pressure applied on the shaft fragment. Occasionally, the epiphyseal fracture becomes a surgical emergency because the shaft fragment impinges upon the popliteal vessels. If there is circulatory embarrassment and the fracture cannot be easily reduced by closed methods, prompt open reduction is indicated. Legs have been lost through delay.

Lateral displacement of the epiphysis of the Type II variety may occur from a valgus force applied to the knee. Closed reduction should be successful with traction and replacement of the epiphysis, followed by immobilization in a single leg plaster spica.

Epiphyseal fractures of the Type III and IV variety may require open reduction and internal pin fixation if closed reduction is unsuccessful. In the Type III fracture, it will be necessary to cross the epiphyseal plate with one or two pins which do not harm the plate. They can be removed after 3 or 4 weeks. In the Type IV fracture, if the metaphyseal fragment is large enough, it is preferable to use this for fixation with pins or a screw. Internal

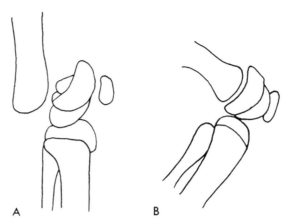

A   B

Figure 17–46   *A*, Epiphyseal fracture of distal femoral epiphysis (Type II) caused by hyperextension of the knee. The popliteal vessels and nerves may be damaged by the posterior displacement of the proximal (shaft) fragment. *B*, Closed reduction is performed with the patient in the prone position. The fragments are distracted by traction-countertraction and the displacement corrected by downward pressure on the proximal (shaft) fragment. The limb is immobilized with the knee flexed in a single-leg plaster spica.

fixation is supplemented by a long-leg plaster cast. Open reduction and internal fixation are justified to restore the anatomy of the knee joint. Care is taken not to damage the epiphyseal plate at operation.

TRAUMATIC DISLOCATION OF THE HIP JOINT

Seldom does a child suffer traumatic dislocation of the hip. When such an injury does occur it is seen more frequently in boys than in girls and occurs equally in each hip, with posterior dislocations predominating. Sciatic nerve injury with posterior dislocation in the child appears to be an infrequent complication. Associated fractures of the acetabulum, femoral head, or trochanter are also less common in the child than in the adult.

The mechanism of injury may be a trivial fall, an athletic injury, or a severe fall or auto accident.

End result studies seem to correlate the importance of the interval between injury and reduction as most important. Reduction within the first 24 hours favors the best result. The factors which seem to influence a poor result are the severity of the trauma, the presence of associated fractures about the involved joint, treatment delayed beyond 24 hours, and possibly open operation. The factors that seem to have no influence on the final result are the age of the patient, the type of nonoperative treatment given, and the period of nonweight bearing.

TREATMENT

Reduction by closed manipulation (see page 274 and Fig. 16–47) under general anesthesia is the treatment of choice followed by immobilization in a plaster spica for a period varying from 4 to 12 weeks or a period of skin traction and bed rest. Open reduction should be reserved for those cases which cannot be reduced closed or in which associated injuries about the hip joint require open reduction. The fact that the results are better with closed manipulation may be due to the fact that open reduction is reserved for complicated cases which influence the end result.

INJURIES OF THE LEG AND ANKLE

FRACTURES OF THE SHAFTS OF THE TIBIA AND FIBULA

Fractures of the shaft of the tibia vary in character with the age of the child. In infants and children up to 6 years, torsion of the foot produces spiral fracture of the tibia with no break of the fibula. There is frequently little or no displacement.

The older child falls with the foot caught and produces the same injury. In children from 5 to 10 years, direct trauma frequently produces a simple transverse fracture of both bones with or without displacement. Among adolescents, sports such as skiing cause comminuted fractures of the middle third with butterfly fragments and marked displacement.

TREATMENT

The spiral fracture of the infant is treated by a long-leg cast from toe to midthigh with the knee flexed. This needs to be worn only 3 weeks.

A similar fracture in an older child with minimal displacement needs immobilization in the same manner for only 4 to 5 weeks. When there is no fracture of the fibula, displacement sufficient to justify reduction is rare. When *both bones* are broken and displaced, manipulation under anesthesia will usually give satisfactory position. A long cast with the knee flexed 30 degrees is the only immobilization that is necessary. When there is gross over-riding with considerable displacement as in highway accidents, skeletal traction through the os calcis may be indicated. The traction device is incorporated in a cast extending to midthigh with the well-padded knee slightly flexed (see Fig. 16–64). As in the case of the femur, over-riding of 1 cm. is considered a favorable position. Overgrowth in the leg occurs less rapidly but as consistently as it does in the femur. All closed leg fractures should be treated nonoperatively in children.

In the adolescent approaching bone maturity it is necessary to fulfill the same requirement of anatomic restoration as in the adult. It is seldom

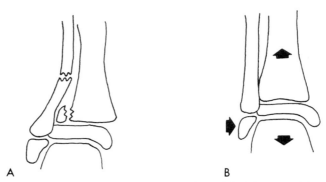

Figure 17–47   *A*, Epiphyseal fracture of the distal tibia (Type II) with separation and lateral displacement of the epiphysis. *B*, Treated by closed reduction. Distraction of the fragments by traction-countertraction and pressure applied to the lateral side of ankle and foot corrects the displacement. Immobilize in a long-leg circular plaster 4 to 6 weeks.

necessary to employ open reduction and internal fixation in fractures of the tibia in an adult and the same applies to children.

EPIPHYSEAL FRACTURES OF THE ANKLE

Fracture separation of the distal tibial epiphysis can occur by torsion and shearing. Treatment consists of manipulative reduction and a long-leg cast for 3 to 4 weeks (Fig. 17–47).

Fracture of the distal fibular epiphysis with displacement may accompany a similar fracture of the distal tibial epiphysis and is treated concomitantly by closed reduction.

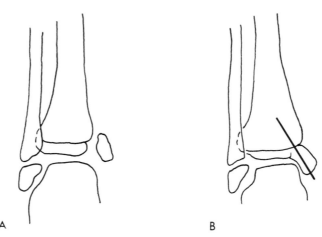

Figure 17–48   *A*, Epiphyseal fracture of the distal tibial epiphysis (Type III) splitting the epiphysis. *B*, Restoration of the integrity of the ankle joint is mandatory. If closed reduction is not successful, open reduction and pin fixation is indicated.

Type III epiphyseal fractures are rare but occur most often at the distal tibial epiphysis with displacement of the medial malleolar component. Accurate reduction is essential to restore the integrity of the ankle joint. If closed reduction is unsuccessful, open reduction and pin fixation is mandatory. The pins are removed in 4 to 6 weeks (Fig. 17–48).

Fracture at the distal fibular epiphysis without displacement is diagnosed on clinical grounds alone. The roentgenogram is normal. The diganosis is established by focal tenderness directly over the epiphyseal plate. A below-knee plaster cast without weight bearing for 3 weeks is the treatment of choice. This injury is often misdiagnosed as an ankle sprain. Accurate diagnosis will lead to proper treatment. Growth disturbance, always a possibility, is rare with this lesion.

Chapter 18

Peripheral Nerves

INTRODUCTION

Loss of peripheral nerve function can result from (1) contusion, stretch, or traumatic devascularization or (2) transection.

Contusion, Stretch, or Traumatic Devascularization: In these instances:

1. The nerve sheath is intact.
2. The reason for the loss of function may be physiological, not anatomical.
3. Function may return through the natural healing process.
4. Early attempts at surgical "repair" are *not* indicated.
5. But the injury must be identified and its location noted in the chart.

Transection: In cases of transection:

1. Surgical repair is indicated either early or late (see below).
2. Axonal regrowth starts a few millimeters proximal to the point of injury and continues across it and distally to the point(s) of innervation.
3. Regrowth takes place at a rate of about 1.5 mm per day (0.4 inches per week).
4. Exact anatomical alignment of uncontused nerve ends promotes regeneration.
5. Malalignment of contused nerve ends impedes regeneration.
6. Tissue between the nerve ends prevents regeneration.

DIAGNOSIS

Peripheral nerve injury must be suspected and searched for carefully whenever an injured extremity is examined. Injury to specific nerves can

378

be identified by evidence of the loss of specific sensory and motor functions as follows:

UPPER EXTREMITY

1. **Median Nerve**
   a. *Sensory* — loss of sensation over the palmar aspect of the thumb, the index and long fingers, and half of the fourth digit (Fig. 18-1).
   b. *Motor* — inability to bring the thumb into a position of opposition with the other digits. Thenar eminence palsy (abductor pollicis brevis, opponens, half flexor pollicis brevis).
   c. *Median injury above the elbow* — inability to flex the thumb and index distal phalanges. Weak digit flexion on radial aspect of the hand. Inability to flex the wrist well or pronate the forearm.
2. **Radial Nerve**
   a. *Sensory* — anesthesia over the radiodorsal aspect of the forearm and the dorsum of the thumb, the index and long fingers, and part of the fourth digit (Fig. 18-1).
   b. *Motor* — dropped wrist with inability to extend the fingers at the metacarpophalangeal joints or the thumb at all joints. High injury — inability to extend the elbow.
3. **Ulnar Nerve**
   a. *Sensory* — anesthesia, both dorsal and palmar, over the little finger and ulnar half of the ring finger (Fig. 18-1).

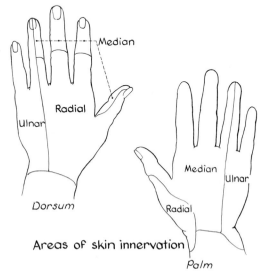

Figure 18-1 Sensory distribution in the left hand for the radial, ulnar, and median nerves.

   b. *Motor*—inability to spread and close the fingers or achieve flexion of the metacarpophalangeal joints without interphalangeal flexion. Weak thumb pinch. Clawing of ulnar 2 digits.
4. **Brachial Plexus**
   a. *Sensory*—mixed area losses.
   b. *Motor*—no clear peripheral nerve distribution, but mixed weakness of the arm, forearm, and hand musculature.

LOWER EXTREMITY

1. **Peroneal Nerve**
   a. *Sensory*—loss of sensation over the dorsum of the foot, most marked adjacent to the great and second toes (Fig. 18-2).
   b. *Motor*—foot drop and an inability to extend the toes.
2. **Tibial Nerve**
   a. *Sensory*—anesthesia over the lateral aspect of the foot (Fig. 18-2).
   b. *Motor*—loss of plantar flexion of the ankle and toes.
3. **Sciatic Nerve**
   Combination of the aforementioned motor and sensory losses for tibial and peroneal nerves.

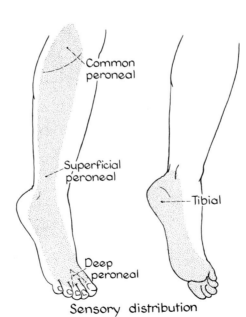

Sensory distribution

Figure 18-2   Sensory distribution in the lower extremity for the peroneal and tibial nerves.

TREATMENT

When it is clear that a peripheral nerve has been transected a decision must be made whether repair should be undertaken *early* or *late*. Immediate suture saves time in regeneration, avoids another operation, and may reduce scar formation at the site of the nerve injury. It is time-consuming, requires accurate identification of "normal" nerve ends, and demands meticulous operative technique. Late repair does not jeopardize the final result of nerve suture.

EARLY REPAIR

The indications for early repair are as follows:
1. A clean wound.
2. A nerve which can be joined without stretch.
3. Available time (from the standpoint of the patient).
4. A surgeon familiar with nerve suture techniques.

Contraindications to early repair are:
1. Gross contamination.
2. Established infection.
3. Extensive contusion, in addition to laceration of the nerve.
4. Inadequate soft tissue covering for sutured nerve.
5. Other injuries requiring lifesaving attention.
6. Other patients requiring the surgeon's attention.

The technique of early repair is as follows:
1. Careful debridement (see Chapter 20, Hand).
2. Adequate identification of the nerve. The cut ends of the nerve and tendons are occasionally confused, particularly in the hand, with the result that one may be sutured to the other. Identification can be readily made according to the criteria in the following table.

Nerve	*Tendon*
a. Soft	a. Firm
b. Friable, capable of stretch	b. Inelastic and tough
c. "Off white" or "light ivory" color	c. White, often "glistening"
d. Has branches	d. No branches
e. No true attachments	e. Attached to bone and muscle

The use of magnifying loupes to aid in identification and precise repair is highly recommended.
3. Debridement of the nerve. With the aid of the magnifying loupe and a razor blade, cut thin transverse sections back to uncontused nerve proximally and distally.
4. Gentle approximation. The nerve ends must come together, lying

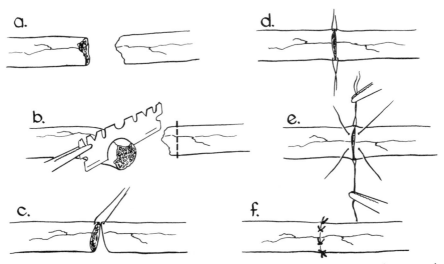

Figure 18–3 Technique for peripheral nerve repair. *a* and *b*, Recut ragged nerve ends. *c*, After lubrication of suture materials in local fat, place primary suture with surface vessels properly aligned. *d*, *e*, and *f*, Sutures in nerve sheath only.

in a clean bed without being stretched. If need be, flex the extremity to accomplish this. Do not pinch the nerve—only the sheath should be handled with fine instruments.

    5. Precise alignment.
        a. Identify position of major funiculi.
        b. Note alignment of blood vessels proximally and distally.
        c. Place one coaptation suture at an identifiable point.
    6. "Atraumatic" suture technique:
        a. Use 6–0 or 7–0 silk.
        b. Pass suture only through the nerve sheath.
        c. Preserve alignment of nerve ends.
        d. Four to six sutures are usually sufficient (Fig. 18–3.).

Immobilization can be established as follows:
1. Place the limb in a position which will relax the sutured nerve.
2. Apply a well-padded splint.
3. Keep the part immobilized for 2 weeks.
4. If necessary extend the limb gradually by reapplying splints with the limb in appropriate position.

AFTERCARE

    1. Avoid injury to the anesthetized parts. The lack of a protective sensation sets the stage for a patient to sustain inadvertent, unrecognized injury.

2. After a period of immobilization, it is essential to provide splinting and passive motion to prevent postparalytic contracture.

3. Electrical stimulation of paralyzed muscles delays denervation atrophy in the period before reinnervation and return of voluntary motor function. However, dynamic splinting with carefully balanced rubber band traction that functions continuously is more effective.

4. Tinel's Sign: About 5 weeks after suture, gently percuss the skin over the course of the severed nerve. Start distally and proceed proximally until the patient reports an "electric shock" sensation in the sensory distribution of the nerve. This is the point to which regeneration has progressed distally from the suture line. Regeneration over a distance of about 2 inches should be apparent 5 weeks after operation.

Chapter 19

Blood Vessels

Advances in vascular surgery have changed our attitude toward injuries of the blood vessels. The time-honored procedures of ligation or amputation were based on the concept of saving life, frequently at the expense of a limb. The modern techniques of direct operative repair and the concept of restoration of blood flow have immensely extended the surgeon's opportunities—and his responsibilities. The techniques of arterial reconstruction should be familiar to every surgeon who may be called upon to deal with major trauma.

URGENCY OF TREATMENT

The time lag from injury to operation, always a basic limiting factor, has taken on new meaning. Prompt treatment is essential not only because there is danger of death from exsanguination but also because the chances for successful restoration of arterial blood flow decrease with each hour's delay in surgical exploration. There is no precise time in which the anoxic damage to tissues that are deprived of blood supply becomes irreversible. Experience has shown that the best results are obtained when vascular repair is accomplished within 10 hours of injury. Limited success is possible after this period, but the chances are less favorable. Adequate assistance and the facilities of a well-equipped operating room are essential for success.

PRIMARY CARE

External hemorrhage should be controlled, if possible, prior to the patient being transferred to the hospital, by direct pressure upon the bleeding point rather than by the encircling occlusion of a tourniquet.

384

The prolonged application of a tourniquet gravely jeopardizes the success of reconstructive surgery, and it makes amputation almost inevitable. A tourniquet is permissible only if elevation, immobilization, and pressure on the site of bleeding are ineffective.

Shock must be combated and any **blood** lost must be replaced. If whole blood is not immediately available, one of the blood substitutes or physiologic salt solution should be infused intravenously during the interval before surgery. If possible, **fluid replacement** should be started prior to or during transportation to a medical facility.

VARIETIES OF ARTERIAL INJURY

The variety of blood vessel injuries often makes diagnosis difficult on a clinical basis. The presence of injury and how extensive it is may be evident only by arteriography or at exploration.

Some injuries involve **profuse external bleeding,** which makes the diagnosis of vascular injury and the need for operation obvious. On the other hand, a major vessel which has been completely severed or contused may have little or no signs of bleeding because of retraction, thrombosis, or vascular spasm of injury.

Contusions of the vessel wall are often associated with **thrombosis** causing obstruction and arterial insufficiency of the distal part.

Bone fragments displaced from nearby fractures or dislocations may cause compression, contusion, or laceration.

The untreated arterial injury may lead, within a matter of days, to the development of **pulsating hematoma** and ultimately a **false aneurysm** or **arteriovenous fistula.**

Signs of arterial injury may be produced by **vasospasm** resulting from minor contusion or injury to adjacent tissues such as bone and muscle. The diagnosis of vasospasm should be made by exclusion, employing arteriography, so that proper surgical therapy is not delayed. Vasospasm may be treated by warming the entire patient with an electric blanket. If operation is being performed for other injuries, hot wet compresses may be applied to the vessel. Operation is not indicated for vasospasm per se.

SIGNS OF INJURY AND INDICATIONS FOR EXPLORATION

Absence of pulsations distal to the site of injury is almost certain evidence of injury.

Pain, pallor, paresthesia, mottling, cyanosis, decreased temperature,

anesthesia, motor weakness, and later, **muscle tenderness** and **rigidity** indicate vascular injury.

A **false aneurysm** is indicated by the presence of an abnormal pulsation or a pulsatile mass. A systolic murmur is frequently present over the site of injury. Distal signs of arterial injury—absent pulses, pallor, and so forth—also may be noted.

Arteriovenous fistula is manifested by the presence of a machinery-like murmur and a thrill over the site of injury. Distal signs of vascular injury also may be present.

Recurrent hemorrhage from a wound indicates vascular injury and the need for immediate operation.

A **wound near vascular structures** should suggest possible vascular injury.

Progressive swelling, particularly of a limb, suggests a concealed hematoma or recurrent bleeding.

Arteriography is the definitive method of diagnosis short of exploration. Arteriography should be performed in most cases to confirm the diagnosis and to determine the location and extent of injury so that the proper operation can be planned. A completely transected artery may show a sharp cutoff of the visualized column without extravasation of the medium and should not be misinterpreted as spasm.

OPERATIVE TREATMENT OF ARTERIAL INJURIES

To control active bleeding, the wound is packed with gauze, and local pressure is applied during induction of anesthesia and the initial preparations for exploration.

The wound of the skin and subcutaneous tissues is usually too small for **exploration and vascular repair**. To control bleeding and provide proper exposure, an incision is made first above and then below the suspected site of vascular injury. The normal vascular structures are exposed through these two small incisions, and soft, noncrushing arterial clamps are applied. With bleeding thus arrested, the two incisions are connected, exposing the site of injury as well as the normal proximal and distal segment of the vessels.

The nature and extent of **arterial injury** are carefully noted. The extent of damage resulting from tearing, crushing, and contusion injuries may not be obvious. In fact, severe intimal laceration and thrombosis may be present without obvious external evidence of damage. Arterial damage is suspected in these cases when absent pulsations and firmness of the arterial wall are noted in the region of injury.

A **thrombus** frequently extends for some distance both proximally and distally to the region of injury. The thrombus is removed by various maneuvers, depending on its length. These include traction with forceps;

massage of the vessel, applied in the direction of the wound; retrograde flush; and aspiration with a catheter. A Fogarty balloon catheter makes the removal of clots much more successful.

To prevent **arterial constriction** and introduction of fibrous tissue into the lumen with the sutures, the adventitia is removed from the arterial edges to be sutured. The damaged, devitalized, surrounding soft tissues are debrided. Excessive debridement is avoided in order to conserve tissue to cover the affected artery, especially the region of repair.

Bone fractures must be reduced and stabilized prior to arterial repair to prevent arterial wound disruption, recurrent injury, or obstruction. Internal fixation is usually the preferred method.

The **repair** of simple, sharply incised wounds can be done by simple suturing of the wound edges. Arterial lesions (wounds), produced by crushing, contusion, tearing, and multiple lacerations, frequently must be excised. The remaining defect, as in cases in which the wounding mechanism has carried away an arterial segment, must be bridged and ligation avoided. Most defects may be bridged by mobilizing the proximal and distal healthy arterial segments between the major important branches. Small muscular arterial branches may be ligated for this purpose. The cut ends of the vessel are brought together by traction on the arterial clamps. Although no tension should exist at the suture line while it is being constructed, considerable tension is well tolerated after construction. Some defects, because of their extent, may require grafting.

False aneurysms and **arteriovenous fistulas** are prevented by early surgical correction of the arterial injury, which otherwise might lead to their development.

Ligation is employed only in the treatment of injuries to small, unimportant arteries, in the presence of established infection, or in a hopelessly mangled limb. Table I shows estimates of loss of limb following ligation in wartime patients. These rates are for young adults and should be revised upward for older patients with arteriosclerosis. Nevertheless, ligation is sometimes the only possible procedure, as in the presence of established infection, an intolerance of protracted operative procedure, or a hopelessly mangled limb. There is no justification for ligating a concomitant vein with an artery unless the vein also is damaged.

TABLE 1. Loss of Limb Following Ligation

Artery Ligated	Per cent of Patients Losing Limb
Brachial below the profunda branch	26
Superficial femoral	35
Axillary or high brachial	45 to 56
Common femoral	81
Popliteal	72 to 100

TECHNIQUE OF ARTERIAL SUTURE

Vasospasm of the artery in the region to be sutured is eliminated by dilating or stretching the vessel in the region of repair, using hemostats or Mixter right angle clamps.

A **continuous suture** is used for repair, the bites being taken through the full thickness of the vessel wall about 1 mm from the margin and 1 mm apart. This coapts the ends and apposes intima to intima. Monofilament polyethylene (No. 4-0 or No. 5-0), swedged on fine, curved, noncutting needles, is used because these materials do not deteriorate and are well tolerated in contaminated wounds.

End-to-end anastomoses are made in a similar manner. Suturing is facilitated by first creating a triangle with the line of suture. This is accomplished by placing, but not tying, three equally spaced interrupted sutures in the prospective anastomosis. With proper traction on these sutures the wound edges are brought together and the "back wall" of the artery is held away from the "front wall" being sutured.

Before the last two or three sutures are placed, the clamps should be temporarily removed to permit bleeding to flush out small thrombi that may have formed during the anastomosis.

After completion of the anastomosis, the clamps are removed and the exposed arteries covered with hot wet sponges to control bleeding at the suture line and to reduce vasospasm. Suture-line bleeding usually stops after 3 to 5 minutes. Persistent bleeding may be controlled by carefully placed interrupted sutures.

It is necessary to *cover the involved artery* with adjacent soft tissue without leaving dead space. Mobilization of adjacent muscle may be required for this purpose.

Distal pulses should be present after successful repair. Should pulses not reappear, an arteriogram should be performed before wound closure, so that proper treatment, such as embolectomy or reanastomosis, may be carried out at this time.

VASCULAR GRAFTING

Autogenous veins are the most practical source of graft material for the surgeon operating in an emergency, since a segment of the patient's saphenous vein is usually available. Whenever possible the graft should be obtained from an uninjured extremity. The normal direction of the vein should be reversed when the vein is inserted as a graft, lest its valves impede blood flow. The vein should be distended with saline to overcome venous spasm. The technique for introducing a vein graft is identical with that described for arterial repair. During the operation, heparin solution is introduced locally to prevent thrombosis.

The relative merits of various textiles as arterial prostheses are still being evaluated. Insertion of these materials requires special skill and experience. Crimped, knitted Dacron tubes are preferable.

ASSOCIATED VASCULAR PROCEDURES

Lumbar sympathectomy is *not* to be employed as a substitute for arterial repair, and it is rarely indicated after a successful repair associated with restoration of peripheral pulses. This procedure is indicated principally in cases in which repair either was not successful or was delayed for 12 to 36 hours, causing pulses to remain absent because of swelling and severe vasoconstriction. A final indication would be following ligation because of wound infection.

Fasciotomy alone may be disappointing. The main indication for this procedure is interstitial hemorrhage, as occurs in gunshot wounds and soft tissue contusion. It may be considered occasionally in patients in whom repair has been delayed. The muscle compartments in such cases may become intensely swollen following restoration of circulation. Early operative decompression may prevent ischemic necrosis of the involved muscle groups.

AFTERCARE OF ARTERIAL REPAIRS AND GRAFTS

Anticoagulant drugs are of little benefit in maintaining patency of an arterial anastomosis.

The **circulation** must be closely observed after arterial surgery. Should pulses disappear or signs of arterial insufficiency appear, an arteriogram should be considered to determine patency because reoperation and a second attempt at repair may be necessary. Should **gangrene** develop despite all efforts at corrective therapy, amputation may be deferred until a line of demarcation appears, so long as there is no evidence of spreading infection or of seriously diminished urinary output.

Immediately after successful arterial surgery, the patient may be covered with an electric blanket to **increase body temperature** and reduce vasospasm. Room temperature is preferable when repair has not been successful.

Affected extremities should be maintained at the level of the heart when swelling occurs, but in the absence of significant swelling, ambulation may be started when general conditions permit. **Splinting** is necessary only in the presence of fractures and dislocations.

Prophylactic antibiotics are advised if the injury occurred under contaminated conditions.

VARIETIES OF VENOUS INJURY

Injury to a vein causes many of the same problems as does injury to an artery.

Profuse **external hemorrhage** may occur if there is a wound which prevents the pressure of the forming hematoma from occluding the lacerated vein. **Internal hemorrhage** of massive size may occur when the superior or inferior vena cava is injured. Bleeding from the great veins is just as life-threatening as bleeding from the major arteries.

Contusion of the wall of a vein may lead to **thrombosis**. **Cyanosis** and **swelling** of the tissue distal to the thrombosis may occur. Elevation of the part and compression bandaging will help to control the acute situation. In most instances collateral venous channels will develop to prevent the situation from becoming chronic. If previous venous disease existed, however, then chronic venous insufficiency following injury to the vein is likely to occur.

Pressure from **bone fragments** of nearby **fractures,** or severe **swelling from hematomata** may cause compression of a vein with subsequent thrombosis.

Venous spasm secondary to injury does occur but never causes major problems for the patient as is occasionally seen with arterial spasm.

SIGNS OF INJURY AND INDICATIONS FOR EXPLORATION

Major hemorrhage, either internal or external, is an indication for immediate exploration. Arterial injury as a cause may be partially excluded in external hemorrhage by the absence of signs of ischemia. However, it must be remembered that serious arterial injury may occur such as a laceration with the peripheral pulses remaining intact. The **approach to major hemorrhage** from arterial or venous sources is the same, so that a preoperative diagnosis is of limited importance. When major arterial injury is found, great care should be taken to explore the concomitant vein which may well be injured. Venous injury may have temporarily caused its bleeding because of a lightly attached clot. Careful exposure of the vein after repair of the artery will usually uncover this possibility and prevent later hemorrhage.

Sudden onset of **massive swelling** of the arm or leg with peripheral color change ranging from ischemia to cyanosis suggests massive **venous thrombosis** of the main vein draining the arm or leg. This situation may be secondary to direct trauma to the venous system at the time of injury. It also is seen as a spontaneous event in the injured patient who has not had a direct injury in the area of thrombosis.

OPERATIVE TREATMENT OF VENOUS INJURY

The methods of managing venous injury are similar to those for managing arterial injury.

Control of active bleeding is achieved by **direct pressure** to the bleeding area. This is easily accomplished with finger pressure in the low pressure venous system. The area is then carefully cleared of blood, the venous injury defined and controlled by suture repair, patch graft, vein graft or ligation. The techniques are identical to those previously described for arterial repair. The great veins should always be repaired if possible. Synthetic prosthetic materials have not had much success in venous repair, so that a defect is best managed by a vein graft or patch from a distant source.

Thrombosis in the major veins is amenable to surgical removal within the first 24 to 48 hours. The vein should be exposed and cleaned out by means of a Fogarty balloon catheter, with proximal control to prevent clots from being broken up and causing embolization. If the vein, such as the leg veins, contains valves, proximal control is obtained, and the clots are milked out the venotomy by manual compression of the leg while it is elevated.

TECHNIQUE OF VENOUS REPAIR

Suture of a lacerated vein is carried out in the same manner as is suture of an artery. A **continuous suture** of fine (5-0) synthetic material swedged on a small, curved noncutting needle is used for the repair.

When the posterior wall of one of the great veins is lacerated, suture is most easily accomplished by opening the anterior wall of the vein and suturing the posterior wall from within, with a running stitch. The suture is tied on the outside of the vein. The anterior wall is then sutured.

End-to-end anastomosis of a vein is best accomplished using the triangular suture technique previously described.

Chapter 20

Hand

INTRODUCTION

The goal of the surgeon in caring for acute hand injuries is to preserve viable and useful parts, restore functional alignment of bones and joints, and attain wound healing without infection. The surgeon aims to restore and retain maximum function of *all* parts with minimal residual permanent disability. He should start with a careful initial evaluation and plan of treatment based on an accurate knowledge of functional anatomy.

EVALUATION AND PLANNING

1. In making the initial evaluation and planning treatment proceed as follows: Assess the total patient for (a) associated injuries, (b) complicating medical conditions, and (c) the risk of anesthesia.

2. Get a detailed history of the mechanism of injury to help determine (a) the severity and extent of the injury, (b) a plan for the initial operation, and (c) the prognosis for final function.

3. Systematically evaluate all injured tissues before an anesthetic is given. Do this examination and evaluation under sterile conditions wearing masks and gloves. Keep the wound covered after inspection of the skin wound. **Digging in the wound gives little information on damage to the deep parts, adds to the chance of infection, and may cause further damage to the deep parts.**

Plan the routine of evaluation and the priority of repair of the parts of the hand in the following order.

Skin: Estimate the skin loss from the injury and that anticipated from excision of the wound and plan the methods of closing the skin wound.

Nerves: Examine the hand for sensory and motor loss in the ulnar, median, and radial nerves.

SENSORY LOSS: Sensory loss in the **ulnar nerve** involves anesthesia in the pad of the little finger.

In the **median nerve,** sensory loss is expressed by anesthesia in the pad of the index finger, while in the **radial nerve** it appears as anesthesia over the dorsum of the thumb web.

MOTOR LOSS: When motor loss occurs in the **ulnar nerve,** there is an inability to adduct and abduct the fingers.

When the **median nerve** is involved the patient is unable to oppose the thumb to the base of the little finger with the nail parallel to the palm of the hand.

Motor loss in the **radial nerve** is seen in the inability to extend the wrist, fingers, and thumb.

Bones and Joints: Evaluate by X-ray with multiple views in preference to unnecessary painful manipulation of injured tissues. X-ray the uninjured hand for comparison.

Tendons: Specifically test individual extensor and flexor tendons to demonstrate tendon or muscle disruption.

Blood Supply: Examine for color and test for capillary return by digital pressure. **The only absolute indication for amputation of a digit is lack of blood supply.**

4. After evaluation, determine the priorities for immediate repair of the parts of the hand. Conditions may preclude immediate repair of one or more of the parts. As a rule, each successive step depends on the preceding.

Skin: Close the skin, if possible, to restore cover to the hand in order to obtain early healing.

Nerves: Repair the nerves because a hand without sensation is dangerous as well as useless.

Bones and Joints: Unless the hand has rigid members with good hinges, the repair of tendons is futile.

Tendons: Repair tendons if conditions are ideal and if the above can be accomplished, otherwise plan a delayed repair.

If two or more of the above parts of one finger are damaged, the value of saving the finger may be questioned. A finger that remains crippled can interfere with the function of the good fingers.

OPERATION

OPERATING ROOM

The sterile techniques, equipment, and assistance available only in an operating room contribute to the quality of the final result. Only simple lacerations of the skin *without* damage to the other tissues should be repaired in an emergency room.

ANESTHESIA

General anesthesia or axillary block of the entire arm are preferred. The choice depends on age, recent intake of food, familiarity with techniques, associated injuries, and the general status of the patient.

TOURNIQUET

Work only in a bloodless field. Inflate a tourniquet on the upper arm to 250 to 300 mm. of mercury after the hand and forearm are emptied of blood by wrapping or by elevation. If the operation is prolonged, deflate the tourniquet for 10 minutes every 90 minutes. Control bleeding and empty the arm of blood before inflating the tourniquet again. Before closing the wound, evaluate the circulation of the skin by releasing the tourniquet and noting the flush of postischemic vasodilatation.

REPAIR OF THE PARTS OF THE HAND

Convert the contaminated wound into a clean wound by irrigating it profusely with an isotonic electrolyte solution. Inspect the depths of the wound carefully. With meticulous care, excise all devitalized tissue and remove all foreign material. Enlarge the wound without hesitation to clean the wound, to identify parts, and to repair parts. **Don't cross flexion creases at right angles. Don't make "T" incisions. Avoid the eminences of the hand.**

Skin: Close the wound, if possible, to obtain early wound healing. If conditions are unfavorable because of the degree of contusion of the wound, the amount of contamination, the presence of dirt or other foreign material that can't be completely removed, or the length of time since injury, plan a delayed closure. **As to sutures, if in doubt, leave them out!**

1. Accurately approximate sharply incised or carefully debrided skin edges to obtain prompt healing, but only if the skin edges are viable and if they can be approximated without tension.

2. Use split-thickness skin as a permanent graft or as a dressing graft to close defects in the skin. A convenient donor site is the proximal volar surface of the forearm.

3. Use direct pedicle flaps over avascular tissues or over moving parts, but *only* if conditions are ideal.

Local pedicle flaps can be rotated up to 45 degrees to cover exposed bones, joints, or tendons. Base such a flap proximally and preserve the vascularity of the distal tip of the flap by careful incision and undermining. A digit with severe, irreversible damage that requires amputation may provide an excellent local pedicle flap after removal of bone and tendon.

Distant pedicle flap grafts from the abdomen or chest are rarely necessary. Such flaps are reserved for coverage of essential deep structures that cannot be covered by split-thickness grafts or local pedicle flaps.

Nerves: Primary nerve repair is often possible. Contraindications include loss of substance, severe stretching or crushing of the nerves, and extensive mutilating injuries that are heavily contaminated.

Accurately align and meticulously but loosely approximate the freshened nerve ends with a few fine (6–0) sutures of nylon or polyethylene through the nerve sheath alone. Nerves may be repaired to the level of the distal interphalangeal joint.

Bones and Joints: Accurate reduction of displaced bones and joints is necessary for ultimate good function of the moving structures of the hand.

In a closed wound, if the reduction cannot be obtained *easily* by manipulation, open reduction and fixation with Kirschner wires are necessary. Immobilize fractures of the hand in a position of function. The major complication of fractures of the hand is stiffness. Nonunion and osteomyelitis are rare. Therefore, for most fractures, the patient may begin active motion 4 weeks after reduction.

In an open fracture, unless the wound is as clean and healthy as an operative wound, avoid internal fixation. Instead, reduce dislocations, mold fragments into place, and hold them in position with a splint and dressing. Close subcutaneous soft tissues over exposed joints and fracture sites.

Tendons: Repair tendons if the wound is sharply incised and other tissue damage is minimal. If conditions are less than ideal, plan a secondary repair using a tendon graft.

Repair extensor tendons using a simple figure-of-eight wire suture brought out through the skin (Fig. 20–1). Or use a horizontal criss-cross suture (Fig. 20–2) or one or more simple horizontal mattress sutures. Relieve tension by extension of the wrist and metacarpophalangeal joints for 3 weeks.

Limit primary repair of flexor tendons to sharp lacerations without associated injuries that can be treated within 8 hours under ideal conditions.

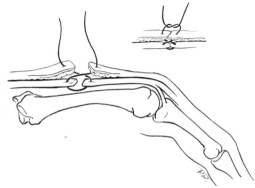

Figure 20–1 Use a simple figure-of-eight suture brought out through the skin to approximate the ends of a divided extensor tendon. Relieve tension by splinting, and dress the wrist and metacarpophalangeal joints in extension.

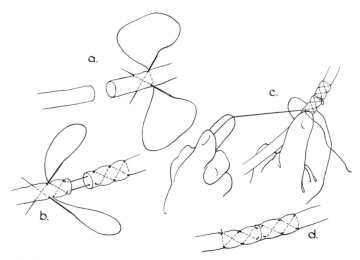

Figure 20–2   Use a horizontal criss-cross suture to approximate the ends of a divided flexor tendon. Relieve tension by splinting the wrist in flexion with the fingers in a position of function.

The best results are achieved in patients under 10 years of age. In patients over 50, the results of primary or secondary repair are less satisfactory.

In the finger, repair a single tendon (either profundus or sublimis) only if this repair will not interfere with the function of the remaining normal tendon. If the profundus tendon is severed at the level of the middle phalanx, repair it by advancement; excise the distal end and suture the proximal end into a short stump of the distal end. This places the repair distal to where the tendon glides. If both tendons are cut, repair the profundus and allow the sublimis to retract into the palm.

In the palm or thumb, the lacerated tendon can usually be repaired without jeopardizing motion of the uninjured tendons.

In the forearm, all tendons should be repaired for optimum balance of the hand, but adherence to other tendons may occur. Therefore, some loss of individual agility of the digits can be anticipated.

Accurate approximation by a horizontal criss-cross suture of 4–0 nylon or polyethylene (Fig. 20–2) is frequently suitable for flexor tendons. Relieve tension by splinting the wrist in 20 degrees of flexion with the fingers in a position of function. Maintain this position for 3 weeks. The suture is not removed.

DRESSING

A bulky pressure dressing, usually with a splint, is useful (1) for compression to minimize edema, (2) for immobilization to decrease pain and aid in the healing of bones, joints, and soft tissues, (3) for protection from contamination, and (4) for maintenance of position of function.

1. Place nonadherent gauze in a single layer over wounds and grafts.

2. Place gauze pads between the fingers to separate them.

3. Place the hand in a position of function, as reaching for a glass, with the wrist extended 20 degrees, the thumb in line with the radius, and the fingers slightly flexed with the tips equidistant from the tip of the thumb.

4. Keep in mind that the nature of the injury or repair may necessitate flexion or extension of the wrist or fingers.

AFTER CARE

The hand should be elevated on pillows or suspended while the patient is in bed (Fig. 20–3). The hand and arm should be supported in a sling

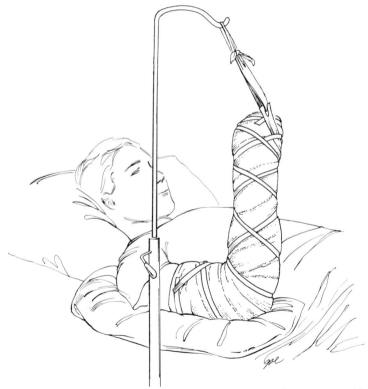

Figure 20–3 *A,* Elevate the hand after operation. Mechanics' waste provides bulk to the dressing. Bias-cut stockinette provides mild pressure, holds the mechanics' waste in place, and holds an incorporated plaster splint in place. A strip of 2-inch adhesive tape fixed to the dressing provides an "eye" for support. Spiral wound ½-inch tape holds the 2-inch tape and the stockinette in place. A strip of 2-inch roller bandage through the "eye" in the 2-inch tape tied to an I.V. stand holds the hand up while the upper arm rests on a pillow. *Illustration continued on opposite page.*

when the patient is up. Undue pain without remission may indicate tightness of the dressing that requires release. After 1 or 2 days, gentle, frequent, active motion should be encouraged in parts not requiring immobilization.

FIRST DRESSING

Unless there are signs of infection (fever, odor, and pain), the initial dressing may be left in place for about 10 days. Sutures can then be removed, wound edges cleansed, and a smaller, sterile dressing applied, usually with a splint to hold the hand in a position of function for another 7 to 10 days. After 3 weeks, dressings are not needed unless there has been a delay in healing or a complex fracture problem.

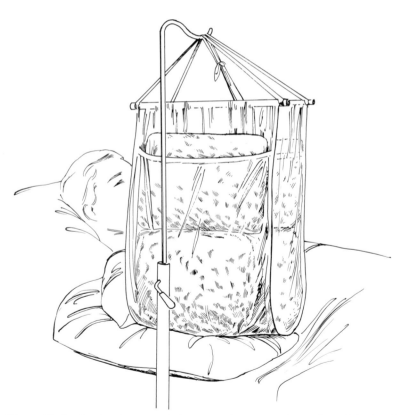

Figure 20–3 *Continued. B,* Use of the jacket shown permits cooling of the hand.

SPECIAL INJURIES

BASEBALL OR MALLET FINGER

This results from a sudden forced flexion of the distal interphalangeal joint that avulses the extensor tendon from the distal phalanx and produces a marked flexion deformity. If the patient is seen early, immobilization of the distal interphalangeal joint in marked hyperextension and the proximal interphalangeal joint in 15 degree flexion usually will result in repair. Maintain the immobilization with a plaster cast for 8 weeks.

BUTTONHOLE DEFORMITY

This results from avulsion of the insertion of the common extensor tendon from the base of the middle phalanx, producing flexion of the proximal interphalangeal joint and extension of the distal interphalangeal joint. Such an injury usually requires operation to reinsert the tendon into the phalanx.

INDELIBLE PENCIL WOUNDS

These injuries cause local tissue necrosis because of the toxic dyes. Excise all of the discolored tissue and leave the wound open.

GREASE GUN INJURIES

These injuries result in the intrusion of grease through planes, spaces, and tendon sheaths. The grease causes an intense chemical reaction and subsequent fibrosis. Serious infection may add to the destruction. Open up all involved planes, spaces, and tendon sheaths and remove as much of the grease as possible. Leave all spaces open, because grease will continue to exude from the depths. This will reduce the chance of infection and the amount of fibrosis.

AMPUTATION OF A FINGER

1. Identify nerves, put them on a stretch, and divide them proximally so they will retract as far as possible.
2. Preserve all possible length of bone, but remove the articular cartilage if the amputation is through a joint.
3. Close the skin defect with a split-thickness skin graft.
4. If the bone is exposed, close the skin defect with a pedicle flap.

WRINGER INJURIES

This serious injury may result in ischemia, necrosis, and damage to the skin, tendon, muscle, and bone.

1. Gently clean the skin.
2. Apply a sterile dressing and a bulky pressure dressing with the hand in the position of function.
3. Elevate the hand.

4. Change the dressing each day.

5. Evacuate fluid, incise the fascia, and debride any necrotic tissue.

CORN PICKER INJURIES

These and similar injuries crush, tear, and avulse skin, nerves, and tendons and cause multiple fractures.

1. Meticulously clean the wound, remove all foreign material, and excise all nonviable tissue, including skin, muscle, tendon, and bone.

2. Mold the fragments into position.

3. Close the wound. The safest method is to cover the wound with a primary or delayed thin, split-thickness skin graft as a dressing. After the wound is healed, one can replace the graft with secondary pedicle flaps and proceed with further reconstruction.

Chapter 21

Traumatic Amputations

Complete traumatic amputations of extremities occur from time to time from various kinds of trauma, such as railroad or other vehicular accidents, entanglements in farm or industrial machinery, or crushes caused by collapsing buildings or falling heavy objects. These same kinds of trauma may lead to "near amputations" in which an extensive comminuted open fracture, a severed major artery, and severe muscle damage are present, yet some continuity of muscle, fascia, and skin remains.

In recent years, a number of efforts have been made to reimplant completely severed limbs by using an expert team approach. Some of these have met with varying degrees of success, particularly when the surgery involved reimplantations or reattachments of upper extremities. The reader is referred to articles in the surgical literature of the past decade for the problems and details of reimplantation surgery. The following outline is provided as a guideline for physicians in a hospital emergency department and for surgeons who are confronted with a patient with a severed extremity for whom reimplantation is considered.

I. *Guidelines Concerning Reimplantation*
   A. *General*
      (Excellent emergency care before the patient and the severed extremity reach the hospital will favor a successful reimplantation. Hemorrhage should be controlled by a sterile massive compression dressing. If tourniquet control appears essential, a broad compression tourniquet such as the cuff of a sphygmomanometer should be used above the elbow. The severed extremity should be wrapped in sterile dressings, if available, otherwise in clean sheets. Ideally, the wrapped extremity would be enveloped in ice cubes held by waterproof material, such as an inflatable air splint or other plastic bag.)
      Reimplantation of an upper extremity only is to be considered.

401

1. If the severed part is not with the patient, advise the transportation personnel to obtain it. If it is not used for reimplantation, skin may be available for necessary grafting.
2. Extremity must have the potential of viability—it must be available within a six-hour time limit. If the extremity is cooled promptly, the time limit for reimplantation is 12 hours.
3. Tissue destruction must not be extensive.
4. The patient, as a rule, must be no older than 40; implantation is contraindicated in the elderly.
5. The patient must have been in good general condition prior to the accident.
6. The plan must be explained to patient and relatives.
7. Two teams should be established: Team A (responsible for patient) and Team B (responsible for severed extremity). The operating team consisting of a vascular surgeon, a neurosurgeon, and an orthopedic surgeon should be available in the emergency department to direct and coordinate Teams A and B (see below).
8. When assignments to Teams A and B have been completed (see below) in the emergency department, the patient and severed extremity are transported to the operating room. If the patient's condition and the hospital's emergency organizational policy warrant, both the patient and the severed extremity may be transported to the operating room immediately on arrival.

B. *Team A (responsible for patient)*
1. Institutes monitoring procedures on the patient.
2. Provides hemostasis necessary for the patient, but avoids use of nonvascular clamps on major vessels.
3. Stabilizes patient with resuscitative measures (see Chapter 3).
4. Orders emergency blood typing and cross-matching of four pints of whole blood for transfusions.
5. Provides tetanus prophylaxis and initiates systemic antibiotic therapy.
6. Copiously irrigates the patient's wound. Resective debridement of patient's wound is not to be performed in emergency department.
7. Identifies structures to be reconstituted, provided this is possible without unwarranted dissection.
8. Provides a sterile dressing for the stump.

C. *Team B (responsible for severed extremity)*
1. Aspirates major arteries and veins.
2. Inserts a tube into the main artery and places a tie over the end of the artery to moderately compress the artery against the tube.   Perfuses the extremity by gravity flow for about 20

minutes with one of the following cooled solutions containing 2000 units of heparin per liter: (a) lactated Ringer's, (b) physiological saline; (c) 10% low molecular weight dextran (Rheomacradex).

3. Repeatedly "milks" the veins of the extremities during the period of the perfusion, from the fingers to the level of the traumatic amputation. This is carried out by gentle manual compression of the extremity, hand(s) above hand(s), until the level of the amputation is reached. Repeat several times.

4. Adds antibiotics to perfusate solution; two million units of aqueous penicillin ordinarily is to be used.

5. Copiously irrigates the tissues. Resective debridement of the wound of the severed extremity is not to be performed in emergency department.

II. *Anatomical Order of Reconstitution in Operating Room*

As first step in operative procedures, adequate debridement of wound stump and severed extremity is carried out. Tissue specimen from each is obtained for culture and sensitivity tests. Then the following steps are carried out.

1. The bone is approximated and stabilized.
2. Circulation, both arterial and venous, is re-established.
3. Anastomosis of the major nerve trunks is carried out.
4. Muscles and tendons are repaired to extent practicable.
5. The skin is sutured to the extent practicable without excessive tension at the operating table or after swelling occurs later.
6. Fasciotomy to the forearm is performed.

III. *Postreimplantation Management*

1. Arterial circulation to the extremity, must be continuously observed.
2. Water, electrolyte, and acid-base balance must be regulated.
3. Satisfactory urine output must be maintained.
4. Systemic administration of antibiotics should be instituted.
5. Low molecular weight dextran should be administered daily.
6. Edema of the extremity must be treated.
7. On signs of gross nonviability, amputation should be carried out without delay.

PARTIAL OR NEAR AMPUTATIONS

Many severely damaged limbs that may be considered "near amputations" have been salvaged during the past two decades largely as a result of widespread surgical knowledge and skills regarding vascular repair, including the use of vein grafts. While restoration of arterial and often venous circulation is crucial in order to avoid amputation in many extensively damaged extremities, other precise surgical procedures are also of great importance. Thorough cleansing of the open wound and debridement of devitalized tissues, particularly muscle, must be carried out to minimize the chances of sepsis which, if present, will jeopardize the vascular repair, may lead to amputation at a higher level and even risk the life of the patient. The surgeon must be familiar with the techniques required to achieve adequate soft part coverage of the sites of vascular repair and with the principles of staged wound closure. Fractures must be treated so as to favor union in satisfactory alignment, yet the method of fracture management must not prejudice vascular repairs and wound healing or predispose to wound sepsis.

Over-zealous efforts to save a "near amputation" must not jeopardize the life of the patient. Moreover, the anticipated function of the salvaged limb must justify not only the risk to the patient but also the prolonged hospitalization, expense, and period of temporary disability which will be necessary. For example, efforts to save a lower extremity would hardly be justified if the injury included a severed femoral artery, a severely comminuted fracture of the femur, and a crushed and severed sciatic nerve which defies repair. The burden of proof rests on the surgeon who undertakes to salvage a limb, particularly a lower extremity, which has sustained severe damage to each essential soft-tissue component and bone, especially in view of the risks involved and the current status of lower-extremity prostheses fitting.

Surgical Procedure for Amputation

Assuming that it is not tenable to try to reimplant a completely severed extremity or to save the extremity with a "near amputation," then complete amputation should be carried out according to several well-established principles of surgery.

PREOPERATIVE CONTROL OF HEMORRHAGE

Hemorrhage must be controlled as an emergency measure. Fortunately exsanguinating life-endangering hemorrhage usually does not occur because the severed blood vessels retract promptly into the muscle mass of the stump and because the normal clotting mechanism goes into effect. Even so, significant shock-producing hemorrhage must be stopped and shock countermeasures instituted by blood-volume replacement using balanced salt solutions and whole blood transfusions (see Chapter 3).

In the usual case, a firm compression dressing over the stump will adequately control the hemorrhage. Briskly bleeding arteries may be clamped prior to application of a compression dressing. As a last resort, a tourniquet may be applied just proximal to the amputation site, but in such instances the tourniquet should be removed as soon as surgical facilities and personnel can be made available for control of hemorrhage but not until intravenous fluids and blood transfusions have been provided to control shock.

DEBRIDEMENT OF STUMP

Following prompt adequate resuscitation of the patient under general or spinal anesthesia (the latter alternative is only for lower extremities), adequate surgery on the open stump must be carried out. All devitalized tissue, particularly muscle, must be excised, and severed major blood vessels must be ligated. Nerve trunks must be identified, pulled downward, cut short with a sharp instrument, and allowed to retract into living muscle.

BONE

The level at which the bone is finally severed identifies the level of amputation. In many instances, projecting bone must be sawed off. In determining the saw line, so-called sites of election for definitive amputations usually should be ignored in traumatic amputations and the bone shortened merely to the level just proximal to the remaining viable muscle mass. The same precautions used in elective amputations should be followed to insure a smooth bony stump without projecting jagged bony spicules. Excess periosteum should be excised, and in some instances a cuff of periosteum may be excised so as to leave the distal one-fourth inch of bone devoid of periosteal covering to minimize the hazard of painful spur formation.

SKIN

Handling of skin is a problem requiring precise surgical judgment. A time-honored guideline, particularly in military surgery, has placed the level of primary amputations resulting from trauma at the lowest level of viable tissue. A companion guideline has called for open circular amputations in such injuries. In a way the two guidelines may be paradoxical. In traumatic amputations, a long flap of healthy viable skin may extend distal to the bone end, particularly after it has been sawed at the level of the remaining viable muscle. If the flap of skin is cut away in order to carry out an open circular amputation, obviously the amputation has not been at the lowest level of viable skin.

TYPES OF AMPUTATION

The surgeon has the choice of performing an open amputation, either open circular or with an open flap or flaps, or a closed amputation with sutured skin flaps. The latter usually is to be avoided in traumatic amputations. Ordinarily, some form of open amputation is preferable by far as it runs less risk of sepsis in the stump because of the open drainage it provides, and, moreover, it furnishes a "second look" at the stump at the optimal time to verify that stump debridement was adequate. In very few traumatic amputations—and practically all of these involve the arm or forearm—is the surgeon justified in primarily closing fashioned flaps of the stump. Even in these, an open amputation has many advantages and provides less risk.

OPEN CIRCULAR AMPUTATION

In traumatic amputations in which the skin has been severed near the level of the postdebridement stump, the open circular amputation usually is indicated. Often called a "guillotine" amputation—erroneously, because it is not a "meat cleaver" procedure—the technique calls for the muscle to be severed at the level to which the circular cut skin retracts, and the saw line of the bone to be at the level to which the muscle retracts. The result is a short inverted cone.

Following an open circular amputation, continuous traction on the skin is mandatory. Following application of a dressing which is limited to the open wound, a few pounds of skin traction may be provided with adhesive strips as in ordinary Buck's traction or as shown in Figure 21–1. The illustrated technique may be used for continuous traction over the foot or side (for upper extremities) of the bed or in a "banjo" cast which permits the patient to turn and be out of bed in a chair. The spreader as shown in Figure 21–1 should be utilized in all forms of skin traction to avoid excessive pressure on the skin against the bone end.

Skin traction must be maintained until the skin has become fixed by healing processes. As edema in the stump decreases and atrophy of the muscle occurs, skin margins often tend to fold over the raw stump, thereby reducing the size of the open wound. Complete healing by scar formation may take place. Regardless, skin traction is required for at least three weeks and often one or two more. Ordinarily skin traction may provide adequate immobilization of the joint above the amputation in the desirable position. At times, however, that joint should be held by a rigid splint.

Open circular amputations usually, but not always, require revision which may include shortening of the bone before fitting of a prosthesis. Reference is made to standard texts and the surgical literature regarding the indications for stump revision following open circular amputations, preferable levels for definitive amputations, and the selection and fitting of prostheses.

OPEN FLAP AMPUTATION

A modified open flap procedure may be indicated following traumatic amputations. Just as in open circular amputations, thorough debridement of the stump, adequate hemostasis, shortening of visible nerve trunks, and perhaps shortening of a projecting bone end are carried out before consideration of flap design. Seldom if ever should bone be shortened to permit flaps to be fashioned. Rather a flap or flaps may be created only from

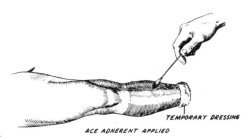

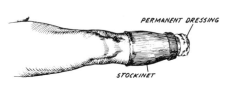

TEMPORARY DRESSING

ACE ADHERENT APPLIED

Figure 21–1 Steps in application of skin traction following amputation in the middle third of the leg. Tincture of benzoin may be used instead of ace adherent. While the sagittal section shows arrangement for continuous traction in a banjo cast, traction may be provided over a pulley at the foot of the bed. (From Hampton, O. P. Jr.: *Wounds of Extremities in Military Surgery*. St. Louis, C. V. Mosby Co., 1951. Reprinted by permission.)

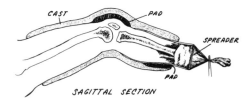

PERMANENT DRESSING

STOCKINET

CAST PAD

SPREADER

PAD

SAGITTAL SECTION

healthy viable skin extending distal to the stump after debridement and shortening of the bone if necessary. Under this concept, standard anterior and posterior flaps are unlikely to be feasible; therefore, a flap or flaps may be asymmetrical and based at unusual places. In summary, a flap or flaps come from healthy viable skin that remains available.

Open flap amputations require careful dressing. Precautions are necessary to avoid torsion of flaps and excessive pressure on them, either of which might jeopardize their viability. Even so, a reasonably snug compression dressing is indicated to minimize edema of the stump. Rigid splinting of the joint above the amputation usually is indicated. The splint should extend a short distance beyond the stump to protect it.

The optimum time for closure of open flap amputations is 3 to 5 days after the initial surgery. Preferably, the dressing applied in the operating room at the end of that surgery remains undisturbed until the patient again is in the operating room and under anesthesia. Only signs and symptoms of infection in the stump justify an earlier dressing. Even under these circumstances, the first dressing preferably is carried out under anesthesia in the operating room set up for any indicated surgery on the wound. Infection in the stump usually demands further debridement. Conversion of the open flap to an open circular amputation may be indicated. If not, after adequate redebridement, the wound is dressed again with the flap or flaps protected.

If the amputation stump is clinically clean when it is exposed in the operating room, the flap or flaps may be sutured so as to close the stump. Drainage with a Penrose drain or drains is usually advisable. A compression dressing and a protective splint completes the reparative surgical procedure.

Chapter 22

Pulmonary Insufficiency
After Trauma

Over the past decade pulmonary insufficiency after severe hemorrhage, trauma, or burn has emerged as a major cause of death in patients in intensive care units. This is not a new syndrome. For many years respiratory distress has been recognized as a complication of trauma and has been referred to under such entities as fat embolism, congestive atelectasis, and traumatic wet lung. However, increased awareness of this problem has emerged, in that improved resuscitative measures have unmasked this syndrome in patients who in earlier times would have succumbed to their injuries.

It is important to appreciate that pre-existing pulmonary disease is usually absent and that the injuries involved are primarily nonthoracic in nature. Wider use of blood gas analysis has been of paramount importance in documenting the frequency and degree of hypoxemia in critically ill patients. Since serious degrees of pulmonary insufficiency may be unsuspected because of a lack of clinical findings, the regular measurement of the arterial blood gases must be a part of the observation of all seriously injured patients.

The specific therapy that follows injury is a major determinant in the subsequent development of pulmonary failure. Ten points related to the prevention and management of post-traumatic pulmonary insufficiency are presented here.

1. Precise resuscitation must be guided by central venous pressure, urine volume, and arterial blood pressure.

2. In addition to the hemodynamic data, indices of tissue perfusion such as urine output, central venous oxygen tension, skin temperature, cerebral responses, and arterial lactate levels should be monitored regularly.

409

3. No single intravenous solution should be relied on for volume replacement. Whole blood will eventually raise the hematocrit and increase blood viscosity. Salt solutions will reduce colloid osmotic pressure and result in edema of peripheral tissues, bowel wall, cerebrum, and lungs. Fluid replacement should reflect the nature and volume of fluids lost, and hematocrit values should be maintained between 35 and 40 per cent.

4. Patients with major injury should be started on antibiotics selected on the basis of the presumed infecting organism. Subsequent antibiotic therapy will be guided by cultures and sensitivity testing.

5. The adequacy of ventilation can only be established by direct measurement of arterial pCO_2.

6. Avoid excessive oxygen tension in the inspired air by employing the lowest concentration compatible with adequate arterial oxygenation.

7. Do tracheostomy promptly for upper airway obstruction, but all other patients should have a test period of endotracheal intubation in order to evaluate the advantages to be derived from tracheostomy. If only temporary respiratory assistance is required, an endotracheal tube will often make it possible to avoid tracheostomy.

8. Strict precautions are essential in order to avoid introducing infection via the airway or vascular cannulae.

9. Heated humidification of the inspired air is essential in tracheostomized patients.

10. Ventilator support is indicated when the respiratory rate rises above 30 and tidal volume falls, when there is CO_2 retention, or when oxygenation is inadequate despite an increased inspired oxygen concentration.

THE CLINICAL SYNDROME

In certain injured patients resuscitation is difficult a refractory low flow state follows. This clinical situation is a frequent setting for the subsequent development of acute pulmonary insufficiency.

These patients often show moderate to severe alterations in acid-base balance. The initial acidosis due to lactic acid accumulation frequently gives way to varying degrees of alkalosis. The alkalosis arises in part from spontaneous but persistent hyperventilation with hypocarbia as well as from the large volumes of citrated whole blood given for resuscitation. Citrated blood has an alkalizing effect and is ultimately as effective a buffer as an equimolar amount of sodium bicarbonate. The cause of hyperventilation is unknown, but may be related to the pain and anxiety of trauma and poor perfusion of the peripheral chemoreceptors in the initial shock phase. After a latent interval, lasting as long as several days, evidence of increasing respiratory distress develops. This is characterized by persistent hyperventilation, hypocarbia, and hypoxemia with veno-arterial shunting.

Chest films are often a poor guide to a patient's pulmonary status at this time since it is frequently possible to demonstrate a marked disparity between x-ray findings and blood gas analysis of pulmonary function. The primary deficit relates to failure in oxygenation of arterial blood. Carbon dioxide retention, characteristic of chronic lung disease, takes place only as a terminal event or if the injury has interfered with the bellows function of the thorax. Arterial desaturation is treated with oxygen; because of this, knowledge of the level of inspired oxygen is essential for proper evaluation of blood gas results. A trial with 100 per cent oxygen inhalation often fails to bring the pO_2 to levels above 500 mm Hg. Respiratory fatigue and problems with maintaining an airway may necessitate ventilatory assistance. The reaccumulation of lactic acid that follows in some patients implies a guarded prognosis. Progressive hypoxemia and a rising pCO_2 then ushers in the final phase of coma, bradycardia, and asystole.

PATHOLOGIC CHANGES IN LUNGS

The postmortem findings of patients who have succumbed to the respiratory insufficiency syndrome are readily evident. In general, the lungs weigh two to three times as much as normal. Pulmonary edema, congestion, atelectasis, alveolar hemorrhage, and pneumonia are frequent findings. Microscopically focal hemorrhage, fibrosis, alveolar cell hypertrophy, and hyaline membrane deposits along with fat droplets and thromboemboli may be visible. These findings are not unique to this clinical syndrome but are seen in hyaline membrane disease of infancy, uremia, radiation and rheumatic pneumonitis, and viral infections.

PATHOGENESIS

INTRAVENOUS FLUID ADMINISTRATION

Saline solutions have received increasingly widespread use in the resuscitation of injured patients because they are inexpensive, available, and stable. It must be realized, however, that these solutions expand extracellular fluid to a greater extent than plasma volume, and overloading of extracellular fluid is not reflected in the central venous pressure. Plasma proteins are diluted by saline solutions so that capillary leakage can take place at lower transcapillary pressures. In the patient in whom blood pressure and flow are only precariously re-established, the possibility of excessive administration is greatly increased. Unloading of the large fluid loads often required for resuscitation is not automatic and a further insidious increase in water loading may take place. The importance of proper fluid therapy in minimizing pulmonary complications cannot be overemphasized. In fact, some attribute the increased incidence of post-traumatic pulmonary insufficiency to the more vigorous use of intravenous solutions that has taken place in recent years. Everyone is well aware that pulmonary edema may follow acute overload of the circulation. However, chronic water retention after resuscitation may be far more commonplace in the pathogenesis of pulmonary complications. Prolonged positive pressure ventilation may reinforce the tendency to water retention. Awareness of changes in body weight makes it possible to recognize progressive fluid loading. Precise fluid therapy, including the use of diuretics, plays a critical role in the proper management of the injured patient.

PULMONARY INFECTION

While bacterial infection always plays a role in the final stages of post-traumatic pulmonary insufficiency, the time sequence is variable. In certain patients a septic focus elsewhere in the body finally seeds the blood stream, and eventually similar organisms are recovered from the lungs. In other patients, respiratory tract infection represents the original area of infection. The significance of organisms in the upper airway is not clear since this can never be a sterile area. Furthermore, bacterial colonization is a constant feature in patients who have multiple incisions, tubes, and catheters and who are also subjected to a changing series of potent antibiotics. When the lower airway is opened up by tracheostomy or an endotracheal tube, the hazards of infection are further increased. Some immunologic injury is also suggested by declining resistance to ambient flora of low virulence. Despite the prevalence of bacteria in these patients their role in the development of respiratory failure continues to be uncertain. Organisms cultured from the surroundings of the patient are similar to those isolated in sputum and urine, but less severely injured patients are better able to withstand similar conditions. Pulmonary infection in this setting may be a secondary manifestation related to poor perfusion and tissue damage in patients with altered immunologic competence.

FAT EMBOLISM

The syndrome of respiratory insufficiency following trauma specifically to the musculoskeletal system has been appreciated for decades. Since autopsy specimens of many individuals who succumbed to trauma have shown lipid accumulation in pulmonary tissue, the term fat embolism has been used.

Clinically significant fat embolism occurs most frequently in patients with multiple fractures of the long bones, pelvis, and ribs. Rough handling, failure to splint, and careless transport increase the incidence of fat embolism in fracture patients. Hypovolemic shock is a synergistic factor and should be avoided or rigorously treated. The diagnosis of fat embolism should be considered seriously in any patient with fractures — particularly fractures of long bones, pelvis, or ribs — in whom an episode of hypovolemic shock has occurred.

Patients with fat embolism commonly exhibit tachypnea and dyspnea as signs of their pulmonary insufficiency. Disturbances of consciousness, ranging from delirium to coma, are frequent. The findings of the classic petechial hemorrhages in the axilla, across the chest and flanks, and in the subconjunctivae establish the clinical diagnosis of fat embolism. Such petechiae are not found in association with other forms of post-traumatic pulmonary insufficiency.

The clinical diagnosis of fat embolism is supported by a variety of laboratory findings. Early after injury there may be fat in the urine, a thrombocytopenia, an anemia, and a decrease in the P_aO_2. An electrocardiogram may demonstrate evidence of right-heart strain. Diffuse pulmonary infiltrates may be visible on the chest x-ray. The serum lipase may become elevated 5 to 7 days after injury.

The pathogenesis of the fat embolism syndrome is poorly understood. Classically, it has been theorized that there is a mechanical release of fat from the marrow elements of bone, that depot lipid is mobilized in response to shock, or that circulating chylomicrons or lipoproteins are altered. The lung is felt to trap this lipid or allow it to escape to the systemic circulation through veno-arterial channels. A "chemical phase" has been postulated by the action of lipoprotein lipase on neutral fat releasing free fatty acids that then damage the lung parenchyma.

At present, however, there is evidence to suggest a more complex pathogenesis of this syndrome. Lipid droplets may be found in the lung of individuals who never developed respiratory insufficiency and died from unrelated causes. Introduction of an intramedullary rod into a femur, a procedure that severely disrupts bone marrow elements, usually is not followed by the fat embolism syndrome. The cerebral manifestations of this syndrome may develop from alterations in acid-base balance. Defective oxygen extraction associated with a leftward shift in the oxyhemoglobin dissociation curve as pH rises, as well as cerebral ischemia resulting from effects of hypocarbia and alkalosis, may produce an irrational, disoriented restless patient.

Recently, it has become apparent that marked alterations in blood coagulation occur following trauma. The pattern that often develops is consistent with nonlethal episodes of disseminated intravascular clotting. These clotting changes may arise from tissue thromboplastin at the injured site, hemolysis of transfused blood, ischemia, formation of endotoxin, and aggregation of platelets. In this process, serotonin is released from platelets and fibrinopeptides from fibrinogen. These substances are potent pulmonary vasoconstrictors and may produce respiratory insufficiency. In the fat embolism syndrome, coagulation alterations suggestive of disseminated intravascular clotting have been noted by several authors. The thrombocytopenia is consistent with this and is the basis for the petechial rash that has been described. Finally, intravascular fibrin deposits have been found in the brain and lungs of patients in whom the diagnosis of fat embolism has been made. It is therefore evident that more is involved in the syndrome of fat embolism than pure embolic fat.

The prevention of fat embolism begins at the scene of the accident with gentle handling, careful splinting, and careful transport. Needless to say, these same precautions in patient handling should be followed after the patient arrives at the hospital. Hypovolemic shock should be prevented or treated by the administration of adequate amounts of fluids and whole fresh blood. Among the fluids to be recommended is 5 per cent dextrose-5 per cent ethanol solution. Support of respiration by means of intubation or tracheostomy and positive pressure respiration with varying concentrations of oxygen may be life-saving. The administration of corticosteroid hormones in full pharmacological dosage for a period of 3 to 5 days is recommended when the pulmonary insufficiency is severe.

OXYGEN TOXICITY

An increasing awareness of anatomic damage to the lung as the result of exposure to high oxygen tensions has led to greater care in the administration of supplemental oxygen. The pulmonary lesions associated with high oxygen concentrations have been well defined in a number of animal species. It is important to appreciate that oxygen injury can take place at normal barometric pressure. One does not need a hyperbaric chamber to see oxygen toxicity. While human tolerance to high concentrations of oxygen are not well defined by experimental work, several studies suggest that the response resembles that seen in experimental animals. It is now accepted that oxygen therapy must be carefully titrated to achieve an adequate level of saturation with the lowest possible concentration of inspired oxygen. It is not possible to achieve injurious levels of inspired oxygen using nasal cannulae or an oxygen tent since these devices rarely exceed an inspired oxygen concentration of 40 per cent. Only a closed system using a cuffed tracheostomy tube is capable of delivering up to 100 per cent oxygen since critically ill patients will not tolerate tight fitting face masks for any length of time. It has become a general rule not to exceed 60 per cent oxygen in the inspired air unless severe desaturation exists. When faced with continued hypoxemia at that level a trial period on 100 per cent oxygen can be used to determine the maximum benefit to be expected from increased airway oxygen. In this way it is possible to define the minimum oxygen tension compatible with an acceptable arterial level.

TREATMENT

A thorough understanding of pulmonary pathophysiology is essential in managing the severely injured patient. The treatment of shock must be prompt and expeditious. Proper fluid replacement and appropriate monitoring of arterial and central venous pressures and urine output with frequent blood gas determinations are important. If evidence of respiratory insufficiency develops, the intelligent use of oxygen is indicated. If mechanical ventilatory support and tracheostomy is necessary, the inherent problems in their use must be appreciated.

Tracheostomy is frequently employed in the management of post-traumatic pulmonary insufficiency. However, upper airway obstruction is rarely the indication. While occasional patients are considered candidates for tracheostomy because of difficulty in clearing secretions, the danger of introducing infection into the lower airway has led to a more cautious approach. Presently, tracheostomy in injured patients usually implies that there is a need for higher levels of oxygen than can be administered without a closed system or that ventilation must be assisted. In both instances the tracheostomy exists to allow ventilator therapy. As a rule, a trial period of endotracheal intubation should precede tracheostomy in order to assess the value of mechanical ventilation in the patient. There is some controversy regarding continued use of endotracheal tubes in a conscious patient but good evidence suggests that the incidence of laryngeal injury starts to rise significantly after 48 hours.

Pressure-cycled and volume-cycled ventilators have been employed in the management of post-traumatic pulmonary insufficiency. Volume ventilators are frequently more effective in patients with secretions and changing levels of pulmonary compliance; thus they have received wisespread use in injured patients.

The diversity of clinical backgrounds in injured patients who develop pulmonary insufficiency provides a therapeutic challenge to physicians. It is unlikely that any single factor is dominant, and proper treatment must take into account the additive effects of multiple factors. Proper treatment clearly depends on the recognition of all the diverse agents that individually or collectively can lead to impairment of pulmonary function.

Chapter 23

Legal Aspects

INTRODUCTION

The purpose of this chapter is to impart a basic understanding of the concepts which the law applies to the physician-patient relationship in an emergency department situation. It is not intended as a guide concerning the laws of any particular state or a guide on how to handle any specific situation. For such guidance, there is no substitute for consulting a local attorney.

The chapter first discusses the creation of the voluntary physician-patient relationship by consent. Topics such as the forms this consent may take, what constitutes "informed consent," and when consent may be given by another person or waived during an emergency are dealt with. We then turn to the legal obligations of the physician after the creation of the voluntary physician-patient relation: the extent of the physician's duty to care for the patient, possible contractual liability, and the legal standards of medical practice. Lastly, problems relating to notification of the next of kin and to autopsies are noted. The references cited throughout the chapter are in accordance with the practice followed in legal writing.

THE REQUIREMENT OF CONSENT

All patients have a right *not* to be treated without their consent. The legal system may look upon any unauthorized treatment as a battery (an unauthorized touching) or an assault (a threat of such touching). Damages for such unauthorized conduct may be granted without regard to whether the physician is negligent. Thus, a physician who acts in the absence of actual informed consent may be liable, even though he relies on the normal

416

practice of the hospital and assumes that it has obtained the consent. Because of this risk, a physician, for his own protection, should be sure that the patient has given his consent. Consent, however, is implied in many circumstances. In the words of one author, ". . . no patient should be allowed to die in the emergency room . . . because there isn't someone available to sign a form."[1]

REQUIREMENTS FOR EFFECTIVE CONSENT IN GENERAL

ORAL v. WRITTEN CONSENT

Physicians need not obtain written consent, but reliance upon oral consent complicates the problem of proving that consent was actually given.[2] Consent also may be implied from circumstances, for example, when a person voluntarily submits himself to treatment although he never expressly gives his consent. But such consent also involves problems of proof.[3] The use of written consent forms is therefore preferable.

SPECIFIC v. GENERAL CONSENT

Physicians should avoid general consent forms, e.g., those which permit physicians "to do anything necessary," because the courts may view such forms as worthless.[4] Consent forms should note the type of disease affecting the patient and the type of treatment authorized.[5]

SCOPE OF PATIENT'S AUTHORIZATION

Generally, authorization for one type of treatment or operation does not grant permission to a physician or surgeon to engage in another type of treatment. If a physician or surgeon decides that such unauthorized treatment is necessary, he should obtain further consent. If for some reason the patient is unable to grant permission—for example, if he is unconscious—then the physician may engage in an unauthorized treatment only if an emergency exists.[6]

INFORMED CONSENT

If consent is to be effective, it must be informed. The physician or surgeon should give a reasonable explanation of the risks inherent in the proposed treatment or operation so that the patient may give an informed and intelligent consent. Not all the possible results need be described, and a medical practitioner may withhold information for therapeutic reasons. Several jurisdictions state that the test of the sufficiency of the explanation is similar to that for malpractice, i.e., the disclosures made must resemble those which reasonable medical practitioners would divulge under the same or similar circumstances.[7]

REQUIREMENTS OF CONSENT FOR ADULT AND CHILD PATIENTS

ADULTS

Conscious Adults: An adult who is capable of giving informed consent is the sole judge of whether or not he is to be given medical treatment. The husband's consent need not be given for treatment of the wife, nor the wife's for the husband's.[8] Nevertheless, several experts in medicolegal matters deem it advisable to obtain the spouse's consent if the treatment or operation involves either danger to life, sterilization or impairment of sexual functions, or the death of an unborn child.[9]

Unconscious or Incompetent Adults: In instances when an adult is unable to give informed consent, either for temporary reasons, such as unconsciousness due to accident or sedation, or for permanent reasons, such as mental illness, consent must be given by another authorized person or waived by emergency in order to allow treatment.

ANOTHER PERSON: Generally, an individual, even a spouse, cannot consent to treatment of another person. One may give consent only if he has been previously authorized to do so by the person undergoing treatment.[10] If a patient has been ruled incompetent by a court, the court-appointed guardian is the one who must give consent.

EMERGENCIES: If no one has been authorized to give consent, an emergency situation must exist in order to allow a physician to treat the unconscious or incompetent patient. The legal definition of "emergency" varies from jurisdiction to jurisdiction. A usual formula speaks of treatment "necessary for the life or health of the patient."[11] A New York case goes as far as finding implied consent where treatment was necessary to alleviate "pain or suffering."[12] Several jurisdictions defer to the judgment of physicians in ruling that a physician may treat unconscious or incompetent adults in cases where the "usual and customary practice among physicians and surgeons in the same locality" is to give immediate treatment.[13]

MINORS

In General: Generally minors cannot either consent to or refuse medical care. This decision is the responsibility of the parent or guardian. The parent's consent also must be an informed one.[14]

Emancipated Minors: Certain minors who are responsible for themselves are "emancipated" — outside of their parents' control. Factors which establish emancipation include marriage, the earning of one's own living, the maintenance of a home separate from one's parents, and psychological maturity.[15] A minor, whether male or female, who is emancipated is treated as an adult, and the aforementioned rules on consent apply.

Emergencies: If a parent or guardian cannot be reached, then the aforementioned rules on emergency care apply. These rules also apply in cases where an emancipated minor is unable to give an informed consent.

EXTENT OF DUTY TO CARE FOR PATIENT

Given expressed or implied consent, the physician has a duty to care for the patient from the initial diagnosis until he withdraws from the case or properly discharges the patient. In an emergency department, there is a duty to treat a patient if an emergency exists.[16] A physician who initially treats a patient is responsible to see that the patient subsequently receives adequate medical care. Surgeons, for example, are generally held responsible for seeing that their instructions concerning postoperative care are carried out.[17] Withdrawal from a case is permissible, but in doing so the physician must give the patient sufficient time to procure other medical attention.[18] A discharged patient should be informed of any further medical care which may be necessary.

CONTRACTUAL LIABILITY

A physician does not have a duty to cure, but instead is held to certain professional standards, which will be discussed in the next section on malpractice. A physician may, however, establish a duty to cure if he contracts with a patient by assuring that a certain result will be achieved or that a specific treatment will be given. A physician does not enter into a contract if he gives such reassurances as "You'll be all right," but he may be bound in contract by specific words of commitment. For example, the words "I will see to it that a Caesarean will be performed" have been interpreted as establishing an obligation to perform that operation.[19]

MALPRACTICE

IN GENERAL

The law imposes standards of professional practice upon physicians. There are several formulations of this standard, the basic variance being in the area from which the standard is derived.

The traditional standard is that the physician "have the learning and skill of physicians in good standing in the same locality and that he use ordinary care and diligence in applying that learning and skill."[20] Another standard is expressed as "that level of care in the same or like locality."[21] Several states give the requisite standard of care to be that of "the average physician under the same or similar circumstances."[22] Recently, several jurisdictions have come to impose a standard based on nationwide practices.[23] Many jurisdictions impose an additional duty on the specialist— that he use "his best judgment and whatever superior knowledge, skill and intelligence he has."[24] Thus, a specialist may be held liable in a situation in which the general practitioner would not be held liable.

These standards do not differ in emergency department situations, although the conditions of the specific situation are considered in determining what constitutes malpractice.

LIABILITY FOR THE MALPRACTICE OR NEGLIGENCE OF OTHERS

In certain instances, a physician may be liable for the acts of others. One is generally liable for the acts of one's employees, and several, but not all, jurisdictions impose liability on physicians for the malpractice or negligence of persons (*e.g.*, nurses) acting under their supervision and control.[25] Another doctrine (again one which is not accepted in all jurisdictions) imposes liability on the surgeon in charge of an operation for any negligence committed by another (*e.g.*, the anesthetist) during the operation.[26] As previously mentioned, the surgeon may be held responsible for his patient's postoperative care.

GOOD SAMARITAN LEGISLATION

A major legislative alteration in medical law has been made by the "Good Samaritan" statutes. These attempt to relieve the physician from at least some of the possible liability that might stem from emergency treatment. No such statute, however, explicitly covers treatment in emergency departments, and no courts have yet applied these laws to such situations. Moreover, it is doubtful that these laws would be construed to relieve physicians from liability for emergency department care. The intent of the Good Samaritan legislation is to protect the physician who gratuitously renders care at a roadside emergency from liability; it does not change the consent and malpractice laws concerning physicians and surgeons practicing in a hospital setting.[27]

DUTY TO INFORM NEXT OF KIN OF DEATH OF PATIENT

Generally, state statutes require only that the attending physician complete a certificate upon the death of a patient.[28] The next of kin should be notified of the death of their relative. Liability has been imposed for preventing a family from viewing the deceased's burial.[29] Autopsies should not be done without the permission of the nearest relatives or without authority from the appropriate public official.[30]

REFERENCES

1. R. Bergen, Informed Consent 13, April 23, 1963 (A.M.A. monograph). (*Note:* The cases and texts cited are not those most authoritative or best reasoned on the point discussed, but are those which fully explain the principle involved.)
2. *Keister v. O'Neil,* 59 Cal. App. 2d 428, 138 P. 2d 723 (1943).

3. *Dicenzo v. Berg*, 340 Pa. 305, 16 A.2d 15 (1940).

4. *Rodgers v. Lumbermen's Mu. Cas. Co.*, 119 So. 2d 649 (La. Ct. of App. 1960).

5. E. Hayt, *Law of Hospital, Physician, and Patient*, 254 (2d. ed. 1952).

6. *Gravis v. Physicians & Surgeons Hosp.*, 427 S.W.2d 310 (Tex. 1968).

7. *Collins v. Meeker*, 198 Kan. 390, 424 P.2d 488 (1967).

8. *Kritzer v. Criton*, 101 Cal. App. 2d 33, 224 P.2d 808 (1950).

9. *A.M.A. Medicolegal Forms with Legal Analysis* 14–15 (1961).

10. *Gravis, supra*

11. *Wells v. McGehee*, 39 So. 2d 196, 202 (La. Ct. of App. 1949).

12. *Sullivan v. Montgomery*, 155 Misc. 448, 279 N.Y.S. 575 (N.Y. City Ct. 1935).

13. *Wells, supra*

14. *Brown v. Wood*, 202 So. 2d 125 (Fla. App. Ct. 1967).

15. *Bach v. Long Island Jewish Hosp.*, 49 Misc. 2d 207, 267 N.Y.S. 2d 289 (Sup. Ct. 1966).

16. *Gen. Hosp. v. Manlove*, 54 Del. 15, 174 A.2d 135 (1961).

17. *Levy v. Kirk*, 187 So. 2d 401 (Fla. App. Ct. 1966).

18. *McManus v. Donlin*, 23 Wis. 2d 289, 127 N.W.2d 22 (1964).

19. *Stewart v. Rudner*, 349 Mich. 459, 84 N.W.2d 833 (1957).

20. E. Hayt, *supra.*, note 5, at 353.

21. *Johnson v. Vaughn*, 370 S.W.2d 591, 596 (Ky. 1963).

22. *Pederson v. Dumouchel*, 72 Wash. 2d 73, 431 P.2d 973 (1967).

23. *Brune v. Belinkoff*, 354 Mass. 102, 235 N.E.2d 793 (1968).

24. *Toth v. Community Hosp.*, 22 N.Y.2d 255, 262–63, 239 N.E.2d 368, 29 N.Y.S. 2d 440 (1968).

25. *Natanson v. Kline*, 186 Kan. 393, 411–413, 350 P.2d 1093 (1960); *cf. Nichter v. Edmiston*, 81 Nev. 606, 610–11, 407 P.2d 721 (1965).

26. *Rockwell v. Stone*, 404 Pa. 561, 173 A.2d 48 (1961); *cf. Grant v. Touro Infirmary*, 254 La. 203, 219–20, 223 So. 2d 148 (1969).

27. See Louisell & Williams, *Medical Malpractice*, ¶¶ 21.01–.42 (1970).

28. (e.g. *Ill. Ann. Stat.* (1970 Supp.) ch. 111-1/2, §73–18(2); *Calif. Health & Safety Code* § 10200).

29. *Spiegel v. Evergreen Cemetery Co.*, 117 N.J.L. 90, 186 A. 585 (1936).

30. *French v. Ochsner Clinic*, 200 So. 2d 371 (La. Ct. of App. 1967).

Chapter 24

Management of Mass Casualties

DISASTER PLAN

When the number of casualties exceeds that which can be handled adequately by the usual resources of a hospital, a disaster plan is needed. The plan should be worked out before the disaster occurs and should include:

1. A system for sorting (triage) patients.
2. Provision for identifying (tagging) patients.
3. Provision for effective means of communication for efficient mobilization of personnel and equipment—telephone, radio, and television.
4. Provisions for security, including traffic control to assure uninterrupted access of necessary vehicles and personnel; an information center, a place away from the treatment area for the press and relatives; and control of unauthorized personnel.
5. An area available for treatment.
6. An area available as a morgue.

SYSTEM FOR SORTING OF MASS CASUALTIES

Patients should be sorted by priorities according to medical requirements. The most experienced surgeon available should control the sorting, basing the process upon diagnosis and prognosis. If possible the sorting should be done near the receiving area. A second area may be established for walking casualties. The sorting process should be continually updated since the physiologic, pathologic, and metabolic conditions of the seriously

TABLE 24–1   FLOW SHEET FOR MONITORING – EVALUATION
(EVERY 15 MINUTES)

Monitor	Evaluation
Pulse rate	Degree of discomfort
Arterial pressure	Level of consciousness
Ventilation-respiration (tidal vol.)	Central nervous system
Central venous pressure	Cavities (chest and abdomen)
Temperature	Vascular system
Hematocrit	Peripheral nerves
Gastric aspirate volume	Soft tissues
and character	Skeletal system
Timed urine volume and	Urinary system
character	Wounds
	Latent diseases

injured patient keep changing. Continuous monitoring should be provided and a flow sheet maintained (See Table 24–1).

In general, the most seriously injured patients should be treated first. If the number of casualties overwhelms the resources of the facility in terms of people, space, equipment, and supplies, those patients most likely to survive should be treated first so that the greatest good can be done for the greatest number.

PRINCIPLES OF SORTING BY PRIORITIES

As previously stated, patients should be sorted according to their needs for medical care. To conserve the emergency resources of the hospital, those patients who have minor injuries, such as minor lacerations and burns, should be given simple care on ambulatory basis.

Hospital Admission: Patients with the following injuries need to be admitted and classified for definitive care and early operation: (1) respiratory obstruction, (2) sucking wounds of the chest, (3) hemorrhage and cardiac tamponade, (4) incomplete amputations, (5) open fractures of major bones, (6) severe crushing wounds of the extremities, (7) perforating abdominal wounds, and (8) severe lacerations.

The second category of patients who need to be admitted for definitive care and possible later operation, are those suffering from severe burns, closed injuries of the head and spine, closed injuries of the chest, hemothorax, pneumothorax, flail chest, closed injuries of the abdomen, closed fractures, labor and complications of pregnancy, serious medical illnesses including psychiatric emergencies, and loss of consciousness.

Finally, some patients may be admitted for observation and evaluation.

Hospital Transfer: Patients may be transferred to another hospital for care when other facilities are less heavily taxed, or when the patient requires the special services of another facility. In some instances a patient may be transferred if he or his family requests it. If the stress of circumstances permits, arrangements for transfer of the patient should be made with another physician selected in consultation with the patient and his family. This physician shall then assume responsibility for continuing care.

No patient should be transferred unless hemorrhage has been controlled, resuscitation has been effected, ventilation has been assured, wounds have been dressed, and fractures have been splinted.

IMMEDIATE CARE

The basic principles of care described in previous chapters apply to the victims of disaster (Table 24–2). The most important steps are: (1) insure adequate ventilation; (2) control hemorrhage; (3) restore blood volume; and (4) care for wounds and prevent tetanus. Roentgenologic studies, as a rule, should be limited to those patients with life-threatening conditions requiring immediate care.

ORGANIZATION OF THE OPERATING ROOM

Organization of the operating room should be part of the disaster plan established by the hospital before disaster strikes. After a disaster, the assignment of personnel and other decisions will follow the dictates of circumstances and availability.

Patients should be sorted again in the operating room according to their needs. An experienced surgeon should do the sorting and assign the

TABLE 24–2   CHECKLIST OF BASIC PROCEDURES OF VALUE
DURING SORTING AND RESORTING PROCESS

Airway and Ventilatory Care	*Wound and Extremity Care*
Removal of foreign bodies	All wounds covered with sterile dressings
Suction removal of blood and secretions	Splints applied to all injured extremities
Oral airway tube	
Endotracheal tube	*Drug Therapy*
Tracheostomy	
Ventilator (hand or mechanical)	Tetanus prophylaxis
Stabilization of flail chest	Intravenous sedation
	Intravenous antibiotics
Hemorrhage	
	Volume Expansion
Pressure dressing	
Temporary individual ligature	Ringer's lactate
Tourniquet (rarely)	Normal saline
	Dextran
	Serum albumin
	Plasma
	Whole blood

patients to the several teams. He should also supervise the activities in the operating room and the recovery room. Regular sterile techniques should be maintained unless major utility services are lost.

Experience suggests that the number of casualties requiring operation during a disaster seldom exceeds the number of operations usually performed in a hospital during a 24-hour period. On this basis a sufficient number of surgeons and nurses should be mobilized to man the necessary number of operating rooms. Two surgeons and two nurses per operating room is the rule.

In disasters, many walking casualties may need care. The use of operating room personnel in the organization and direction of surgical activities in the outpatient department can help to insure the use of good surgical principles and techniques in the treatment of the walking wounded.

Index